Beyond the Barriers: Transforming Public Health in Nigeria and Developing Nations

Authored by

Jalal-Eddeen Abubakar Saleh

World Health Organization

Nigeria

Beyond the Barriers: Transforming Public Health in Nigeria and Developing Nations

Author: Jalal-Eddeen Abubakar Saleh

ISBN (Online): 979-8-89881-573-8

ISBN (Print): 979-8-89881-574-5

ISBN (Paperback): 979-8-89881-575-2

Published by Bentham Science Publishers Pte. Ltd. Singapore, in collaboration with Eureka Conferences, USA.

First published in 2026.

Bentham Science Publishers Pte. Ltd.
No. 9 Raffles Place
Office No. 26-01
Singapore 048619
Singapore
Email: subscriptions@benthamscience.net

BENTHAM SCIENCE

CONTENTS

PREFACE

In recent decades, the world has witnessed unprecedented advancements in healthcare, resulting in remarkable improvements in life expectancy and quality of life. However, these achievements have not been evenly distributed. In many developing nations, particularly Nigeria, public health systems face formidable challenges that threaten to reverse the progress made thus far. The barriers to effective healthcare in these regions are numerous and complex, ranging from weak governance and political instability to poverty, insecurity, and inadequate infrastructure. These obstacles not only impede access to essential health services but also perpetuate a cycle of poor health outcomes and underdevelopment.

Beyond the Barriers: Transforming Public Health in Nigeria and Developing Nations is a follow-up to my earlier work, **Resilient Communities: Navigating Public Health Challenges in Developing Nations**, which was intended to empower local health actors to drive resilience and innovation in health service delivery. This new book is a culmination of my experiences, observations, engagements with government officials and development partners, and personal reflections as a public health professional committed to tackling these challenges.

Over the past three decades, I have worked in the health sector—15 years as a clinician and the subsequent 15 as a public health expert with the World Health Organization—focusing on immunization and disease prevention and control. Throughout this journey, I have witnessed firsthand the struggles of underserved and hard-to-reach communities, communities that are often overlooked and left behind by conventional health systems. I have seen the toll that poverty, conflict, and systemic neglect take on human lives. Yet, I have also witnessed the incredible resilience of those who work tirelessly to overcome these barriers.

This book is not merely an analysis of the problems; it is a call to action. It is an invitation to policymakers, health professionals, community leaders, and international partners to rethink and reimagine our approach to public health in Nigeria and other developing countries. It urges us to go beyond the barriers that have held us back for too long and to seek innovative, sustainable solutions that can transform the health landscape of the developing world.

Each chapter explores a specific aspect of Nigeria's public health challenges, offering insights, case studies, and practical recommendations. I hope that this book will serve as a valuable resource for those who are committed to improving the lives of millions who continue to suffer from preventable diseases, inadequate healthcare, and systemic neglect.

Transforming public health in Nigeria and other developing nations is not merely a possibility; it is an imperative. I invite you to join me on this journey as we work together to build a healthier, more equitable future for all.

Jalal-Eddeen Abubakar SALEH
World Health Organization
Nigeria

Disclaimer: The views expressed in this book are solely my own and do not reflect the official positions or policies of the World Health Organization. The content of this book is objective, non-partisan, and was not influenced by my affiliation with WHO.

Dedication

To the unsung heroes of public health—those who tirelessly work behind the scenes, from bustling urban clinics to remote village outposts. May your dedication continue to light the path toward a healthier, more equitable world.

ACKNOWLEDGEMENTS

I wish to acknowledge that in the final stages of refining this book, I chose to use ChatGPT as an editorial aid and an intellectual companion. While the ideas, arguments, lived experiences, and analytical processes presented in these pages are entirely my own, I deliberately used ChatGPT as a powerful tool for grammar, reflection, flow, and clarity. This has helped to sharpen the language, strengthen the structure, and enhance the content without diluting authorial intent. I appreciate the intellectual capacity of ChatGPT to engage critically with complex concepts, suggest alternative framings, and streamline dense material, which mirrors the evolving role of Artificial Intelligence (AI) not as a substitute but as an enabler of human creativity. I leveraged this advanced technology thoughtfully and responsibly, bridging insight with expression more efficiently. This has reaffirmed that when AI is used with discernment, ChatGPT and the like can expand the reach of human thought, scholarship, and storytelling, and not entirely replace them.

GLOSSARY

In this comprehensive glossary, we provide key terms and their definitions that have been introduced and discussed throughout this handbook. The glossary provides definitions for key terms and concepts discussed throughout the book, helping readers to better understand the context and significance of the topics addressed.

Access to Healthcare: The ability of individuals to obtain and make use of appropriate health services on time, influenced by factors such as cost, geography, availability, and cultural acceptability.

Accountability: The obligation of individuals or organizations to report, explain, and be answerable for their actions, particularly in the management of resources or in public service.

Anti-Corruption Initiatives: Programs or strategies are implemented to prevent, detect, and punish corruption, particularly in public sectors such as health and education.

Brain Drain: The emigration of trained and talented health professionals from their home country to more developed regions, often due to better working conditions, pay, or security.

Case Study: A detailed examination of a specific instance or event used to illustrate broader principles, strategies, or outcomes, often utilized to draw lessons in public health interventions.

Community-Driven Health Initiatives: Health programs or interventions that are led and implemented by local communities, emphasizing local knowledge, participation, and ownership.

Community Health Workers (CHWs): Trained public health workers who provide healthcare services, health education, and referrals at the community level, especially in underserved or hard-to-reach areas.

Conflict Zones: Geographic areas experiencing armed conflict or insecurity, often resulting in disrupted health services and increased public health risks.

Corruption: The abuse of entrusted power for private gain can undermine the effectiveness of public health services and hinder equitable access to healthcare.

Crisis Situations: Emergency or unstable situations, such as natural disasters, pandemics, or armed conflicts, that severely impact health infrastructure and service delivery.

Development Goals: Specific targets set by international bodies, such as the United Nations, aimed at improving global health, reducing poverty, and fostering sustainable development. The Sustainable Development Goals (SDGs) are the most prominent example.

Economic Determinants of Health: Factors related to economic conditions—such as income, employment, and financial stability—that influence individual and community health outcomes.

Equity in Health: The fair distribution of health resources, opportunities, and services across different populations ensures that everyone has the opportunity to attain their full health potential.

Health Budget: The allocation of financial resources by a government or organization to fund health services, programs, and infrastructure.

Health Governance: The processes, structures, and institutions through which decisions about health systems and policies are made and implemented at national, regional, and local levels.

Health Information Systems (HIS): Systems that collect, analyze, and disseminate health-related data to support evidence-based policy-making and health program management.

Health Literacy: The capacity of individuals to obtain, process, and understand basic health information and services to make informed health decisions.

Health Promotion: Activities aimed at enhancing health and preventing disease by enabling people to increase control over and improve their health.

Health Systems Strengthening (HSS): Efforts to improve the performance of health systems, focusing on components such as healthcare delivery, financing, workforce, information systems, and governance.

Immunization Coverage: The proportion of a population that has received specific vaccines, often used as an indicator of access to essential health services.

Innovative Financing Mechanisms: New or creative financial tools and strategies are designed to mobilize resources for health initiatives, often involving partnerships between the public and private sectors.

International Partnerships: Collaborations between countries or international organizations aimed at addressing global challenges, including health crises, through shared knowledge, resources, and strategies.

Malnutrition: A condition resulting from inadequate or imbalanced nutrient intake, which significantly affects public health, especially among vulnerable populations.

Mental Health and Psychosocial Support (MHPSS): Services that address emotional, psychological, and social well-being, especially important in settings affected by conflict or disaster.

Mobile Health (mHealth): The use of mobile devices and technology to deliver health information, services, and interventions, particularly in remote or underserved areas.

Monitoring and Evaluation (M&E): A systematic process of collecting, analyzing, and using data to assess the performance of health programs or interventions and guide decision-making.

Nutrition-Sensitive Interventions: Public health programs that address the underlying causes of malnutrition by integrating nutrition objectives into sectors like agriculture, education, and social protection.

Policy Implementation: The process of putting health-related policies into action through programs, regulations, and practices at various levels of governance.

Post-Conflict Recovery: The process of rebuilding and restoring health systems, infrastructure, and services in areas affected by conflict or disasters.

Primary Health Care (PHC): Essential healthcare based on scientifically sound and socially acceptable methods, made universally accessible to individuals and families in the community.

Public-Private Partnerships (PPPs): Collaborative agreements between government entities and private sector companies to deliver public services or infrastructure, such as healthcare, while sharing risks and rewards.

Resilient Health Systems: Health systems capable of preparing for, responding to, and recovering from shocks such as disease outbreaks or natural disasters while maintaining essential services.

Social Determinants of Health: The non-medical factors that influence health outcomes, including education, housing, employment, income, and social support networks.

Social Protection Systems: Policies and programs designed to reduce poverty and vulnerability by promoting efficient labor markets, diminishing people's exposure to risks, and enhancing their capacity to manage economic and social risks.

Surveillance Systems: Mechanisms for the continuous collection, analysis, and interpretation of health data for planning, implementation, and evaluation of public health practices.

Sustainable Development Goals (SDGs): A collection of 17 global goals set by the United Nations in 2015, aimed at ending poverty, protecting the planet, and ensuring prosperity for all by 2030. Goal 3 focuses on good health and well-being.

Technological Innovations in Healthcare: The application of advanced technologies, such as digital tools, telemedicine, and mobile health applications, to improve the delivery of healthcare services.

Transparency: The practice of making information accessible and understandable to the public, particularly regarding government actions, budgets, and decision-making processes in the health sector.

Universal Health Coverage (UHC): A health system goal ensuring that all individuals receive the health services they need without suffering financial hardship.

Zero-Dose Children: Children who have not received any basic vaccines are particularly vulnerable to vaccine-preventable diseases.

CHAPTER 1

The Foundation of Health: Political Will and Governance

Abstract: The chapter delves into the critical role that political leadership and governance play in shaping health outcomes in Nigeria and other developing nations. It explores the multifaceted impact of political will on public health, emphasising how effective leadership can drive the formulation and implementation of health policies that are essential for sustainable health systems. The chapter is structured to provide a comprehensive analysis, beginning with the role of political leadership in health and governance structures at the federal, state, and local levels. It then examines the processes involved in health policy formulation and implementation, highlighting key successes and failures through various case studies. The chapter further discusses the detrimental effects of political instability on health programs and concludes by proposing pathways to strengthen political commitment, thereby fostering an environment conducive to improved health outcomes. Through a blend of theoretical insights and practical case studies, this chapter underscores the necessity of robust political engagement to overcome the barriers hindering health system development in Nigeria.

Keywords: Case studies, Federalism, Governance structures, Health systems, Health governance, Health policy, Health reform, Health programs, Leadership, Nigeria, Political instability, Political will, Public health.

INTRODUCTION

Public health is a reflection of a nation's commitment to the well-being of its people. It encompasses not only the prevention and treatment of diseases but also the broader socio-economic and environmental factors that contribute to overall health. In developing countries like Nigeria, the state of public health is intricately tied to leadership, political will, and governance structures that drive decision-making as well as resource mobilisation and allocation. Without strong political leadership and effective governance, even the most well-intentioned health initiatives can falter, leaving communities vulnerable and underserved.

This chapter delves into the crucial role of political leadership and governance in shaping Nigeria's health landscape. It will explore how political will, or the lack

Jalal-Eddeen Abubakar Saleh

thereof, influences health outcomes and the effectiveness of health systems. Through an examination of governance structures at the federal, state, and local levels, it will analyse how these layers of government interact to formulate and implement health policies. Additionally, it will present case studies that highlight both the successes and failures of health governance in Nigeria, offering insights into the challenges that must be overcome to achieve sustainable health improvements. Finally, it will discuss the impact of political instability on health programs and propose pathways to strengthen political commitment to health in Nigeria and other developing nations.

THE ROLE OF POLITICAL LEADERSHIP IN HEALTH

Political leadership is a cornerstone of public health systems worldwide. It is the driving force that shapes health policies, mobilises resources, and creates an enabling environment for effective healthcare delivery. In the context of developing nations, such as Nigeria, the role of political leadership is even more critical. The health challenges faced by these countries - ranging from inadequate infrastructure and workforce shortages to infectious disease outbreaks and chronic underfunding - require strong, visionary leadership that prioritises health as a fundamental pillar of national development [1 - 3].

Globally, health transformation by governments of countries is dependent on the interplay between political will and governance. The term Political Will is considered to be that commitment demonstrated by political leaders in prioritising, resourcing, and sustaining actions that advance public health goals, which sometimes may be difficult or unpopular. The measurable indicators are actions that link the decisions to outcomes, and this includes budgetary allocations to health, policy enactment and enforcement of policies, establishing accountability mechanisms, and consistency of priorities across political transitions [1 - 5].

Governance, on the other hand, refers to a set of structures, processes, and relationships through which power is exercised in the management of public affairs, including health. The measurable indicators include transparency, policy coherence, responsiveness to evidence, coordination efficiency, and equity in service delivery. Thus, ensuring that the health of citizens remains a non-negotiable priority across political cycles, there is a need to have strong governance that transforms good intentions into operational realities.

Given that developing nations have health systems that are often fragile and fragmented, political will and governance in health are non-negotiable dimensions, as they help in determining whether public health programs achieve sustainable impact or are trapped in cycles of systemic relapse and short-term success [1 - 6].

Political Leadership as a Catalyst for Health Reform

Effective political leadership has the power to transform health systems and drive meaningful reform. Leaders who prioritise health not only shape policy but also inspire national momentum, allocate critical resources, and mobilise cross-sectoral support. Their commitment can elevate health on the political agenda, foster innovation, and push through reforms that otherwise stall in bureaucratic inertia. In many successful global health stories, strong and visionary political leadership has been the defining factor behind progress [1, 2].

1. **Setting the Health Agenda:** Political leaders have the power to set the national health agenda, determining the priorities and focus areas of public health efforts. In Nigeria, where the burden of disease is high and health outcomes are often poor, the importance of a clear and robust health agenda cannot be overstated. Effective political leadership involves not only identifying key health challenges but also articulating a strategic vision for overcoming them. This vision must be rooted in a commitment to universal health coverage, equitable access to care, and the reduction of health disparities across different population groups.
2. **Mobilising Resources and Ensuring Accountability:** One of the most significant roles of political leadership in health is the mobilisation of resources. In many developing nations, healthcare systems suffer from chronic underfunding, which hampers their ability to deliver quality services. Political leaders must advocate for increased investment in health, both from domestic sources and through international partnerships. This includes ensuring that health budgets are adequate and that funds are allocated efficiently and transparently. Moreover, political leaders must establish mechanisms for accountability to prevent corruption and ensure that resources are used effectively to achieve health outcomes.
3. **Health Policy Formulation and Implementation:** Political leadership is crucial in the formulation and implementation of health policies that address the specific needs of the population. In Nigeria, this involves creating policies that are responsive to the diverse health challenges facing the country, from infectious diseases like Tuberculosis, Malaria, and HIV/AIDS to the rising burden of non-communicable diseases. Effective policies must be evidence-based, inclusive, and adaptable to changing circumstances. Political leaders play a key role in ensuring that these policies are not only well-designed but also implemented with the necessary resources, infrastructure, and human capacity.

The Intersection of Politics and Health Outcomes

Health outcomes are deeply influenced by political decisions, whether in budgeting, legislation, or emergency response. Political ideologies, governance styles, and institutional priorities shape the distribution and quality of health services. Where political environments are stable and health is treated as a public good, outcomes tend to improve. Conversely, politicisation of health or neglect of vulnerable populations can deepen inequities and undermine progress. Understanding this intersection is key to designing interventions that are both technically sound and politically viable [2 - 4].

1. **Health as a Political Priority:** The degree to which health is prioritised on the political agenda has a direct impact on health outcomes. When political leaders prioritise health, it leads to the development of stronger health systems, better access to services, and improved public health outcomes. Conversely, when health is not a political priority, it often results in neglected health systems, inadequate funding, and poor health indicators. In Nigeria, the political will to prioritise health has varied over time, reflecting broader economic, social, and political contexts. A sustained political commitment to health is essential for achieving long-term improvements in health outcomes.
2. **Leadership in Crisis Situations:** The role of political leadership becomes even more pronounced during public health crises, such as disease outbreaks, natural disasters, or humanitarian emergencies. In these situations, the ability of political leaders to respond swiftly and effectively can mean the difference between containment and widespread disaster. Effective crisis leadership involves clear communication, rapid mobilisation of resources, and coordination with international and local partners. The Ebola outbreak in West Africa, for example, highlighted the importance of strong political leadership in coordinating a comprehensive response that ultimately brought the epidemic under control.
3. **Promoting Equity and Social Justice:** Political leadership in health is not only about managing resources and policies but also about promoting equity and social justice. In many developing nations, health disparities are closely linked to social determinants such as poverty, education, and gender. Political leaders have a responsibility to address these social determinants through inclusive policies that ensure all citizens have access to the resources and opportunities needed to live healthy lives. This includes addressing the root causes of health inequities and implementing targeted interventions to improve health outcomes for marginalised and vulnerable populations.

Challenges to Effective Political Leadership in Health

Despite its importance, political leadership in health is often constrained by competing priorities, short-term political cycles, limited technical understanding, and systemic corruption. In some contexts, health is overshadowed by more politically expedient sectors, receiving inadequate attention until crises arise. Additionally, leadership transitions can disrupt continuity, while weak accountability systems may discourage bold or reformative action. Overcoming these challenges requires deliberate capacity-building and sustained political engagement with the health agenda [4, 5].

1. **Political Instability and Governance Issues:** One of the most significant challenges to effective political leadership in health is political instability. In countries like Nigeria, frequent changes in leadership in the 70s through the 90s, political turmoil, and weak governance structures contributed to the disruption of health initiatives and undermined progress. Political instability often leads to inconsistent health policies, underfunding, and a lack of continuity in health programs. Strengthening governance and ensuring political stability are, therefore, essential for sustained health improvements.
2. **Corruption and Mismanagement:** Corruption is a pervasive issue that affects many aspects of public health, from the allocation of resources to the delivery of services. Political leaders have a crucial role in combating corruption and ensuring that health resources are used effectively and transparently. This involves implementing strong anti-corruption measures, promoting accountability, and fostering a culture of integrity within the health sector. Without strong political leadership to address corruption, health systems will continue to suffer from inefficiencies and poor outcomes.
3. **Balancing Competing Priorities:** Political leaders often face the challenge of balancing competing priorities, particularly in countries with limited resources. In Nigeria, where economic development, education, security, and health are all pressing concerns, political leaders must make difficult decisions about how to allocate resources. Ensuring that health remains a priority in the face of competing demands requires strong advocacy, strategic planning, and a commitment to the long-term benefits of investing in health.

The Way Forward: Strengthening Political Leadership for Health

To strengthen political leadership in health, countries must invest in leadership development, foster a culture of accountability, and create mechanisms that encourage long-term commitment to health priorities. Building alliances with health professionals, civil society, and the media can amplify health issues and hold leaders to their promises. Furthermore, embedding health targets within national development plans and linking them to political performance metrics can incentivise sustained political action. True progress will come when leaders recognise that a healthy population is both a moral obligation and a strategic imperative for national development [4 - 6].

1. **Building Political Will:** Strengthening political leadership for health requires building and sustaining political will at all levels of government. This involves engaging political leaders in a dialogue about the importance of health, demonstrating the link between health and economic development, and creating incentives for political leaders to prioritise health. Civil society, international organisations, and the private sector all have roles to play in advocating for stronger political leadership in health.
2. **Investing in Leadership Development:** Developing the capacity of political leaders to effectively lead health initiatives is essential for long-term success. This includes providing training and support for health policy-making, leadership skills, and crisis management. Investing in leadership development can help ensure that political leaders are equipped to address the complex health challenges facing their countries and lead their nations toward better health outcomes.
3. **Promoting Accountability and Transparency:** Ensuring that political leaders are accountable for their actions in the health sector is crucial for building trust and achieving sustainable health improvements. This involves implementing mechanisms for transparency in health budgeting, expenditure, and policy implementation. By promoting accountability, political leaders can build public confidence in the health system and ensure that health resources are used effectively to improve health outcomes.
4. **Fostering Partnerships and Collaboration:** Effective political leadership in health also involves fostering partnerships and collaboration across sectors and with international partners. Health is not the sole responsibility of the health ministry; it requires a whole-government approach that involves education, finance, infrastructure, and other sectors. Political leaders must work collaboratively with other government ministries, the private sector, civil society, and international organisations to achieve shared health goals.

CONCLUSION

The role of political leadership in health care cannot be overstated. It is the driving force behind the formulation and implementation of health policies, the mobilisation of resources, and the creation of an enabling environment for effective healthcare delivery. In Nigeria and other developing nations, where health challenges are complex and multifaceted, strong political leadership is essential for achieving sustainable health improvements. By prioritising health, promoting equity, and building strong, accountable health systems, political leaders can lay the foundation for a healthier future for all.

GOVERNANCE STRUCTURES: FEDERAL, STATE, AND LOCAL LEVELS

Nigeria's federal structure operates across three tiers. The health policies are formulated, implemented, and monitored across three administrative tiers: federal government (FMOH, NPHCDA, NCDC), state government (SMOH, SPHCDA), and local government (health authority). This three-tier arrangement aims to foster decentralisation and responsiveness in the healthcare sector. While the FMOH, the first tier, provides overall policy direction, coordination, and regulation guiding the states and local governments in service delivery, the two lower tiers often have some overlapping mandates and weak accountability mechanisms that often blur responsibilities, resulting in policy fragmentation, adversely affecting quality service delivery.

Effective governance structures are fundamental to the success of any public health system. In a country as large and diverse as Nigeria, the distribution of power and responsibility across federal, state, and local levels is crucial in shaping health outcomes. These governance structures determine how health policies are formulated, implemented, and monitored, and they significantly impact the efficiency and effectiveness of health service delivery [6 - 10]. This section explores the roles and responsibilities of federal, state, and local governments in Nigeria's health sector, the challenges they face, and the opportunities for strengthening governance to improve public health outcomes.

Table **1** outlines the distinct roles and responsibilities of Nigeria's three tiers of government, federal, state, and local, in managing health systems. The federal level is tasked primarily with policy formulation, national coordination, and funding of overarching programs, particularly in tertiary healthcare and disease control. The state governments, in contrast, are responsible for delivering healthcare services, managing budgets, and overseeing secondary care facilities. Meanwhile, local governments are at the frontline, ensuring primary healthcare delivery and community engagement. While this layered structure allows for specialisation and targeted intervention, it also introduces challenges in coordination, funding equity, and capacity. Similarly, the table highlights how each level faces unique obstacles: the federal tier grapples with policy implementation gaps, states are hindered by financial and human resource limitations, and local governments often lack the operational capacity to meet healthcare demands. Understanding these distinctions is critical for designing reforms that assign appropriate roles while enhancing collaboration and accountability across the governance spectrum [6 - 10].

Table 1. Health governance structure in nigeria.

Tier of Government	Key Responsibilities	Health Services Provided	Challenges	Key Indicators
Federal Government (FMOH, NPHCDA, NCDC, NHIA)	Policy formulation, regulation, coordination, emergency preparedness, funding mechanisms (*e.g.*, BHCPF)	National programs, tertiary care	Policy implementation gaps	National health policy updates, budgetary allocation (% GDP), coordination of disease surveillance and response
State Governments (SMOHs, SPHCBs)	Adaptation and implementation of federal policies, service delivery oversight, human resource management, and co-funding of primary care	Secondary care	Resource limitations	State budgetary allocation to health, implementation of PHC under one roof (PHCUOR), % immunization coverage, and health worker density/Human Resources.
Local Governments (Primary Healthcare Centres)	Basic healthcare service delivery, quality data generation and reporting, and community mobilization	Primary healthcare, outreach services	Capacity constraints	Functioning primary healthcare facilities, timeliness/completeness of data, and community participation mechanisms

The Federal Government: Policy, Coordination, and Oversight

The federal government serves as the bedrock of health governance, providing national leadership, setting policy direction, and coordinating intergovernmental and intersectoral efforts. Through institutions such as the Federal Ministry of Health and related agencies, it formulates health strategies, allocates resources, establishes regulatory frameworks, and ensures alignment with global health standards. Effective oversight mechanisms are essential to ensure equity, accountability, and responsiveness in health service delivery across the federation [6 - 10].

1. **Centralised Health Policy and Strategic Planning:** The federal government plays a central role in shaping Nigeria's overall health policy framework. It is responsible for developing national health policies, strategies, and plans that set

the direction for the entire health system. These policies are designed to address the major health challenges facing the country, such as high maternal and child mortality rates, infectious diseases, and the rising burden of non-communicable diseases. The Federal Ministry of Health (FMoH) is the primary body responsible for formulating these policies and ensuring that they align with international health goals, such as the Sustainable Development Goals (SDGs).

2. **Regulation and Standard Setting:** In addition to policy formulation, the federal government is responsible for setting standards and rules for the health sector. This includes establishing guidelines for service delivery, quality of care, and the accreditation of health facilities and professionals. The FMoH collaborates closely with regulatory bodies, including the Medical and Dental Council of Nigeria (MDCN), the Nursing and Midwifery Council of Nigeria (NMCN), and the National Agency for Food and Drug Administration and Control (NAFDAC), to ensure that health services meet the required standards of safety and effectiveness.
3. **Coordination of National Health Programs:** The federal government also coordinates national health programs, such as immunisation campaigns, disease surveillance, and emergency response efforts. This coordination is essential for ensuring that health interventions are implemented consistently across the country and that resources are allocated efficiently. For example, the National Primary Health Care Development Agency (NPHCDA) oversees primary healthcare programs, including routine immunisation, while the Nigeria Centre for Disease Control (NCDC) is responsible for disease surveillance and outbreak response.
4. **Funding and Resource Allocation:** While health service delivery is largely the responsibility of state and local governments, the federal government plays a critical role in funding the health sector. The federal budget includes allocations for national health programs, federal health institutions, and specific interventions such as the procurement of vaccines and essential medicines. Additionally, the federal government is responsible for mobilising external resources from international donors and development partners, which are crucial for funding large-scale health initiatives. However, the equitable distribution of these resources across states and local governments remains a significant challenge, often resulting in disparities in health service delivery.

Nigeria's public health trajectory provides several instances where strong political will and coordinated governance produced measurable outcomes. These three examples are particularly instructive [6 - 10].

The 2012 Presidential Task Force on Polio Eradication

In responding to the global concern about Nigeria's status as one of the last reservoirs of wild poliovirus, the President inaugurated a high-level task force that brought together the three tiers into play: federal, state, and local government. This effort, a clear demonstration of how top-level political leadership can overcome bureaucratic inertia in delivering results, translated into intensified disease surveillance, community engagement, and accountability mechanisms that reduced wild poliovirus cases by over 95% between 2012 and 2015 [11, 12].

The 2014 Ebola Virus Disease (EVD) Response

In July 2014, after Nigeria recorded its first Ebola case, decisive governance structures were immediately activated. Under the leadership of the Federal Ministry of Health (FMOH), the Nigerian Centre for Disease Control (NCDC) established an Emergency Operations Centre (EOC) to coordinate multi-sectoral efforts in containing the outbreak. The support from the political leadership was unprecedented, aligning efforts, resources, and communication. The level of coordination and commitment resulted in halting transmission within three months, recording only 20 cases and 8 deaths. This level of commitment has earned Nigeria international commendation, demonstrating how *governance and political will* can contain an epidemic and avert a potential crisis [13, 14].

The 2020–2022 COVID-19 Response

In 2020, when COVID-19 struck, Nigeria's response to the pandemic showcased both progress and persistent governance gaps. The COVID-19 Presidential Committee, inaugurated by the President, coordinated a national effort to contain the outbreak, addressing public health crises through lockdown and ensuring economic continuity. However, because of underfunded subnational response teams, there was variable compliance. This experience showcased that political will must be matched by institutional capacity and sustained financing to achieve equitable outcomes [15].

State Governments: Implementation and Adaptation of Health Policies

State governments act as critical intermediaries between federal directives and local realities, bearing the primary responsibility for translating national health policies into actionable programs within their jurisdictions. Given the diverse socioeconomic and cultural contexts across states, the ability to adapt policies to local needs while maintaining fidelity to national goals is vital. State ministries of health thus play a pivotal role in resource planning, health workforce management, and program execution, often determining the success or failure of public health interventions. Nigeria's health governance landscape has evolved and been guided by key policy instruments that codify political will into legal and institutional frameworks. The two policy documents that provide the structural basis for aligning political will with measurable governance outcomes across federal and state levels are the National Health Act (2014) and the National Health Policy (2016) [9, 10].

It was the NHA (2014) that established the *Basic Health Care Provision Fund (BHCPF)*, which aims to guarantee a minimum package of services at the primary health care level through predictable funding. Similarly, the NHP (2016) reaffirmed the government's commitments to attaining universal health coverage, equity, and intergovernmental collaboration. It also emphasised the principles of accountability and underscored citizen participation. These two policies have transformed the landscape, operationalised governance ideals into measurable commitments, and provided a framework through which political intent is translated into health system performance [9, 10].

However, the challenge remains in the implementation, where federal vision is not always mirrored by the states. However, bridging this divide requires aligning incentives, strengthening subnational accountability, and institutionalising health leadership beyond individual personalities or electoral cycles.

1. **Health Policy Adaptation and Implementation:** State governments are primarily responsible for implementing national health policies within their jurisdictions. They have the authority to adapt federal health policies to meet the specific needs of their populations, taking into account local health challenges, cultural contexts, and available resources. This flexibility allows states to design and implement health programs that are more responsive to the needs of their communities. However, the effectiveness of these programs depends on the capacity of state governments to manage and oversee their health systems.
2. **Management of State Health Systems:** State Ministries of Health (SMoH) are responsible for managing the health system within their states. This includes overseeing secondary healthcare facilities, such as general hospitals, as well as coordinating with local governments to support primary healthcare services. State governments also play a key role in the recruitment, training, and deployment of healthcare workers, ensuring that there is an adequate and well-distributed workforce to meet the health needs of the population. Furthermore, states are responsible for managing health budgets, which are funded through state allocations, federal transfers, and internally generated revenue.

3. **Health Financing and Budgeting:** One of the most significant responsibilities of state governments is health financing. State budgets must allocate sufficient resources to fund health services, including infrastructure development, healthcare worker salaries, and the procurement of medical supplies. However, many states face challenges in generating adequate revenue, leading to underfunded health systems and poor service delivery. The ability of state governments to effectively manage and allocate resources is crucial for improving health outcomes, particularly in states with high levels of poverty and disease burden.
4. **Challenges in Health Governance at the State Level:** State governments often face significant challenges in health governance, including limited financial resources, weak health infrastructure, and a shortage of skilled healthcare workers. In some cases, political instability and corruption further undermine the capacity of state governments to deliver quality health services. Additionally, disparities in governance capacity between states can lead to unequal health outcomes, with some states performing significantly better than others in terms of health indicators. Addressing these challenges requires a concerted effort to strengthen state-level governance, build capacity, and ensure that health resources are used efficiently and transparently.

Local Governments: The Frontline of Health Service Delivery

Local governments represent the closest tier of governance to the people, and their role in public health is both foundational and transformative. As the frontline providers of primary healthcare services, local authorities are tasked with managing health facilities, mobilising communities, and responding to immediate health needs. Strengthening local government capacity is essential for achieving universal health coverage, improving maternal and child health outcomes, and ensuring resilience in the face of public health emergencies [16, 17].

1. **Primary Healthcare Delivery:** Local governments are the frontline providers of primary healthcare services in Nigeria. They are responsible for managing primary healthcare centres (PHCs), which are the first point of contact for most Nigerians seeking health services. These centres provide essential health services, including maternal and child health care, immunisation, treatment of common illnesses, and health education. Local governments are also tasked with implementing community-based health initiatives and engaging with local communities to promote health and prevent disease.
2. **Community Engagement and Participation:** Local governments play a crucial role in engaging with communities to promote health and encourage the use of healthcare services. This involves working closely with community leaders, civil society organisations, and other stakeholders to raise awareness

about health issues, encourage health-seeking behavior, and ensure that health services are accessible and acceptable to the local population. Effective community engagement is essential for building trust in the health system, increasing the uptake of health services, and addressing social determinants of health.

3. **Health Infrastructure and Workforce Management:** The management of health infrastructure and the health workforce at the local level is a critical responsibility of local governments. This includes maintaining and upgrading PHC facilities, ensuring the availability of essential medicines and medical supplies, and managing the recruitment, training, and retention of healthcare workers. However, many local governments struggle with inadequate infrastructure, a shortage of healthcare workers, and limited financial resources, which can lead to poor service delivery and low utilisation of healthcare services.
4. **Challenges in Local Health Governance:** Local governments face several challenges in delivering effective health services, including inadequate funding, poor infrastructure, and limited administrative capacity. In many cases, local governments are heavily reliant on federal and state transfers to fund their health services, leading to financial instability and uncertainty. Additionally, local governments often lack the technical expertise and resources needed to manage health services effectively and address the health needs of their populations. Strengthening local health governance requires building the capacity of local governments, improving resource allocation, and enhancing coordination between local, state, and federal levels of government.

Strengthening Governance Structures for Better Health Outcomes

Robust governance structures are indispensable for the effective delivery of health services and the realisation of equitable health outcomes. Fragmented roles, weak institutional capacities, and poor intergovernmental coordination often hinder progress. Strengthening governance involves building transparent systems, enhancing accountability, fostering cross-sectoral collaboration, and empowering health institutions at all levels. A well-structured governance framework is key to aligning efforts, optimising resource utilisation, and achieving sustainable health development [16 - 18].

1. **Improving Coordination and Collaboration:** Effective governance in the health sector requires strong coordination and collaboration between federal, state, and local governments. This includes clear communication channels, joint planning and decision-making processes, and mechanisms for sharing resources and best practices. Strengthening intergovernmental collaboration can help

ensure that health policies are implemented consistently across the country and that resources are allocated efficiently to meet the needs of all Nigerians.

2. **Building Capacity at All Levels of Government:** Capacity building is essential for improving governance at all levels of government. This includes training government officials in health policy and management, enhancing the technical capacity of health ministries and departments, and developing the skills of healthcare workers. Investing in capacity building can help ensure that governments are equipped to manage their health systems effectively and respond to emerging health challenges.
3. **Ensuring Accountability and Transparency:** Accountability and transparency are critical for effective health governance. This involves implementing mechanisms for monitoring and evaluating health programs, ensuring that health budgets are spent efficiently, and addressing corruption and mismanagement. By promoting accountability and transparency, governments can build trust in the health system, improve the quality of health services, and achieve better health outcomes.
4. **Enhancing Community Involvement in Health Governance:** Engaging communities in health governance is essential for ensuring that health services are responsive to the needs of the population. This includes involving communities in the planning and decision-making processes, encouraging community participation in health programs, and promoting health literacy. By enhancing community involvement, governments can increase the uptake of health services, improve health outcomes, and address the social determinants of health.

CONCLUSION

Effective governance structures are the foundation of a strong and resilient health system. In Nigeria, the distribution of power and responsibility across federal, state, and local levels plays a crucial role in shaping health outcomes. By strengthening governance at all levels, improving coordination and collaboration, and promoting accountability and transparency, Nigeria can build a health system that is capable of delivering quality health services to all its citizens. As the country continues to face significant health challenges, the importance of effective governance in achieving sustainable health improvements cannot be overstated.

HEALTH POLICY FORMULATION AND IMPLEMENTATION

The formulation and implementation of health policies are critical processes that shape the effectiveness of any healthcare system. In a country as complex and diverse as Nigeria, the development of sound health policies requires a nuanced understanding of the country's demographic, economic, and cultural landscape.

This section delves into the intricacies of health policy formulation and implementation, examining the key actors involved, the challenges faced, and the strategies needed to ensure that policies translate into tangible improvements in public health outcomes [19 - 24].

The Health Policy Formulation Process

The formulation of health policy is a complex yet critical process that involves identifying public health priorities, consulting stakeholders, analysing data, and crafting evidence-based strategies. Ideally, this process is participatory and inclusive of communities, professional bodies, civil society, and development partners. A sound policy formulation process ensures that health interventions are contextually appropriate, culturally sensitive, and strategically aligned with national and global health goals [19, 20].

1. **Identifying Health Priorities:** The first step in health policy formulation is identifying the most pressing health issues that need to be addressed. In Nigeria, this process is informed by a variety of data sources, including national health surveys, disease surveillance reports, and health systems assessments. Key health priorities often include reducing maternal and child mortality, combating infectious diseases like malaria and HIV/AIDS, and addressing the growing burden of Non-Communicable Diseases (NCDs). The identification of these priorities requires input from a wide range of stakeholders, including government agencies, healthcare professionals, civil society organisations, and the communities affected by these health issues.
2. **Stakeholder Engagement and Consensus Building:** Effective health policy formulation involves engaging with a broad spectrum of stakeholders to build consensus on policy goals and strategies. This includes consultations with government ministries, health professionals, Non-Governmental Organisations (NGOs), donor agencies, and the private sector. Stakeholder engagement is crucial for ensuring that policies are inclusive, culturally sensitive, and aligned with the needs of the population. In Nigeria, the National Council on Health (NCH) serves as a key platform for stakeholder engagement, bringing together representatives from the federal, state, and local levels to discuss and approve national health policies.
3. **Policy Design and Development:** Once health priorities have been identified and stakeholder consensus has been achieved, the next step is the design and development of the policy. This involves outlining the policy objectives, strategies for achieving these objectives, and the roles and responsibilities of various actors. The policy design process must also consider the resources required for implementation, including financial, human, and infrastructural

resources. In Nigeria, the FMoH plays a central role in drafting health policies, often in collaboration with international partners such as the World Health Organisation (WHO) and other development agencies.

4. **Legislative Approval and Enactment:** After a policy has been developed, it may require legislative approval before it can be implemented. This is particularly true for policies that involve significant changes to existing laws or the creation of new regulatory frameworks. In Nigeria, health policies often need to be approved by the National Assembly, which scrutinises the policy's objectives, feasibility, and budgetary implications. The legislative process can be lengthy and complex, with various committees and stakeholders providing input before the policy is enacted into law.

Challenges in Health Policy Formulation

Despite the strategic importance of health policy, its development is frequently beset by challenges ranging from political interference and inadequate data to limited stakeholder engagement and bureaucratic inertia. In many developing contexts, policy decisions are reactive rather than proactive, often driven by crises rather than long-term planning. Addressing these obstacles requires institutional reforms, improved data systems, and fostering a culture of policy-driven leadership [21, 22].

1. **Fragmentation and Lack of Coordination:** One of the major challenges in health policy formulation in Nigeria is the fragmentation of the health system, with responsibilities spread across federal, state, and local levels. This fragmentation can lead to a lack of coordination and consistency in policy development, with different levels of government pursuing conflicting or overlapping health initiatives. Additionally, the involvement of multiple stakeholders, each with their own priorities and interests, can complicate the policy formulation process and make it difficult to reach a consensus on key issues.
2. **Political Interference and Instability:** Political interference is another significant challenge in the formulation of health policies in Nigeria. Policies are sometimes influenced by political considerations rather than evidence-based assessments of public health needs. This can result in the adoption of policies that are not aligned with the best interests of the population. Furthermore, political instability and frequent changes in government can disrupt the policy formulation process, leading to delays or the abandonment of important health initiatives.
3. **Resource Constraints:** Resource constraints are a pervasive challenge in the formulation of health policies in Nigeria. Limited financial resources, coupled with inadequate infrastructure and a shortage of skilled health workers, can

restrict the scope and ambition of health policies. Policymakers must often make difficult decisions about how to allocate scarce resources, balancing the need to address immediate health crises with the long-term goal of building a resilient health system. This scarcity of resources can also lead to reliance on external funding, which may come with conditions that influence the direction of health policies.

4. **Data Limitations and Health Information Systems:** Accurate and timely data are essential for informed health policy formulation. However, in Nigeria, the health information system is often characterised by data gaps, inconsistencies, and delays in reporting. These limitations can hinder the ability of policymakers to accurately assess the health needs of the population, identify emerging health threats, and monitor the impact of existing policies. Strengthening health information systems is, therefore, a critical priority for improving the quality of health policy formulation in Nigeria.

Health Policy Implementation: Turning Policy into Action

Transforming well-crafted policies into tangible health outcomes requires a robust implementation framework. This phase bridges the gap between intent and impact, involving logistics, resource mobilisation, capacity building, and ongoing monitoring. Effective implementation depends not only on technical efficiency but also on political will, institutional synergy, and community participation. It is here that the real test of a policy's value and viability unfolds [22 - 24].

1. **Developing Implementation Plans:** Once a health policy has been approved, the next step is to develop a detailed implementation plan. This plan outlines the specific actions that need to be taken to achieve the policy's objectives, the timeline for implementation, and the resources required. It also identifies the key stakeholders responsible for carrying out these actions, including government agencies, healthcare providers, and community organisations. In Nigeria, implementation plans are often developed at the federal level but require adaptation at the state and local levels to reflect regional variations in health needs and resources.
2. **Capacity Building and Training:** Effective policy implementation requires a well-trained and capable health workforce. Capacity building and training are, therefore, essential components of the implementation process. This includes training healthcare workers on new protocols and procedures, strengthening the management and leadership skills of health administrators, and building the technical expertise of health professionals in areas such as disease surveillance and health information management. Capacity-building efforts must also extend to the community level, where local health workers and volunteers play a critical role in delivering health services and promoting health education.

3. **Resource Mobilisation and Allocation:** The successful implementation of health policies depends on the availability of adequate resources. This includes not only financial resources but also human resources, medical supplies, and health infrastructure. In Nigeria, resource mobilisation is often a collaborative effort involving the federal government, state governments, donor agencies, and the private sector. Effective resource allocation is crucial for ensuring that resources are directed to where they are most needed and used efficiently to achieve the desired health outcomes.
4. **Monitoring and Evaluation:** Monitoring and evaluation (M&E) are critical components of the policy implementation process, allowing policymakers to assess the effectiveness of health interventions, identify challenges, and make necessary adjustments. In Nigeria, M&E systems are often weak, with limited capacity for data collection, analysis, and reporting. Strengthening M&E systems is essential for improving accountability, ensuring that policies are implemented as intended, and providing evidence for future policy development. The use of digital tools and technology can enhance M&E efforts by enabling real-time data collection and analysis.
5. **Community Engagement and Participation:** Community engagement is a key factor in the successful implementation of health policies. Policies that are developed and implemented without input from the communities they are intended to serve are less likely to be effective. In Nigeria, involving communities in the implementation process can help to build trust, ensure that health services are culturally appropriate, and increase the uptake of health interventions. Community health workers, traditional leaders, and civil society organisations all play a vital role in mobilising communities and ensuring that policies are responsive to local needs.

Overcoming Barriers to Effective Implementation

Barriers to health policy implementation are numerous, ranging from financial constraints and workforce shortages to weak infrastructure and resistance to change. Overcoming these challenges demands a multifaceted approach that includes improving governance, ensuring adequate funding, fostering innovation, and building resilient health systems. Strategic partnerships, adaptive leadership, and continuous learning are also crucial to navigating the complexities of implementation in dynamic and resource-limited settings [23, 24].

1. **Strengthening Governance and Leadership:** Strong governance and leadership are essential for overcoming barriers to effective policy implementation. This includes ensuring that there is clear accountability for policy outcomes, reducing bureaucratic inefficiencies, and promoting transparency in the use of resources. In Nigeria, efforts to strengthen

governance should focus on enhancing the capacity of health ministries and departments at all levels of government, improving coordination between federal, state, and local authorities, and fostering a culture of accountability and integrity in the health sector.

2. **Addressing Political and Economic Instability:** Political and economic instability can significantly disrupt the implementation of health policies. In Nigeria, efforts to improve the stability and predictability of the political environment are crucial for ensuring that health policies can be implemented consistently and effectively. This may involve advocating for greater political commitment to health, promoting the integration of health goals into broader national development plans, and working to build a more resilient economy that can withstand external shocks.
3. **Improving Health Infrastructure:** Inadequate health infrastructure is a major barrier to effective policy implementation in Nigeria. Many health facilities, particularly in rural areas, lack the basic amenities needed to provide quality care, such as clean water, reliable electricity, and adequate medical supplies. Investing in health infrastructure is therefore critical for enabling the effective delivery of health services and ensuring that policies have the desired impact on health outcomes. Public-Private Partnerships (PPPs) and innovative financing mechanisms can play a key role in mobilising the resources needed to upgrade health infrastructure across the country.
4. **Enhancing Health Information Systems:** Robust health information systems are essential for monitoring the implementation of health policies and assessing their impact. In Nigeria, there is a need to invest in the development of integrated health information systems that can provide accurate, timely, and comprehensive data on health indicators, service delivery, and health outcomes. This will require improvements in data collection, storage, analysis, and dissemination, as well as the training of health workers in the use of digital health tools and technologies.

CONCLUSION

The gap between policy formulation and effective implementation remains a significant challenge in Nigeria's health sector. While the country has made progress in developing comprehensive health policies, the translation of these policies into practice is often hampered by a range of factors, including governance challenges, resource constraints, and weak health systems. Bridging this gap requires a concerted effort to strengthen the capacity of health institutions, improve coordination and collaboration between stakeholders, and ensure that policies are grounded in reality.

CASE STUDIES

Successes and Failures in Health Governance

Understanding the successes and failures in health governance provides valuable insights into the factors that contribute to effective public health systems and the challenges that hinder progress. This section explores notable case studies from Nigeria and other developing nations, analysing both successful and unsuccessful health governance initiatives. By examining these case studies, we can draw lessons that inform future health governance strategies and improve overall health outcomes [25 - 31].

Case Study 1: The Nigeria Polio Eradication Initiative

Background: The Polio Eradication Initiative in Nigeria represents a remarkable success in health governance and disease control. Nigeria was once one of the world's last strongholds of wild poliovirus, but through a concerted effort involving multiple stakeholders, the country made significant progress toward eradicating the disease.

Governance Strategies and Actions

1. ***Strong Political Will:*** The initiative received high-level political commitment from the Nigerian government, with leaders actively supporting vaccination campaigns and allocating resources to the effort.
2. ***Collaborative Approach:*** The initiative involved collaboration between the federal and state governments, international organizations such as the WHO and UNICEF, and local communities. This multi-faceted approach ensured broad support and effective coordination.
3. ***Robust Surveillance Systems:*** A comprehensive surveillance system was established to monitor polio cases and detect outbreaks swiftly. This system included active surveillance in communities and routine immunization data collection.
4. ***Community Engagement:*** Community-based strategies were employed to raise awareness about the importance of vaccination and address local concerns. Traditional and religious leaders played a crucial role in mobilizing communities.

Outcomes

- Nigeria was certified polio-free in 2020, marking a significant achievement in global public health.

- The success of the initiative demonstrated the effectiveness of a well-coordinated, multi-stakeholder approach to disease eradication.

Lessons Learned

- Political will and commitment are critical for the success of large-scale health initiatives.
- Collaborative efforts between governments, international organizations, and local communities can achieve significant health outcomes.
- Effective surveillance and monitoring systems are essential for early detection and response.

Case Study 2: The Nigerian Maternal and Child Health (MCH) Program Challenges

Background: Despite significant investments in maternal and child health programs in Nigeria, the country has faced persistent challenges in improving maternal and child health outcomes. The MCH program has experienced several governance-related issues that have hindered its effectiveness.

Governance Challenges and Issues

1. ***Fragmented Implementation:*** The MCH program suffered from fragmentation, with inconsistent implementation across states and local governments. This led to variations in service delivery and quality.
2. ***Insufficient Funding:*** Inadequate and inconsistent funding for MCH programs limited their scope and impact. Budget constraints often led to shortages of essential supplies and resources.
3. ***Weak Monitoring and Evaluation:*** Weak M&E systems hindered the ability to track progress, identify gaps, and make necessary adjustments. This lack of oversight affected program effectiveness and accountability.
4. ***Lack of Community Engagement:*** Insufficient community involvement in program design and implementation resulted in a lack of awareness and acceptance of MCH services.

Outcomes

1. Maternal and child health indicators did not improve as expected, with high rates of maternal and infant mortality persisting.
2. The fragmented and underfunded program struggled to achieve its objectives and deliver consistent services.

Lessons Learned

1. Fragmentation and inconsistent implementation can undermine the effectiveness of health programs.
2. Adequate and reliable funding is essential for sustaining health interventions and ensuring access to necessary resources.
3. Strong M&E systems are crucial for tracking progress, identifying challenges, and improving accountability.
4. Engaging communities in health programs enhances service uptake and effectiveness.

CONCLUSION

By analysing and learning from case studies one and two, reflecting on successes and failures in health governance, stakeholders can develop more effective strategies to address public health challenges and achieve sustainable improvements in health outcomes. The key takeaways are as follows:

Key Takeaways

1. Successful health governance requires a combination of political commitment, collaborative approaches, strategic planning, and community engagement.
2. Failures in health governance often stem from issues such as fragmentation, inadequate funding, weak monitoring systems, and political instability.
3. Drawing lessons from both successes and failures can inform the development of more effective health governance strategies and improve overall health outcomes.

The Impact of Political Instability on Health Programs

Political instability is a significant factor that can profoundly impact the effectiveness and sustainability of health programs. It can disrupt the delivery of health services, undermine governance structures, and exacerbate existing health challenges. This section explores the various ways in which political instability affects health programs, using case studies to illustrate these impacts and discussing strategies for mitigating the adverse effects of political turmoil on health systems [32 - 37].

Political instability refers to a state of uncertainty or disruption in governance and political processes that can manifest in various forms, including:

1. ***Political Violence:*** Armed conflicts, civil unrest, and terrorism can damage health infrastructure and disrupt services.

2. ***Governance Breakdown:*** Weak or failing state institutions, corruption, and lack of effective leadership undermine the implementation of health policies.
3. ***Economic Instability:*** Fluctuating economic conditions, such as inflation and unemployment, can impact funding for health programs and access to resources.
4. ***Policy Inconsistency:*** Frequent changes in government and shifting policy priorities can lead to inconsistent or poorly coordinated health interventions.

Additionally, political instability affects health programs through multiple mechanisms, including:

1. ***Disruption of Health Services:*** Conflicts and violence can damage health facilities, destroy medical supplies, and disrupt supply chains, leading to interruptions in service delivery.
2. ***Undermining Governance:*** Weak governance structures can result in the poor management of health programs, inefficiencies, and corruption, reducing the effectiveness of interventions.
3. ***Economic Challenges:*** Economic instability can limit the financial resources available for health programs, leading to reduced access to healthcare services and worsening health outcomes.
4. ***Policy Volatility:*** Frequent changes in government and shifting policy priorities can create uncertainty and hinder the continuity of health programs.

Case Study 3: The Impact of the Syrian Civil War on Health Services

Background: The ongoing Syrian civil war has had a devastating impact on the country's health system. The conflict has created a complex humanitarian crisis, with widespread damage to health infrastructure and severe disruptions in health services.

Impact on Health Programs

1. ***Destruction of Health Facilities:*** Hospitals and clinics have been targeted and destroyed in the conflict, severely reducing the capacity to provide medical care.
2. ***Disruption of Supply Chains:*** The war has disrupted supply chains for medical supplies and pharmaceuticals, leading to shortages of essential medicines and equipment.
3. ***Health Workforce Challenges:*** Many healthcare professionals have fled the country, leading to a shortage of trained personnel and a collapse of health services.

4. ***Increased Health Needs:*** The conflict has resulted in a surge in health needs, including trauma care, treatment for chronic diseases, and mental health support, which the fragmented health system struggles to address.

Lessons Learned

1. Political instability can lead to the complete collapse of health systems and infrastructure.
2. Humanitarian interventions and international support are crucial for addressing health needs in conflict-affected areas.
3. Building resilient health systems and establishing emergency response mechanisms are essential for mitigating the impacts of conflict on health services.

Case Study 4: The Effect of Political Instability on Health Programs in Venezuela

Background: Venezuela has experienced significant political and economic instability in recent years, leading to a severe crisis in the healthcare system. The country's economic collapse and political turmoil have had profound effects on health programs.

Impact on Health Programs

1. **Healthcare System Collapse:** Economic instability has led to a lack of funding for health services, resulting in the collapse of the healthcare system. Hospitals face shortages of essential supplies, medicines, and equipment.
2. **Increased Disease Burden:** The deterioration of health services has led to a resurgence of previously controlled diseases, such as malaria and diphtheria, and a decline in the management of chronic conditions.
3. **Migration and Brain Drain:** Political instability and economic hardship have driven many healthcare professionals to leave the country, exacerbating the shortage of medical personnel.
4. **Public Health Crisis:** The crisis has led to widespread malnutrition and a decline in overall public health, with increased mortality rates and deteriorating health indicators.

Lessons Learned

- Economic and political instability can lead to a severe breakdown of health systems and deteriorating health outcomes.
- Addressing health crises in unstable environments requires coordinated international support and effective emergency response strategies.

- Strengthening health system resilience and improving resource management are critical for mitigating the impacts of instability on health services.

Case Study 5: The Effect of Political Instability on HIV/AIDS Programs in Zimbabwe

Background: Zimbabwe has faced political instability and economic challenges over the past decades, which have affected the implementation of its HIV/AIDS programs.

Impact on Health Programs

1. **Funding Constraints:** Political and economic instability has led to fluctuations in funding for HIV/AIDS programs, affecting the availability of antiretroviral therapy (ART) and other critical services.
2. **Disruption of Services:** Inconsistent policy implementation and governance issues have resulted in disruptions in the delivery of HIV/AIDS services, including testing, treatment, and prevention programs.
3. **Healthcare Worker Shortages:** Economic hardships and political instability have led to a migration of healthcare professionals and a decline in the quality of care provided.
4. **Impact on Vulnerable Populations:** Political instability has exacerbated the vulnerability of marginalised groups, including sex workers and people living with HIV, who face increased stigma and reduced access to services.

Lessons Learned

- Political and economic instability can undermine the effectiveness of health programs, particularly those targeting chronic diseases like HIV/AIDS.
- Consistent and reliable funding, along with strong governance and leadership, are essential for sustaining health programs in challenging environments.
- Addressing the needs of vulnerable populations requires targeted interventions and support to mitigate the impacts of instability.

The key recommendations are as follows:

Recommendations

1. Strengthen political commitment and leadership to drive health initiatives and reforms.
2. Foster collaboration between the government, international organisations, and local communities to enhance the effectiveness of health programs.
3. Invest in robust monitoring and evaluation systems to ensure accountability and continuous improvement.

4. Address governance challenges, such as fragmentation and corruption, to create a more cohesive and effective health system.

Strategies for Mitigating the Impact of Political Instability on Health Programs: Political instability poses a significant threat to the continuity and effectiveness of health programs, often leading to disrupted services, funding gaps, and weakened institutional performance. In contexts where governance is fragile or frequently shifting, proactive strategies are essential to safeguard health interventions. These strategies include decentralising program management, embedding health initiatives within community structures, and creating contingency plans that ensure service delivery can withstand political shocks and transitions [38, 39].

1. **Strengthening Health System Resilience:** Building resilient health systems is crucial for mitigating the impacts of political instability. This involves:
    - **Improving Infrastructure:** Investing in robust and adaptable health infrastructure that can withstand disruptions.
    - **Enhancing Supply Chains:** Developing resilient supply chains and stockpiling essential medicines and supplies to ensure continuity of care.
    - **Capacity Building:** Training and retaining healthcare workers to maintain service delivery during periods of instability.
2. **Ensuring Flexible Funding Mechanisms:** Flexible funding mechanisms can help health programs adapt to changing political and economic conditions. Strategies include:
    - **Diversifying Funding Sources:** Seeking funding from multiple sources, including international donors, private sector partners, and philanthropic organisations.
    - **Emergency Funds:** Establishing emergency funds and contingency plans to address immediate health needs during crises.
3. **Strengthening Governance and Accountability:** Effective governance and accountability mechanisms are essential for managing health programs in unstable environments. This includes:
    - **Improving Transparency:** Enhancing transparency and accountability in the management of health resources and programs.
    - **Anti-Corruption Measures:** Implementing anti-corruption measures to reduce the impact of political instability on health program implementation.
4. **Fostering International Collaboration:** International collaboration and support are critical for addressing health challenges in politically unstable contexts. Strategies include:

- **Humanitarian Assistance:** Coordinating international humanitarian assistance to address immediate health needs and support affected health systems.
- **Partnerships:** Building partnerships with international organisations, NGOs, and other stakeholders to leverage resources and expertise.

5. **Engaging Communities:** Community engagement is crucial for maintaining health services and promoting resilience in unstable environments. This involves:
   - **Community-Based Interventions:** Implementing community-based health interventions to reach affected populations and maintain service delivery.
   - **Local Leadership:** Empowering local leaders and organisations to play a role in managing and delivering health services.

CONCLUSION

Political instability poses significant challenges to health programs, disrupting service delivery, undermining governance, and exacerbating health issues. However, by understanding the impacts of instability and implementing strategies to build resilience, manage resources effectively, and foster collaboration, it is possible to mitigate the adverse effects on health systems and improve health outcomes.

The lessons learned from case studies of both successful and failed health programs in unstable environments highlight the importance of strong governance, flexible funding, and community engagement. Addressing political instability and its impact on health programs requires a coordinated effort from governments, international organisations, and local communities to ensure that health services continue to reach those in need and that health systems are better equipped to withstand future challenges.

PATHWAYS TO STRENGTHENING POLITICAL COMMITMENT

Political commitment is essential for the successful implementation and sustainability of public health initiatives. It encompasses the dedication of political leaders to prioritise health issues, allocate necessary resources, and ensure effective governance. Strengthening political commitment involves fostering an environment where health becomes a central concern in policy-making, supported by robust institutional frameworks and collaborative partnerships. This section explores various pathways to strengthen political commitment to health, drawing on strategies and best practices from around the world [40 - 43].

Building Political Will through Evidence-Based Advocacy

Political will is a critical enabler of public health progress. However, it does not emerge spontaneously; it must be cultivated through deliberate, evidence-based advocacy. Presenting policymakers with compelling data, human stories, and cost-benefit analyses can shift perceptions and priorities. Effective advocacy aligns public health goals with political agendas, demonstrating how health investments contribute to economic development, social stability, and national prosperity.

1. **Evidence-Based Advocacy:** Political leaders are more likely to commit to health initiatives when presented with compelling evidence demonstrating the benefits and necessity of such programs. Effective advocacy involves:
   - **Data-Driven Arguments:** Utilising health data and research findings to highlight the burden of diseases, the impact of health interventions, and the return on investment in health.
   - **Success Stories:** Showcasing successful health programs and interventions from other regions or countries to illustrate the potential for positive outcomes and inspire action.
   - **Cost-Benefit Analyses:** Providing detailed analyses that show the economic benefits of investing in health, including reduced healthcare costs, increased productivity, and improved quality of life.
2. **Engagement with Policymakers:** Engaging policymakers directly through meetings, briefings, and presentations is crucial for advocacy efforts. Strategies include:
   - **Personalised Approaches:** Tailoring messages and data to the specific interests and priorities of policymakers to make the case for health initiatives more relevant.
   - **Policy Briefs:** Preparing concise and informative policy briefs that outline key issues, proposed solutions, and the benefits of health investments.
   - **Building Relationships:** Developing and maintaining relationships with key decision-makers to facilitate ongoing dialogue and support for health issues.

Strengthening Institutional Frameworks for Health

Strong institutions form the backbone of resilient health systems. When health governance structures are coherent, well-resourced, and empowered, they can deliver quality services, coordinate stakeholders, and sustain long-term reforms. Strengthening institutional frameworks involves enhancing legal mandates, improving organisational structures, investing in workforce development, and fostering leadership at all levels. Institutional stability, more than individual charisma or short-term initiatives, ensures sustainable public health outcomes.

1. **Creating Strong Health Institutions:** Institutional frameworks play a critical role in ensuring that health policies are effectively implemented. Key components include:
   - **Dedicated Health Ministries:** Establishing or strengthening dedicated health ministries or departments with clear mandates, sufficient resources, and authority to drive health initiatives.
   - **Intersectoral Coordination:** Promoting coordination between health ministries and other relevant sectors, such as education, finance, and agriculture, to address the broader determinants of health.
   - **Decentralised Governance:** Implementing decentralised governance structures that empower local authorities to take ownership of health programs and tailor interventions to local needs.
2. **Capacity Building:** Building the capacity of health institutions and personnel is essential for the effective implementation of health policies. This involves:
   - **Training Programs:** Providing training and professional development opportunities for health officials and staff to enhance their skills and knowledge.
   - **Resource Allocation:** Ensuring that health institutions have the necessary resources, including funding, equipment, and personnel, to carry out their functions effectively.

Engaging Civil Society and Community Leaders

Civil society organizations and community leaders are powerful allies in public health advancement, especially in settings marked by mistrust or limited state presence. Their deep-rooted connections to local populations position them as trusted messengers and mobilizers. Engaging these actors promotes inclusiveness, fosters cultural sensitivity, and enhances program legitimacy. Their participation also encourages accountability and bridges the gap between policy and grassroots realities.

1. **Involving Civil Society Organisations:** Civil society organisations (CSOs) can play a critical role in advocating for and supporting health initiatives. Strategies for engagement include:
   - **Partnerships:** Forming partnerships with CSOs to leverage their networks, expertise, and grassroots connections in advocating for health policies.
   - **Community Mobilization:** Supporting CSOs in mobilizing communities to advocate for health issues, participate in health programs, and hold leaders accountable.
   - **Feedback Mechanisms:** Establishing mechanisms for CSOs and community members to provide feedback on health programs and policies, ensuring that their perspectives are considered in decision-making.

2. **Empowering Community Leaders:** Community leaders can influence political commitment by:
   - **Local Advocacy:** Encouraging community leaders to advocate for health issues at local and national levels, using their influence to garner support from policymakers.
   - **Health Champions:** Identifying and supporting health champions within communities who can lead local health initiatives and advocate for improved services.

Leveraging International Support and Partnerships

Global health initiatives thrive on collaboration. International partners, ranging from multilateral agencies and donor governments to philanthropic foundations and global NGOs, offer financial resources, technical expertise, and strategic guidance. Leveraging these partnerships effectively requires strong domestic ownership, alignment with national priorities, and mechanisms that ensure coordination and sustainability. When well-managed, international support can accelerate progress, foster innovation, and strengthen the resilience of health systems.

1. **International Organisations and Donors:** International organisations and donors can provide technical assistance, funding, and advocacy support to strengthen political commitment. Strategies include:
   - **Global Advocacy Campaigns:** Engaging in global advocacy campaigns led by organisations such as the WHO and the United Nations to highlight health priorities and mobilise political will.
   - **Funding and Grants:** Securing funding and grants from international donors to support health programs and demonstrate the importance of health investments to national governments.
   - **Technical Assistance:** Collaborating with international organisations for technical assistance in areas such as health policy development, implementation, and evaluation.
2. **Regional Cooperation:** Regional cooperation can enhance political commitment by:
   - **Sharing Best Practices:** Facilitating regional platforms for sharing best practices, experiences, and successes in health policy and program implementation.
   - **Joint Initiatives:** Collaborating on regional health initiatives and programs that address common health challenges and promote collective action.

Fostering Accountability and Transparency

Without accountability and transparency, health systems become vulnerable to inefficiency, corruption, and public disillusionment. Establishing robust accountability mechanisms, from performance audits and public reporting to whistleblower protections, ensures that resources are used wisely and services reach intended beneficiaries. Transparency builds trust, empowers citizens, and enhances responsiveness. A culture of accountability not only deters malpractice but also drives continuous improvement in health governance.

1. **Transparency Measures:** Ensuring transparency in health governance is crucial for building political commitment and public trust. Measures include:
   - **Public Reporting:** Requiring regular public reporting on health program performance, expenditures, and outcomes to enhance accountability.
   - **Open Data Initiatives:** Promoting open data initiatives that make health data accessible to the public, enabling citizens to monitor and hold leaders accountable.
2. **Accountability Mechanisms:** Implementing accountability mechanisms to ensure that political commitments translate into effective action includes:
   - **Independent Audits:** Conducting independent audits of health programs and expenditures to identify and address inefficiencies and corruption.
   - **Oversight Committees:** Establishing oversight committees composed of representatives from government, civil society, and the private sector to monitor health program implementation and performance.

Building Consensus and Political Support

Achieving sustainable health reforms often requires building consensus among a diverse array of stakeholders, government actors, legislators, professional bodies, private sector partners, and the public. Consensus-building is a strategic process that involves negotiation, compromise, and inclusive dialogue. It ensures that health initiatives are politically feasible, socially acceptable, and widely supported. Political support built on consensus creates stability, enables legislative backing, and shields reforms from abrupt reversals.

1. **Broad-Based Support:** Building broad-based political support for health initiatives requires:
   - **Multi-Stakeholder Engagement:** Engaging a wide range of stakeholders, including government officials, legislators, civil society organizations, and the private sector, to build consensus on health priorities and policies.

- **Public Awareness Campaigns:** Running public awareness campaigns to educate citizens about health issues and generate public demand for political action.

2. **Long-Term Commitment:** Ensuring long-term political commitment involves:
   - **Sustained Advocacy:** Continuously advocating for health issues and maintaining pressure on policymakers to prioritise health in their agendas.
   - **Policy Integration:** Integrating health considerations into broader policy frameworks and development plans to ensure that health remains a central focus.

Comparative Insight: Political Leadership and Health Outcomes – Nigeria *vs.* Rwanda

In exemplifying how sustained political commitment can translate into measurable health gains, Rwanda's post-2000 health transformation demonstrates how consistent political commitment that aligns with evidence-based governance can yield rapid gains. The government introduced community-based health insurance, ensured strong district-level accountability, and achieved performance-based financing in over 90% immunisation coverage, a 60% reduction in maternal mortality, and a national community-based health insurance scheme for more than 80% of the population [44, 45].

In contrast, Nigeria's progress has been uneven, with diverse political interests influencing health priorities across 36 states and the federal capital territory, resulting in fluctuating political will, weak intergovernmental coordination, and inconsistent financing. However, some programmes recorded localised successes, such as the near elimination of polio and improvements in malaria control by the malaria interventions. This comparison highlights that political will must be institutionalised to ensure consistency in health system performance, and that leadership and governance matter throughout the continuum of governance.

In summary, as with other developing nations, political governance remains the cornerstone of health system performance and the effectiveness of Nigeria's health system. Institutionalising political will through policy coherence, sustained financing, and accountability mechanisms measurably improves health outcomes. Various evidence from national initiatives and regional comparisons affirm that leadership continuity determines the trajectory of public health transformation that serves the populace and in attaining universal health coverage for all. Where governance is weak, even well-designed interventions falter under the weight of inefficiency and fragmentation. Therefore, in Nigeria and other developing nations, transforming public health requires strong governance across all tiers as a measurable determinant of health, and tracking political will and commitment through budgetary allocations and releases, evaluating policy implementation fidelity, and holding leaders accountable for outcomes. Thus, governance and political will are not abstract concepts but are the scaffolding upon which the health and resilience of nations are built. Therefore, strengthening governance and institutionalising political will across all tiers is not a mere administrative process, but it is part of the public health intervention [46, 47].

CONCLUSION

Strengthening political commitment to health is a multifaceted process that requires effective advocacy, strong institutional frameworks, and active engagement of civil society and international partners. By building evidence-based cases for health investments, fostering accountability and transparency, and leveraging regional and international support, it is possible to enhance political will and ensure that health remains a priority in policy-making. The pathways outlined in this section provide a roadmap for strengthening political commitment and achieving sustainable health outcomes. By addressing the challenges and opportunities associated with political commitment, countries can create an environment where health programs thrive, ultimately leading to improved health and well-being for their populations.

REFERENCES

[1] Frenk J, Moon S. Governance challenges in global health. N Engl J Med 2013; 368(10): 936-42. [http://dx.doi.org/10.1056/NEJMra1109339] [PMID: 23465103]

[2] Kickbusch I, Lister G, Told M, Drager N. Global Health Diplomacy: Concepts, Issues, Actors, Instruments, Fora and Cases. Springer Science & Business Media 2012.

[3] Oleribe OE, Momoh J, Uzochukwu BSC, *et al.* Identifying Key Challenges Facing Healthcare Systems In Africa And Potential Solutions. Int J Gen Med 2019; 12: 395-403. [http://dx.doi.org/10.2147/IJGM.S223882] [PMID: 31819592]

[4] Gilson L. Health Policy and Systems Research, a Methodology Reader. Alliance for Health Policy and Systems Research and World Health Organization, 2012. https://www.who.int/alliance-hpsr/alliancehpsr_reader.pdf Available form: https://www.who.int/alliance-hpsr/alliancehpsr_reader.pdf

[5] World Health Organization (WHO). Primary Health Care on the Road to Universal Health Coverage: 2019 Monitoring Report. WHO; 2021.

[6] Chukwuma JN, Obi FA. A political economy analysis of health policymaking in Nigeria: the genesis of the 2014 National Health Act. Health Policy Plan 2025; 40(4): 459-70. [http://dx.doi.org/10.1093/heapol/czaf007] [PMID: 39882935]

[7] Othman MF, Othman N, Shehu I. Nigerian federalism: an overview of its imperatives and impediments. J Int Stud 2021; 17: 183-209. [http://dx.doi.org/10.32890/jis2021.17.8]

[8] Smith DJ. The State and Health Policy in Nigeria. University of Rochester Press 2014.

[9] Meribole EC, Makinde OA, Oyemakinde A, *et al.* The Nigerian health information system policy review of 2014 : the need, content, expectations and progress. Health Info Libr J 2018; 35(4): 285-97. [http://dx.doi.org/10.1111/hir.12240] [PMID: 30417971]

[10] Croke K, Ogbuoji O. Health reform in Nigeria: the politics of primary health care and universal health coverage. Health Policy Plan 2024; 39(1): 22-31. [http://dx.doi.org/10.1093/heapol/czad107] [PMID: 37978878]

[11] Global Polio Eradication Initiative. (2016). Nigeria: Annual status, surveillance & immunisation activities 2010-2015 (IMB report). Geneva: GPEI. Available from: https://polioeradication.org/wp-content/uploads/2016/07/7.5_6IMB-1.pdf

[12] World Bank. (2015, April 10). World Bank supports Nigeria to end polio and sustain routine immunisation [Press release]. Washington, DC: World Bank. Available from: https://www.worldbank.org/en/news/press-release/2015/04/10/world-ba-k-supports-nigeria-to-end-polio-and-sustain-routine-immunization

[13] Shuaib F, Gunnala R, Musa EO, *et al.* Ebola virus disease outbreak - Nigeria, July-September 2014. MMWR Morb Mortal Wkly Rep 2014; 63(39): 867-72. [PMID: 25275332]

[14] Oleribe OO, Crossey MM, Taylor-Robinson SD. Nigerian response to the 2014 Ebola viral disease outbreak: lessons and cautions. Pan Afr Med J 2015; 22 Suppl 1(Suppl 1):13. [http://dx.doi.org/10.11694/pamj.supp.2015.22.1.6490]

[15] Bolu O, Mustapha B, Ihekweazu C, *et al.* Effect of Nigeria Presidential Task Force on COVID-19 Pandemic, Nigeria. Emerg Infect Dis 2022; 28(13): S168-76. [http://dx.doi.org/10.3201/eid2813.220254] [PMID: 36502390]

[16] Abubakar I, Dalglish SL, Angell B, *et al.* The Lancet Nigeria Commission: investing in health and the future of the nation. Lancet 2022; 399(10330): 1155-200. [http://dx.doi.org/10.1016/S0140-6736(21)02488-0] [PMID: 35303470]

[17] Adeoye MI, Obi FA, Adrion ER. Stakeholder perspectives on the governance and accountability of Nigeria's Basic Health Care Provision Fund. Health Policy Plan 2024; 39(10): 1032-40. [http://dx.doi.org/10.1093/heapol/czae082] [PMID: 39185602]

[18] National Bureau of Statistics (NBS). Health Expenditure Review of Federal. State, and Local Governments in Nigeria 2021.

[19] Buse K, Mays N, Walt G. Making Health Policy. 2nd ed., UK: McGraw-Hill Education 2012.

[20] Dodgson R, Lee K, Drager N. Global Health Governance; a Conceptual Review. Centre on Global Change & Health, Department of Health and Development, London School of Hygiene and Tropical Medicine, London and World Health Organization, Geneva, 2002.

[21] Shiffman J, Smith S. Generation of political priority for global health initiatives: a framework and case study of maternal mortality. Lancet 2007; 370(9595): 1370-9. [http://dx.doi.org/10.1016/S0140-6736(07)61579-7] [PMID: 17933652]

[22] Kana MA, Doctor HV, Peleteiro B, Lunet N, Barros H. Maternal and child health interventions in Nigeria: a systematic review of published studies from 1990 to 2014. BMC Public Health 2015; 15(1): 334. [http://dx.doi.org/10.1186/s12889-015-1688-3] [PMID: 25881020]

[23] Ruger, J. P., & Yach, D. (2009). The Global Role of the World Health Organisation. Global Health Governance: The Scholarly Journal for the New Health Security Paradigm, 2(2), 1. Available from: https://pmc.ncbi.nlm.nih.gov/articles/PMC3981564/

[24] National Health Policy 2016. Promoting the Health of Nigerians to Accelerate Socio-economic Development Federal Ministry of Health, September 2016.

[25] Patel M, Cochi S. Addressing the Challenges and Opportunities of the Polio Endgame: Lessons for the Future. J Infect Dis 2017; 216 (Suppl. 1): S1-8. [http://dx.doi.org/10.1093/infdis/jix117] [PMID: 28838196]

[26] Chukwuma JN. Implementing Health Policy in Nigeria: The Basic Health Care Provision Fund as a

Catalyst for Achieving Universal Health Coverage? Dev Change 2023; 54(6): 1480-503. [http://dx.doi.org/10.1111/dech.12808]

[27] World Health Organisation & Alliance for Health Policy and Systems Research. (2017). Primary health care systems (primasys): case study from Nigeria. World Health Organisation. Available from: https://iris.who.int/handle/10665/341137 License: CC BY-NC-SA 3.0 IGO

[28] Otu A, Ameh S, Osifo-Dawodu E, Alade E, Ekuri S, Idris J. An account of the Ebola virus disease outbreak in Nigeria: implications and lessons learnt. BMC Public Health 2018; 18(1): 3. [http://dx.doi.org/10.1186/s12889-017-4535-x] [PMID: 28693453]

[29] Ogundeji YK, Tinuoye O, Bharali I, *et al.* Is Nigeria on course to achieve universal health coverage in the context of its epidemiological and financing transition? A knowledge, capacity and policy gap analysis (a qualitative study). BMJ Open 2023; 13(3): e064710. BMJ Open 2023. [http://dx.doi.org/10.1136/bmjopen-2022-064710]

[30] Oleribe OO, Crossey MME, Taylor-Robinson SD. Nigerian response to the 2014 Ebola viral disease outbreak: lessons and cautions. Pan Afr Med J 2015; 22(Suppl 1) (Suppl. 1): 13. [http://dx.doi.org/10.11604/pamj.supp.2015.22.1.6490] [PMID: 26740841]

[31] Ekwebelem OC, Nnorom-Dike OV, Aborode AT, Ekwebelem NC, Aleke JC, Ofielu ES. Eradication of wild poliovirus in Nigeria: Lessons learnt. Public Health in Practice 2021; 2: 100144. [http://dx.doi.org/10.1016/j.puhip.2021.100144] [PMID: 36101607]

[32] Murray CJL, King G, Lopez AD, Tomijima N, Krug EG. Armed conflict as a public health problem. BMJ 2002; 324(7333): 346-9. [http://dx.doi.org/10.1136/bmj.324.7333.346] [PMID: 11834565]

[33] Macrae J, Zwi A. War and Hunger: Rethinking International Responses to Complex Emergencies. Zed Books 1994.

[34] Oladayo NA. The impact of conflict on health outcomes: a systematic evidence from sub-saharan Africa. Mgbakoigba: Journal of African Studies 2018; 8(1): 88–100. Available from: https://www.ajol.info/index.php/mjas/article/view/187375

[35] Owhor GA, Adekoya OO, Ezenwafor CC, Okoli EA, Chikezie NC, Shomuyiwa DO. How africa's political challenges impede healthcare advancement. Nigerian Health Journal 2024; 24(4): 1641-6. [http://dx.doi.org/10.60787/tnhj.v24i4.831]

[36] United Nations Development Programme (UNDP). Assessing the impact of conflict on development in northeast Nigeria, 2019.

[37] Saleh S, Fouad FM. Political economy of health in fragile and conflict-affected regions in the Middle East and North Africa region. J Glob Health 2022; 12: 01003. [http://dx.doi.org/10.7189/jogh.12.01003] [PMID: 35959965]

[38] Kickbusch I, Gleicher D. Governance for Health in the 21st Century.. WHO Press 2012.

[39] Stuckler D, Basu S. The Body Economic: Why Austerity Kills. Basic Books, 2013.

[40] Yisa SS, Ogunniyi TJ, Dine RD. Strengthening primary health care in Nigeria: a means to achieve universal health coverage. BMJ Global Health 2025; 10: e018486. [http://dx.doi.org/10.1136/bmjgh-2024-018486] [PMID: 41151829]

[41] Aregbeshola BS. Enhancing Political Will for Universal Health Coverage in Nigeria. MEDICC Rev 2017; 19(1): 42-6. [http://dx.doi.org/10.37757/MR2017.V19.N1.8] [PMID: 28225545]

[42] UHC 2030. (2024). 2024–2027 Strategic Framework. African Union Commission. (2019). Africa Leadership Meeting: Investing in Health.

[43] Saleh J-EA. Resilient Communities: Navigating Public Health Challenges in Developing Nations. Bentham Science Publishers 2025. [http://dx.doi.org/10.2174/97898153056091250101]

[44] Boerma T, Ercumen A. Why is Rwanda an exemplar? Exemplars in Global Health: Primary Health Care. Seattle, WA: Exemplars in Global Health 2024; pp. 45-62.

[45] Uwimana, A., & Mbabazi, J. (2025). How Rwanda enhances mother, child health through community engagement. AllAfrica. Available from: https://allafrica.com/stories/202503040425.html

[46] World Health Organisation. (2024). Nigeria Country Cooperation Strategy 2023–2027: Progress on health outcomes. Abuja: WHO Nigeria. WHO | Regional Office for Africa

[47] Wollum A, Burstein R, Fullman N, Dwyer-Lindgren L, Gakidou E. Benchmarking health system performance across states in Nigeria: a systematic analysis of levels and trends in key maternal and child health interventions and outcomes, 2000–2013. BMC Med 2015; 13(1): 208. [http://dx.doi.org/10.1186/s12916-015-0438-9] [PMID: 26329607]

CHAPTER 2

Poverty and Public Health: Addressing Socio-Economic Barriers

Abstract: This chapter examines the profound influence of poverty on health outcomes in Nigeria and other developing nations. The chapter delves into the interconnectedness of poverty and health, exploring how economic constraints hinder access to healthcare and exacerbate malnutrition, particularly among vulnerable populations. By evaluating the impact of poverty reduction programs and social protection systems, this chapter sheds light on the successes and limitations of current initiatives aimed at improving public health. Additionally, it discusses the importance of empowering communities through economic development as a sustainable solution to break the cycle of poverty and enhance health outcomes. Through a detailed analysis of the socio-economic barriers to health, this chapter provides insights into strategies that can be employed to create a healthier and more equitable society.

Keywords: Economic development, Health inequities, Healthcare access, Malnutrition, Nigeria, Poverty reduction programs, Poverty, Public health, Social protection systems, Socio-economic barriers, Vulnerable populations.

INTRODUCTION

Poverty is one of the most significant determinants of health outcomes in developing countries. The intricate relationship between poverty and public health is a cycle that perpetuates vulnerability, where the poor are disproportionately affected by disease, malnutrition, and lack of access to healthcare. In Nigeria and other developing nations, the socio-economic barriers created by poverty pose immense challenges to achieving universal health coverage and improving overall public health.

According to the World Bank's national-poverty estimates, the proportion of Nigerians living below both national and international poverty lines has risen significantly in recent years; extreme poverty increased from 34.7 per cent in 2018/19 to 41.8 per cent in 2022/23, based on the international poverty line of $3.00 per person per day (2021 PPPs). These figures reflect economic shocks, high food inflation, and conflict-driven displacement. Additionally, there are sub-

Jalal-Eddeen Abubakar Saleh

national regional differences within the country. In 2022/23, the poverty rate in the northern region was 57.4 per cent, while in the southern region it was 21.2 per cent, up from 44.7 per cent and 14.9 per cent, respectively, in 2018/19. Globally, Nigeria's under-five and infant mortality rates remain among the highest. The data from UNICEF and the World Bank indicate that under-five mortality stands at approximately 105 per 1,000 live births, with neonatal mortality around 34 per 1,000, well above regional averages, with northern and rural states experiencing disproportionately higher child mortality and malnutrition rates as compared to the southern region [1 - 7].

This chapter delves into the nexus between poverty and health, exploring how economic constraints affect access to healthcare, the impact of malnutrition, and the effectiveness of poverty reduction programs. By examining social protection systems and community empowerment initiatives, this chapter aims to present strategies that can mitigate the adverse effects of poverty on health, ultimately fostering a more equitable and healthy society.

THE NEXUS BETWEEN POVERTY AND HEALTH

The intricate relationship between poverty and health is a central concern in public health, particularly in developing nations like Nigeria. Poverty is not merely an economic condition; it is a multifaceted phenomenon that impacts every aspect of life, including health. The nexus between poverty and health is a vicious cycle where each perpetuates the other, making it a significant barrier to achieving equitable health outcomes [8 - 10]. Income inequality could amplify disease burden through these three mechanisms:

1. **Deprivation of basic amenities:** households with poor income lack food, safe water, sanitation, and access to affordable healthcare, increasing exposure and vulnerability to infectious diseases and malnutrition.
2. **Barrier to accessing preventive care:** out-of-pocket costs and opportunity costs (lost wages, travel time) reduce access and utilisation of antenatal care services, immunisation services, and early treatment of basic ailments.
3. **Social determinants of health:** societal inequality results in weaker social cohesion and psychosocial stress, worse maternal and child health outcomes, and predisposition to chronic diseases.

Empirically, income-inequality metrics (*e.g.*, Nigeria's Gini and poverty gap measures) correlate with lower service coverage and higher child mortality across states; the World Bank's inequality and poverty briefs show Nigeria's persistent Gini and rising poverty rates, which are linked in the literature to poorer population health [2].

Poverty as a Determinant of Health

Poverty is a powerful social determinant of health, shaping exposure to risks, access to care, and overall well-being. It limits access to nutritious food, safe housing, clean water, and healthcare services, while increasing vulnerability to disease and reducing life expectancy. In Nigeria and other Low- and Middle-Income Countries (LMICs), poverty is more than a lack of income; it dictates health outcomes from birth onward. Poor communities are disproportionately affected by infectious diseases such as malaria, tuberculosis, and HIV/AIDS, which thrive in overcrowded settings with inadequate sanitation and limited preventive tools. Poverty also delays or prevents healthcare-seeking due to costs, leading to worse health outcomes. Addressing poverty is therefore essential not only for economic development but also for improving public health and achieving health equity. Some of these consequences include [8]:

1. **Limited Access to Healthcare Services:** Poverty restricts individuals and households from accessing healthcare when they need it most. Many impoverished families cannot afford consultation fees, transportation to health facilities, or the cost of medications. In the absence of functional health insurance systems, out-of-pocket expenditures become catastrophic, often leading to delayed care, self-medication, or complete abandonment of treatment. This results in poor health-seeking behaviour, late presentation of illnesses, and higher mortality rates, especially among children and mothers.
2. **Poor Living Conditions and Environmental Hazards:** Poor communities often reside in overcrowded, poorly ventilated, and unsanitary environments that increase susceptibility to communicable diseases. Lack of access to clean water, proper sanitation, and waste management exposes residents to cholera, typhoid, and parasitic infections. In urban slums and rural settlements, inadequate housing infrastructure and environmental degradation further worsen health outcomes through increased exposure to air pollution, vector-borne diseases, and climate-related health risks.
3. **Nutritional Deficiencies and Food Insecurity:** Poverty is closely tied to undernutrition and food insecurity, which disproportionately affect children and pregnant women. Malnutrition weakens immunity, stunts growth, and increases vulnerability to disease and death. Inadequate diets among the poor often lack essential nutrients, leading to conditions such as anaemia, kwashiorkor, and rickets. Moreover, food insecurity may also contribute to obesity in low-income populations through reliance on cheap, calorie-dense but nutrient-poor foods, creating a paradox of undernutrition and obesity within the same populations.
4. **Educational Inequality and Health Literacy:** Poverty often goes hand-i--hand with low educational attainment, which in turn affects health literacy.

Individuals with limited education may lack the knowledge to prevent disease, understand medical advice, or navigate health systems. Women and girls, in particular, bear the brunt of this intersection, with consequences that reverberate through maternal and child health. A lack of health education perpetuates harmful practices, hinders uptake of preventive services like immunization, and reduces compliance with treatment regimens.

5. **Psychosocial Stress and Mental Health Burden:** Living in poverty is a chronic stressor. The constant struggle to meet basic needs - such as food, shelter, and safety - takes a toll on mental health. Anxiety, depression, and other stress-related conditions are more prevalent among the poor, yet mental health services are rarely accessible or affordable. In many cultures, stigma further impedes access to care. The psychological burden of poverty can also exacerbate physical health conditions, creating a vicious cycle of worsening health and deepening poverty.
6. **Intergenerational Transmission of Poor Health:** Poverty is not just a present-day challenge - it is intergenerational. Children born into poverty are more likely to suffer from preventable diseases, drop out of school early, and grow up in environments that undermine their development. Their health outcomes are significantly worse than those of their more affluent peers. Without targeted interventions, these disadvantages compound across generations, entrenching cycles of poor health and economic stagnation.
7. **Structural Inequalities and Systemic Disempowerment:** The relationship between poverty and health is not merely individual or household-based; it is systemic. In many societies, health systems are structured to disadvantage the poor through regressive financing mechanisms, geographical inaccessibility, or exclusionary policies. The marginalisation of poor communities from political processes means their voices are often unheard in health policy formulation, perpetuating neglect and underinvestment in their health needs.

Poor Health as a Contributor to Poverty

Ill health imposes significant financial strain on individuals and families, disrupting livelihoods, reducing productivity, and deepening poverty. In countries like Nigeria, where many rely on informal employment without health insurance, a single illness can devastate household finances. The absence of universal health coverage and social protection systems means that out-of-pocket healthcare costs often force families to sell assets, incur debt, or sacrifice essentials such as food and education. This not only worsens immediate hardship but also limits future access to care, creating a vicious cycle of poverty and poor health. Chronic illnesses, disabilities, and the long-term care needs of the elderly further intensify this burden, as ongoing treatment costs are often unaffordable for low-income households. Breaking this cycle requires systemic reforms that improve access to affordable, quality healthcare and strengthen social safety nets [9].

1. **Catastrophic Health Expenditures and Out-of-Pocket Payments:** A significant portion of the population in developing nations relies on out-o--pocket payments to access health services. When individuals fall ill and need care, especially for chronic conditions, surgeries, or maternal complications, the cost can be overwhelming. These catastrophic expenditures often result in the sale of household assets, borrowing at high interest rates, or diverting funds from essential needs like education and food. The financial impact of even a single hospitalisation can be devastating, leading to long-term indebtedness and a downward spiral into poverty.
2. **Loss of Income and Reduced Productivity:** Poor health directly affects a person's ability to work, earn, and support their family. In agrarian and informal economies, where income is closely tied to physical labour and daily engagement, illness or injury translates into immediate income loss. Chronic diseases, disabilities, and untreated infections limit productivity not only for the affected individuals but often for their caregivers as well, who may have to forgo economic activities to provide support. For breadwinners, this loss of income can destabilize entire households, especially in the absence of health insurance or employer benefits.
3. **Impacts on Education and Future Earning Potential:** When children or adolescents experience frequent illnesses or malnutrition, their school attendance and performance are compromised. Additionally, when family income is drained by health expenses, education is often one of the first sacrifices made. Early dropout rates, particularly among girls, are frequently linked to the economic consequences of poor health within the family. This disruption in education diminishes future earning potential, entrenching a cycle where today's poor health leads to tomorrow's economic marginalisation.
4. **Economic Burden of Disability and Long-Term Care:** Chronic conditions, mental health issues, and disabilities carry long-term implications for individuals and families. Without inclusive healthcare and disability support systems, families are left to shoulder the costs of care, rehabilitation, and necessary home modifications. In many low-resource settings, this can mean that entire families become economically unproductive as caregiving demands increase. Moreover, people with disabilities often face employment discrimination, further limiting income-earning opportunities and reinforcing economic exclusion.
5. **Gendered Implications: The Burden on Women and Girls:** Women disproportionately bear the brunt of health-related poverty in many cultures. They are often primary caregivers, sacrificing their education or employment to

care for sick family members. Maternal ill-health, complications from childbirth, or lack of access to reproductive health services severely affect women's health and economic participation. In households where resources are scarce, the health needs of women and girls are often deprioritised, reinforcing cycles of gendered poverty and disempowerment. The female gender often suffers from anaemia, constrained access to services, and caregiving burdens that reduce health-seeking. High rates of female anaemia are linked directly to adverse birth outcomes, low birthweight, and child stunting. Similarly, rural populations face steeper barriers to accessing health as compared to their urban counterparts. Some of the reasons include fewer functional primary health centres, longer travel times to access healthcare services, and higher exposure to food insecurity and conflict. The urban poor, though closer to the healthcare facilities, face overcrowded, under-resourced informal settlements with poor water, hygiene, and sanitation, making them vulnerable to severe health consequences.

6. **The Vicious Cycle of Ill Health and Economic Insecurity:** The bidirectional link between poverty and poor health creates a self-perpetuating cycle. Individuals fall sick, lose income, and incur debt, which in turn increases vulnerability to further illness due to malnutrition, stress, and lack of access to preventive care. This cycle is particularly stark in conflict-affected or rural areas where health infrastructure is weak, social safety nets are nonexistent, and employment opportunities are limited. For millions, ill health is both a symptom and a cause of poverty, a feedback loop that is difficult to escape without deliberate, systemic intervention.
7. **Weak Health Systems as Economic Drains:** On a broader scale, underinvestment in public health services affects national productivity. Poorly functioning health systems reduce the health and capacity of the labour force, hinder economic development, and increase national healthcare costs over time. A country that fails to invest in health essentially mortgages its future growth potential. Healthy populations are not only more productive but also better able to contribute to innovation, governance, and societal progress.

Socio-Economic Inequities and Health Disparities

Socio-economic inequities are major drivers of health disparities in Nigeria and other developing nations. Health outcomes often follow a social gradient, with poorer populations facing higher disease burdens, limited access to care, and worse overall health. These disparities are rooted in structural inequalities in wealth, education, housing, and political representation. Rural communities, women, children, and marginalised groups are particularly vulnerable, especially in areas with weak healthcare infrastructure. For instance, maternal and child health outcomes are significantly poorer in impoverished regions with limited access to skilled birth attendants and essential medicines. The urban-rural divide further widens these gaps, compounded by systemic issues such as corruption, underfunding, and poor governance. Tackling health disparities thus requires more than healthcare provision; it calls for addressing the broader social and economic determinants of health [10].

1. **The Social Determinants of Health: A Framework for Understanding Disparities:** The WHO defines social determinants of health as the conditions in which people are born, grow, live, work, and age. These conditions are shaped by the distribution of money, power, and resources. Individuals from lower socio-economic backgrounds are more likely to live in overcrowded housing, lack clean water and sanitation, have limited access to education, and engage in precarious employment - all of which increase vulnerability to poor health. This framework helps public health practitioners understand that health disparities are not simply the result of individual choices but are influenced by broader societal structures.
2. **Access to Health Services: A Divided Landscape:** Socio-economic status often determines access to quality healthcare. In Nigeria and many developing nations, urban elites benefit from proximity to well-equipped private hospitals and specialists, while rural and impoverished communities depend on under-resourced public health facilities, if any exist at all. Financial barriers such as user fees, transportation costs, and informal payments further exclude the poor. These access disparities mean that treatable conditions go unmanaged, immunization coverage remains inconsistent, and maternal and child health outcomes diverge sharply along income and geographic lines.
3. **Education and Health Literacy: A Compounding Inequality:** Education is a critical determinant of health. People with higher levels of education are more likely to understand health information, navigate healthcare systems, and adopt preventive behaviors. Conversely, low levels of education and health literacy can lead to delayed treatment, poor disease management, and low uptake of essential services like immunization, antenatal care, and family planning. In communities where educational opportunities are limited, especially for girls, the compounded effect of ignorance and poverty further entrenches poor health outcomes.
4. **Employment, Informal Work, and Occupational Hazards:** The nature of employment is a major driver of socio-economic health disparities. Those in informal or low-paying jobs often lack health insurance, paid sick leave, or occupational protections. They are more likely to work in environments with physical risks, chemical exposures, and poor sanitation. Furthermore, informal workers rarely have access to employer-sponsored healthcare or retirement

benefits, leaving them vulnerable to both short-term health crises and long-term economic insecurity due to ill health.

5. **Gender Inequities and Intersectionality:** Socio-economic inequities intersect with gender to exacerbate health disparities. Women, particularly those in rural or traditional settings, often have lower economic power, limited decision-making autonomy, and restricted access to health services. Cultural norms and discriminatory practices may prevent women from seeking care, particularly for reproductive and sexual health. For girls and women living in poverty, these overlapping disadvantages result in high maternal mortality rates, low contraceptive use, and increased exposure to gender-based violence, all of which impact their health outcomes and life prospects.
6. **Regional and Ethnic Disparities:** In Nigeria, regional and ethnic disparities are evident in health indicators. The North East and North West regions consistently report higher rates of infant and maternal mortality, lower immunisation coverage, and poorer nutritional outcomes compared to the South. These disparities often reflect historical marginalisation, underinvestment in infrastructure, insecurity, and socio-political neglect. Ethnic minorities and nomadic populations may also face linguistic and cultural barriers to accessing services, further entrenching health inequities.
7. **Health Inequities as a Threat to National Development:** Beyond the moral imperative, health inequities have profound economic and social consequences. A society in which large segments of the population are unhealthy cannot maximise its human capital or drive sustainable development. Unequal health outcomes contribute to lower productivity, higher healthcare costs, and social instability. Bridging the health equity gap is therefore essential not just for justice but also for economic growth and national cohesion.
8. **Strategies to Address Socio-Economic Health Disparities:** Tackling socio-economic inequities in health requires a multi-sectoral approach:
   - **Universal Health Coverage (UHC):** Expanding access to affordable, quality health services, especially for the poor and marginalised.
   - **Pro-poor Health Financing:** Removing user fees, providing subsidies, and investing in community-based health insurance.
   - **Investing in Social Determinants:** Improving education, housing, sanitation, nutrition, and employment conditions.
   - **Community Engagement:** Ensuring marginalised voices are included in health planning and implementation.
   - **Targeted Interventions:** Using disaggregated data to identify high-risk groups and allocate resources accordingly.

Breaking the Cycle: Policy Implications

Poverty and poor health create a vicious cycle, each reinforcing the other. Breaking this cycle is essential for sustainable development and requires integrated, equity-focused policies. Governments must address both the social determinants of health and the health consequences of poverty through systemic reforms across sectors. A multifaceted approach is needed, one that improves healthcare access while simultaneously reducing poverty. Social protection programs like health insurance, cash transfers, and food security initiatives can shield vulnerable populations from the economic impact of illness. Equally important is investment in health infrastructure, especially in underserved regions, to ensure equitable access to essential services. Strengthening primary healthcare, promoting preventive care, and enhancing health literacy are vital to long-term success. A rights-based, pro-poor policy framework grounded in data and inclusiveness can help disrupt the intergenerational transmission of poverty and ill health [9, 10].

1. **Prioritising Universal Health Coverage (UHC) for the Poor:** One of the most impactful policy measures to break the poverty-health cycle is the full implementation of Universal Health Coverage. Poor populations are often deterred from seeking healthcare due to out-of-pocket costs, distance, or low trust in public systems. UHC ensures that all individuals, particularly the most vulnerable, can access needed health services without suffering financial hardship. In practical terms, this entails scaling up the Basic Healthcare Provision Fund (BHCPF) in Nigeria, strengthening the National Health Insurance Authority (NHIA), and ensuring that pro-poor targeting mechanisms are embedded in coverage schemes.
2. **Investing in Primary Health Care as the First Line of Defence:** Primary Health Care (PHC) remains the cornerstone of an equitable health system. Strengthening PHC infrastructure in underserved areas, especially rural communities, improves access, reduces the burden on secondary and tertiary facilities, and enables early detection and management of diseases. Policy should support the training and deployment of community health workers, robust supply chains for essential medicines, and the integration of preventive and promotive health into PHC platforms. Equitable PHC delivery must be funded, monitored, and protected from political interference.
3. **Multi-Sectoral Policy Coordination:** Because the determinants of poverty and ill health span beyond the health sector, breaking the cycle demands a Health in All Policies (HiAP) approach. This means integrating health equity considerations into the policies of education, agriculture, housing, water and sanitation, labor, and social protection. For instance, agricultural subsidies

targeting food security, safe housing policies, investments in clean water infrastructure, and expanded educational access, especially for girls, each play a role in shaping health outcomes. A national policy framework must institutionalize cross-sector collaboration to address these interlinked drivers effectively.

4. **Enhancing Social Protection for the Most Vulnerable:** Social protection systems such as conditional cash transfers, school feeding programs, and unemployment support can cushion the economic impact of illness and build household resilience. In Nigeria, the expansion and institutionalization of the National Social Investment Program (NSIP) can be leveraged to ensure the poor are not pushed deeper into poverty by health-related shocks. Policy must ensure transparency, community participation, and continuous evaluation in the design and delivery of such programs to maximize impact.
5. **Targeted Policies to Address Marginalized Populations:** Policies must recognize and respond to the needs of specific populations who are disproportionately affected by poverty and health burdens, such as internally displaced persons (IDPs), persons with disabilities, ethnic minorities, and people in conflict zones. These groups often fall through the cracks of mainstream health and welfare systems. Deliberate inclusion through tailored interventions, mobile outreach services, and legal protections is essential to closing equity gaps and preventing further marginalization.
6. **Data-Driven Policymaking and Monitoring:** Breaking the cycle requires precise, disaggregated data to identify where the gaps are and how best to target interventions. Strengthening national health information systems, integrating poverty and health indicators, and promoting the routine use of data in policy design and evaluation will enhance transparency and accountability. This also enables the creation of localized strategies responsive to regional disparities in Nigeria's diverse socio-economic landscape.
7. **Education as a Transformative Health Policy Tool:** Educational attainment is one of the most powerful predictors of long-term health outcomes. Policies that promote universal access to quality education, particularly for girls, lay the groundwork for improved health literacy, better health behaviors, delayed childbearing, and higher economic productivity. Linking health and education policies, such as integrating sexual and reproductive health into school curricula, can yield cross-cutting benefits for both sectors.
8. **Economic Empowerment and Livelihood Support:** Health policy must recognize the economic roots of vulnerability. Integrating health with livelihood interventions, such as microfinance, skills training, and youth employment initiatives, empowers families to afford care, make healthier choices, and reduce dependence on external aid. For women, economic empo-

werment is especially critical, as it enhances autonomy in health decision-making and investment in child health and nutrition.

9. **Governance and Political Commitment:** Ultimately, breaking the cycle hinges on political will. Governments must institutionalize equity and health justice as core principles of governance, reflected in budgets, policies, and practice. Stronger intergovernmental coordination, decentralized planning that empowers local governments, and robust civil society engagement are necessary to ensure that policies translate into impact on the ground.

CONCLUSION

Breaking the cycle between poverty and poor health requires bold, inclusive, and sustained policy action. Health must be recognized not only as a fundamental human right but also as a powerful tool for poverty reduction and social transformation. Achieving health equity demands investments in universal health coverage, strengthened primary care, social protection, and education, particularly for the most vulnerable. These are not merely health interventions; they are nation-building strategies. By placing the health of the poor at the centre of development agendas, Nigeria and other developing nations can transform a vicious cycle of poverty and ill health into a virtuous one of opportunity, productivity, and resilience.

ACCESS TO HEALTHCARE: ECONOMIC DETERMINANTS

Access to healthcare is a fundamental human right, yet economic barriers prevent millions in Nigeria and other developing countries from receiving timely and quality care. Low income, unemployment, lack of insurance, and high out-o--pocket costs force many to choose between healthcare and basic needs like food or education. These economic constraints deepen poverty and create a cycle of ill health and financial hardship. Beyond income, systemic issues, such as underfunded health systems and poor distribution of health workers, further limit access and quality of care. Addressing these economic determinants is vital for improving health equity and outcomes. This requires more than expanding services; it demands pro-poor financing models, robust social protection schemes, and policy reforms that prioritise vulnerable populations. Ensuring equitable healthcare access is not just a health goal; it's a socio-economic necessity for sustainable development [11 - 13].

Income and Healthcare Access

In Nigeria, income remains one of the most powerful determinants of healthcare access. With over 40% of the population living below the poverty line, low income limits the ability of individuals to seek care, especially in rural and peri-urban areas. Out-of-pocket payments dominate healthcare financing, pushing families into deeper poverty. The poor are often forced to choose between healthcare and basic needs like food, housing, and education. This financial strain creates a vicious cycle where poverty breeds poor health, and illness entrenches poverty. To achieve equitable healthcare access, it is essential to address the financial barriers that income disparities create [11].

1. **Out-of-Pocket Spending and Catastrophic Costs** Over 70% of healthcare expenditure in Nigeria is paid directly by individuals at the point of service. Costs include consultations, medicines, diagnostics, transportation, and lost income from caregiving or illness. For low-income households, even minor ailments can result in catastrophic health spending, forcing them to sell assets or forgo treatment entirely.
2. **Limited Financial Risk Protection** The lack of widespread health insurance coverage worsens financial vulnerability. While the National Health Insurance Authority (NHIA) has expanded formal sector coverage and launched community-based initiatives, most informal sector workers, who make up a large portion of the population, remain uninsured. Barriers include irregular income, lack of documentation, and limited access to reliable service delivery under the schemes.
3. **Income-Driven Inequities in Health-Seeking Behavior** Income disparities affect not just access but health-seeking behavior. The poor are less likely to pursue preventive care and more likely to delay or avoid treatment, leading to poorer health outcomes and increased risk of early death. These patterns undermine public health efforts and perpetuate inequality.
4. **Compounding Effects of Social and Geographic Inequalities** Income-related health barriers are amplified by gender, geography, and social exclusion. Women-headed households, rural dwellers, and internally displaced persons often face greater challenges in accessing healthcare. Children in poor families are particularly vulnerable to preventable diseases due to the unaffordability of services, even when subsidies exist.
5. **Policy and Systemic Solutions** Reducing income-related barriers requires pro-poor health financing reforms, targeted subsidies, and expanded social protection schemes. Strengthening public investment in affordable and quality healthcare, particularly for underserved populations, is essential. These measures are vital for achieving Universal Health Coverage (UHC) and safeguarding the right to health for all Nigerians.

Employment and Health Insurance

Employment is a critical determinant of healthcare access, not only by shaping income but also through health insurance availability and workplace benefits. In many systems, formal employment provides a gateway to health services, financial protection, and occupational health programs. However, in Nigeria, where informal employment dominates, this link is weak. Over 80% of the labour force works outside the formal sector, often without job security, employer-provided insurance, or healthcare entitlements. As a result, many Nigerians are left to bear healthcare costs alone, worsening inequalities in access and outcomes. Closing this gap is essential for achieving Universal Health Coverage (UHC) [12].

1. **Informal Employment and Health Insecurity** The vast majority of Nigerians, artisans, traders, farmers, and other informal workers lack access to employer-sponsored insurance or health benefits. Without job contracts or stable income, these individuals often turn to self-medication, delay care, or depend on unregulated providers, increasing the risks of poor health outcomes and financial shocks.
2. **Weak Uptake of Informal Sector Insurance Initiatives** Efforts by the NHIA to include informal workers through community-based and contributory health insurance platforms have had limited success. Challenges include erratic income, low public trust, poor awareness, and the unavailability of accredited health providers, especially in remote areas. These systemic issues continue to limit coverage and protection.
3. **Inequities Within the Formal Sector** Even among formally employed Nigerians, disparities persist. Government employees and staff of multinational firms often enjoy comprehensive insurance and private healthcare access. In contrast, workers in small and medium enterprises (SMEs), which dominate the private sector, frequently lack employer-sponsored coverage, leaving them exposed despite being in paid work.
4. **The "Missing Middle" Problem** Many SME employees earn too much to qualify for government subsidies but too little to afford private insurance. This "missing middle" falls through the cracks of Nigeria's fragmented insurance landscape. Without targeted interventions, they remain vulnerable to both health and financial crises.
5. **Occupational Status and Access to Benefits** Job roles further influence healthcare access. Senior professionals often benefit from group insurance plans and quality care, while casual, temporary, and gig workers, who are growing in number, typically receive no benefits. The rise of precarious work models threatens to widen existing access gaps unless protections are broadened.
6. **Gender and Employment-Linked Disparities** Women are disproportionately affected by employment-related health inequities. Many are engaged in unpaid or informal work, or are concentrated in low-wage formal roles with few or no

benefits. This limits access to maternal and reproductive health services, with long-term effects on women's health and societal well-being.

7. **Decoupling Health Insurance from Employment** To reduce disparities, health insurance must be made independent of employment status. Expanding public insurance subsidies, strengthening state-level health plans, incentivizing SME participation, and tailoring schemes for informal workers are all vital. Such reforms would help ensure that all Nigerians can access care, regardless of how they earn a living.

Geographic and Economic Disparities

Geographic and economic factors deeply shape healthcare access in Nigeria. Where a person lives often determines not only how close they are to healthcare facilities, but also the quality, affordability, and timeliness of care available. Stark contrasts between rural and urban areas, and within cities themselves, reflect entrenched inequalities. While rural regions suffer from poor infrastructure and scarce services, urban poor communities face systemic neglect and cost barriers. These disparities reflect a broader failure to design an equitable health system and require deliberate action to ensure healthcare is accessible for all, regardless of location or income [12, 13].

1. **Rural Areas and Structural Barriers to Access** Rural and remote communities often lack functional health facilities due to underdevelopment, poor roads, limited electricity, and insufficient communication infrastructure. Many primary health centres are understaffed, ill-equipped, or inactive, forcing residents to travel long distances to seek care, often at great personal cost and risk.
2. **Economic Hardship in Rural Communities** Rural households, largely dependent on subsistence farming or informal trade, struggle to afford healthcare. Even when services are available, indirect costs such as transport, accommodation, and lost income make access unaffordable. As a result, many delay treatment, rely on traditional medicine, or forgo care altogether.
3. **Unequal Urban Access and the "Two-Tier" System** In cities, healthcare services are more abundant but deeply unequal. While wealthier residents enjoy access to premium private clinics and specialist hospitals, the urban poor, especially those in slums, rely on overcrowded, under-resourced public facilities or unregulated providers. Income remains the key determinant of healthcare quality in urban Nigeria.
4. **Urban Slums: High Need, Low Access** Densely populated informal settlements face heightened health risks due to poor sanitation and overcrowding. Yet, public health services in these areas often suffer from medicine stock-outs, long wait times, and stigma from providers. The cost of

private care is prohibitive, leaving residents with few safe options for treatment.

5. **Vulnerable Groups and Compounded Disadvantage** Women, children, older adults, and people with disabilities are disproportionately affected by both geographic and economic barriers. These groups often require frequent healthcare but face greater challenges in reaching or affording care, especially in rural areas or urban slums with limited resources and discriminatory practices.
6. **The Digital Divide in Health Access** Digital innovations like telemedicine and health apps are reshaping care delivery, but unevenly. Wealthier, urban, educated populations benefit most, while rural and low-income groups often lack internet, smartphones, or digital literacy. Without targeted interventions, digital health may deepen existing disparities rather than close them.
7. **Toward Equitable Health Access** Addressing these disparities requires systemic reforms, including:
   - Investing in rural health infrastructure and revitalising PHCs through the BHCPF;
   - Deploying and retaining skilled health workers in underserved areas *via* incentives.
   - Upgrading urban primary care to meet the needs of slum communities;
   - Designing inclusive insurance schemes for the poor and the informal sector.
   - Expanding digital health access for marginalised populations;
   - And embedding equity into every stage of health policy and program design.

The Role of Health System Financing

Health system financing forms the backbone of equitable healthcare delivery. It dictates how resources are mobilised, distributed, and utilised across the sector, directly shaping access, affordability, and quality of care. In Nigeria, health financing remains a critical weakness, with public underinvestment, high out-o--pocket costs, and ineffective financial protection mechanisms. These structural deficiencies not only deepen health inequalities but also place disproportionate burdens on the poor and vulnerable. Addressing this issue is fundamental to building a resilient and inclusive health system [12, 13].

1. **Chronic Underfunding of the Health Sector** Nigeria consistently allocates far less than the Abuja Declaration's 15% health budget benchmark. Recent allocations linger around 4–6%, reflecting a long-standing neglect of the sector. This underinvestment translates into poorly maintained facilities, medicine shortages, outdated equipment, and staff deficits, especially in rural areas where public health systems are often the only lifeline.

2. **Overreliance on Out-of-Pocket Payments** Over 70% of healthcare costs in Nigeria are paid directly by households at the point of service. This model leaves low-income families particularly vulnerable, forcing them to choose between medical care and necessities. It also leads to delayed care-seeking, untreated illnesses, and increased mortality, trapping families in cycles of ill health and poverty.
3. **Inequities in Access and the Two-Tiered Health System** Nigeria's financing system fosters inequality. Wealthier individuals can access better-quality private care, while the poor depend on overstretched and poorly funded public services. Those in the informal sector, lacking employer-based insurance, face the full brunt of healthcare costs, reinforcing a dual-track system where financial capacity dictates health outcomes.
4. **The Need for Increased and Efficient Public Spending** Boosting health sector investment is a necessary first step. However, it's equally important to ensure funds are used transparently and efficiently. Strengthening accountability, procurement systems, and expenditure tracking can maximize the impact of increased funding, build public trust, and improve service delivery outcomes.
5. **Strengthening the National Health Insurance Authority (NHIA)** The NHIA was created to achieve universal health coverage but remains limited in reach, especially among informal and rural populations. Reforming the NHIA to simplify enrollment, extend coverage, and integrate with other social protection programs is essential. A robust NHIA can pool risk, lower individual costs, and make care more accessible.
6. **Leveraging Community-Based Health Insurance (CBHI)** CBHI schemes offer a low-cost solution tailored to rural and informal communities. By pooling community resources, they provide basic health coverage and financial protection. Successful models in Rwanda and Ghana demonstrate their potential. In Nigeria, scaling up CBHI will require government support and strategic alignment with national financing frameworks.
7. **Exploring Innovative Financing Mechanisms** To diversify and strengthen health sector funding, Nigeria can adopt innovative approaches such as:
   - Health taxes on tobacco, alcohol, and sugary drinks;
   - Public-Private Partnerships to leverage private capital and expertise;
   - Performance-based financing to incentivise improved service delivery. These tools, if equitably designed and implemented, can enhance revenue, promote health, and boost efficiency.
8. **Financing as a Tool for Equity** Ultimately, health financing is more than a budgetary exercise; it is a tool for achieving social justice. By prioritising the needs of the poor, underserved, and vulnerable in financing reforms, Nigeria

can build a more equitable and resilient health system that ensures no one is left behind.

Economic Empowerment and Health Access

Economic empowerment is a fundamental driver of health access, particularly in low-resource settings like Nigeria. When individuals and families have stable incomes, access to financial services, and improved financial literacy, they are better equipped to afford and utilise health services. Economic security enhances resilience to health shocks and promotes timely care-seeking, leading to improved health outcomes and reduced inequalities. Strengthening economic empowerment strategies can, therefore, serve as a powerful catalyst for achieving universal health coverage [12, 13].

1. **Breaking the Cycle of Poverty and Ill Health** Poverty both drives and results from poor health. Without economic means, many Nigerians delay seeking care until illnesses worsen, resulting in higher treatment costs, lost productivity, and preventable deaths. Economic empowerment enables timely access to preventive, routine, and chronic care services, interrupting this vicious cycle and fostering long-term health and productivity.
2. **Microfinance as a Tool for Health Access** Microfinance initiatives, such as small loans to low-income earners and entrepreneurs, enhance household financial stability and enable greater healthcare spending. Some programs link loans to health education and insurance, creating integrated platforms that support financial inclusion and health improvement simultaneously.
3. **Vocational Training and Job Creation** Skills development programs and employment initiatives, especially targeting youth and women, raise income levels and improve access to care. Individuals with stable income are more likely to afford medications, transport, and insurance premiums. Job creation also boosts community resilience and reduces health disparities linked to unemployment and financial insecurity.
4. **Social Protection and Health Security** Conditional cash transfers, food support programs, and unemployment benefits act as crucial safety nets. When tied to health or education benchmarks, like school attendance or child immunizations, such programs not only alleviate poverty but also incentivize proactive health-seeking behavior, particularly in vulnerable households.
5. **Addressing Gender Disparities in Economic Empowerment** In Nigeria, women face systemic barriers in employment, finance, and decision-making. Most are engaged in informal or unpaid labor with limited access to credit or property ownership. These gender gaps undermine their ability to seek and pay for healthcare for themselves and their families, perpetuating health inequities.

6. **The Multiplier Effect of Empowering Women** Evidence consistently shows that women reinvest income in their families' health, education, and nutrition. Empowering women through credit access, savings groups, cooperative societies, and entrepreneurship training not only boosts household health outcomes but also uplifts communities and accelerates national development.
7. **The Role of Financial Literacy in Health Access** Financial literacy, understanding budgeting, saving, and responsible borrowing, empowers individuals to plan for medical expenses, avoid debt traps, and make informed choices about health insurance and service utilization. It enhances participation in formal financial systems and promotes health-conscious financial planning.
8. **Economic Empowerment as a Pathway to UHC** Ultimately, economic empowerment is not just a social development objective; it is essential for achieving universal health coverage. Integrated policies that link health and economic systems can reduce inequities, build community resilience, and ensure that no one is denied healthcare due to financial constraints.

Policy Recommendations

To address the economic determinants of healthcare access, a multifaceted approach is needed. Policymakers should prioritise the following strategies [11 - 13]:

1. **Increasing Public Investment in Health:** Enhance government funding for healthcare to reduce the reliance on out-of-pocket payments and improve the availability and quality of health services, particularly in underserved areas.
2. **Expanding Health Insurance Coverage:** Strengthen and expand the NHIA to cover more individuals, including those in the informal sector, and implement targeted subsidies for low-income households.
3. **Promoting Economic Empowerment:** Implement programs that increase household income, provide stable employment, and support financial literacy, with a focus on empowering women and marginalised communities.
4. **Innovative Financing Mechanisms:** Explore and implement innovative health financing models, such as community-based health insurance schemes, to provide financial protection and improve healthcare access for vulnerable populations.

CONCLUSION

Economic determinants are crucial in shaping healthcare access, especially in low- and middle-income countries like Nigeria. Factors such as income inequality, health system financing, and geographic disparities intersect to determine who receives care and under what conditions. Addressing these issues requires a holistic, multisectoral approach involving policymakers, healthcare providers, community leaders, and international partners. By tackling economic barriers through increased public investment, health financing reforms, poverty alleviation, and empowerment initiatives, we can eliminate longstanding health inequities. Promoting economic resilience at both the household and national levels will not only improve healthcare access but also foster broader social and economic development. Achieving equitable healthcare is an attainable goal that can transform lives and communities, guiding Nigeria and other nations toward a healthier, more just future. The key lies in recognising health as both a driver and an outcome of economic development.

MALNUTRITION AND ITS IMPACT ON PUBLIC HEALTH

Malnutrition is a pervasive public health challenge that has far-reaching consequences for individuals and communities, particularly in developing nations like Nigeria. It is both a cause and a consequence of poverty, and its impact on public health is profound, affecting physical, cognitive, and economic well-being across all stages of life. Understanding the various dimensions of malnutrition and its public health implications is crucial for devising effective interventions and policies to combat this issue [14 - 16].

Globally, Nigeria ranks among the top countries with a high burden of stunting in children under five – 31–32% stunted, with an estimated ~2 million children suffering severe acute malnutrition (SAM). Similarly, wasting and maternal anaemia remain major problems, with over half of women of reproductive age having anaemia. The key drivers for malnutrition in Nigeria are food insecurity because of inflation, disrupted agriculture, conflict-driven displacement (especially in the north), poor infant and young child feeding practices, limited access to timely treatment for severe acute malnutrition, and anaemia and undernutrition among mothers [6, 7].

The Dimensions of Malnutrition

Malnutrition encompasses a range of conditions, including undernutrition (wasting, stunting, and underweight), micronutrient deficiencies, and overnutrition (overweight and obesity). Each of these conditions has distinct causes and consequences, but they often coexist within the same communities and even within the same individuals [14].

1. **Undernutrition:** This form of malnutrition is characterised by insufficient intake of calories and nutrients, leading to wasting (low weight for height), stunting (low height for age), and being underweight (low weight for age). In

Nigeria, undernutrition remains a critical concern, particularly among children under five, where it contributes to high rates of morbidity and mortality.

2. **Micronutrient Deficiencies:** Also known as "hidden hunger," micronutrient deficiencies occur when individuals do not get enough essential vitamins and minerals, such as vitamin A, iron, iodine, and zinc. These deficiencies can lead to severe health issues, including impaired immune function, cognitive delays, and increased susceptibility to infections.
3. **Overnutrition:** Overnutrition, often manifesting as overweight and obesity, is increasingly prevalent in urban areas of Nigeria, driven by changes in dietary patterns and lifestyles. This condition is associated with the rise in non-communicable diseases (NCDs), such as diabetes, hypertension, and cardiovascular diseases, which place a significant burden on the public health system.

The Impact of Malnutrition on Public Health

The impact of malnutrition on public health is multifaceted, affecting individuals' health outcomes, the healthcare system, and the broader socio-economic fabric of society [15].

1. **Childhood Development:** Malnutrition, particularly undernutrition and micronutrient deficiencies, has devastating effects on childhood development. Stunting, for example, not only affects physical growth but also impairs cognitive development, leading to long-term deficits in learning, school performance, and future economic productivity. Children who suffer from malnutrition are more susceptible to infections and illnesses, such as diarrhoea and pneumonia, which further exacerbate their nutritional status and overall health.
2. **Maternal Health:** Malnutrition in women, particularly during pregnancy, has serious consequences for both maternal and child health. Undernourished mothers are at higher risk of complications during pregnancy and childbirth, including preterm birth, low birth weight, and maternal mortality. Additionally, maternal micronutrient deficiencies, such as iron-deficiency anaemia, can lead to adverse pregnancy outcomes and affect the health of the newborn.
3. **Increased Disease Burden:** Malnutrition weakens the immune system, making individuals more vulnerable to infections and diseases. In Nigeria, where infectious diseases like malaria, tuberculosis, and HIV/AIDS are prevalent, malnutrition exacerbates the severity and spread of these diseases. Malnourished individuals are less likely to recover fully from illnesses, leading to prolonged health issues and increased demand on the healthcare system.
4. **Economic Consequences:** The economic impact of malnutrition is significant, both at the individual and national levels. Malnutrition reduces productivity by

impairing physical and cognitive function, leading to lower earning potential and economic hardship for individuals and families. At the national level, the economic costs of malnutrition include increased healthcare expenditures, reduced workforce productivity, and hindered economic growth. In Nigeria, where a large proportion of the population is engaged in labour-intensive work, the effects of malnutrition on productivity and economic development are particularly pronounced.

The Double Burden of Malnutrition

Nigeria, like many developing nations, faces the "double burden" of malnutrition, where undernutrition and overnutrition coexist within the same population. This dual challenge complicates public health efforts, as strategies must address both ends of the malnutrition spectrum. The rise in overweight and obesity, particularly in urban areas, is driven by the nutrition transition, a shift from traditional diets to diets high in processed foods, sugars, and unhealthy fats. This transition, coupled with sedentary lifestyles, has led to an increase in NCDs, adding to the already significant burden of infectious diseases and undernutrition. Addressing malnutrition in Nigeria requires a comprehensive and integrated approach that targets its root causes and promotes sustainable solutions. Key policy recommendations include [14 - 16]:

1. **Strengthening Nutrition-Specific Interventions:** Implement targeted interventions that directly address malnutrition, such as breastfeeding promotion, micronutrient supplementation, and food fortification programs. These interventions should prioritise vulnerable groups, including pregnant women, infants, and young children.
2. **Enhancing Nutrition-Sensitive Interventions:** Address the underlying determinants of malnutrition by integrating nutrition goals into sectors such as agriculture, education, and social protection. For example, promoting the cultivation and consumption of nutrient-rich crops can improve dietary diversity, while school feeding programs can enhance children's nutritional status and educational outcomes.
3. **Improving Public Awareness and Education:** Increase public awareness of the importance of nutrition through community-based education programs and mass media campaigns. Educating communities about healthy eating practices, the benefits of breastfeeding, and the risks of overnutrition can help shift behaviors and improve nutritional outcomes.
4. **Strengthening Health Systems:** Build the capacity of healthcare systems to detect, treat, and prevent malnutrition. This includes training healthcare workers, improving nutrition surveillance, and ensuring the availability of essential nutrition services and supplies at all levels of care.

5. **Promoting Multi-Sectoral Collaboration:** Foster collaboration between government agencies, non-governmental organisations, and the private sector to create a coordinated response to malnutrition. Multi-sectoral approaches that leverage the strengths of various stakeholders can lead to more effective and sustainable outcomes.

Example Model Box — Community Nutrition and Livelihoods: The Integrated Community Approach In several Nigerian states and other neighbouring countries, a successful model in addressing nutrition combines community health worker-led screening and Community-based Management of Acute Malnutrition (CMAM) with small-scale conditional cash transfers or livelihood packages (seed/fertiliser, poultry) to help restore household food production and income. When this model is implemented with reliable supply chains for ready-to-use therapeutic foods and linked behaviour change communication, the outcome is faster SAM recovery rates, reduced relapse, and improved household food security over 12 months. However, rigorous monitoring and community ownership were critical to sustainability [4 - 7].

CONCLUSION

Malnutrition is a critical public health issue that requires urgent attention and action. By addressing malnutrition in all its forms, Nigeria can improve health outcomes, reduce healthcare costs, and promote socio-economic development. The fight against malnutrition is not just a health imperative but a moral and economic necessity for the future of the nation.

POVERTY REDUCTION PROGRAMS: EVALUATING THEIR IMPACT ON HEALTH

Poverty reduction programs are essential for addressing the socio-economic barriers that hinder access to health and well-being. These programs aim to alleviate poverty by providing financial support, improving access to education, healthcare, and employment opportunities, and addressing structural inequalities. In Nigeria and other developing nations, the effectiveness of these programs is crucial in determining their impact on public health outcomes. This section evaluates the impact of various poverty reduction programs on health, highlighting successes, challenges, and the way forward [17 - 19].

Overview of Poverty Reduction Programs in Nigeria

Nigeria has implemented several poverty reduction initiatives over the years, targeting different aspects of socio-economic development aimed at poor households. These initiatives collectively reflect Nigeria's policy evolution toward inclusive growth and social protection. Some of the key programs include [17]:

1. **National Social Investment Program (NSIP):** Launched in 2016, NSIP is one of the largest social welfare programs in Nigeria, aimed at reducing poverty and improving the living conditions of vulnerable populations. The program aims to address poverty and vulnerability through social protection, job creation, and human capital development through N-Power (youth employment and empowerment), Conditional Cash Transfer (CCT), Government Enterprise and Empowerment Programme (GEEP), and Home-Grown School Feeding Programme (HGSFP).
2. **National Poverty Eradication Programme (NAPEP):** Established in 2001, NAPEP targeted income and employment generation through various sectors, including agriculture, health, and education. It was designed to eradicate poverty by providing vocational training, microcredit, and other forms of support to unemployed and underprivileged citizens.
3. **The Presidential Initiative on Job Creation:** This initiative focuses on creating jobs through entrepreneurship and skills development, particularly for youth and women. It aims to reduce unemployment and provide economic opportunities for the marginalised population.
4. **Community-Based Health Insurance (CBHI):** CBHI programs have been introduced in various states to improve access to healthcare for low-income populations, focusing on financial risk protection in health. These programs are designed to provide affordable health insurance, particularly for informal sector workers and rural communities.

Impact of Poverty Reduction Programs on Health

The impact of poverty reduction programs on health outcomes is multifaceted, influencing various aspects of public health. Some of the key impacts include [18]:

1. **Improved Access to Healthcare:** Poverty reduction programs, particularly those that include healthcare components like CBHI, have improved access to healthcare services for low-income populations. By reducing financial barriers, these programs enable more people to seek medical care when needed, leading to better health outcomes. For example, the introduction of CBHI in some Nigerian states has led to increased utilisation of healthcare services, particularly maternal and child health services, reducing mortality rates.
2. **Enhanced Nutrition and Food Security:** Programs like NHGSFP and CCT have had a positive impact on nutrition and food security among vulnerable

populations. NHGSFP, which provides free meals to school children, has improved school attendance and reduced malnutrition rates among participating children. Similarly, CCT programs, which provide financial support to low-income families, have enabled beneficiaries to afford better quality food, contributing to improved nutritional status and overall health.

3. **Reduction in Child and Maternal Mortality:** By addressing the socio-economic determinants of health, poverty reduction programs have contributed to a decline in child and maternal mortality rates. For instance, the NHGSFP has not only improved nutritional outcomes but also increased the likelihood of children receiving vaccinations and other essential health services, which are critical for reducing child mortality. Additionally, CCT programs that incentivise healthcare utilisation during pregnancy and childbirth have led to increased antenatal care visits and skilled birth attendance, reducing maternal mortality.
4. **Economic Empowerment and Mental Health:** Poverty reduction programs that focus on economic empowerment, such as N-Power and GEEP, have had a positive impact on mental health. Economic insecurity is a significant contributor to stress, anxiety, and depression. By providing employment opportunities and financial support, these programs have alleviated economic stress for many beneficiaries, leading to improved mental health and well-being.

Challenges and Limitations

Despite the successes of poverty reduction programs in Nigeria, several challenges and limitations hinder their full potential in improving health outcomes [19]:

1. **Limited Coverage and Reach:** Many poverty reduction programs have limited coverage, reaching only a fraction of the target population. For example, CBHI programs are not available in all states, and where they exist, enrollment rates are often low. Similarly, CCT programs often struggle to identify and reach the most vulnerable populations, limiting their impact.
2. **Sustainability and Funding:** The sustainability of poverty reduction programs is a significant concern, as many are heavily dependent on government funding, which can be inconsistent. Economic downturns, budget cuts, and political changes can lead to the scaling back or discontinuation of these programs, undermining their long-term impact on health.
3. **Program Implementation and Monitoring:** Effective implementation and monitoring of poverty reduction programs are critical to their success. However, in Nigeria, there are challenges related to program management,

including corruption, inefficiencies, and a lack of transparency. These issues can lead to misallocation of resources, delays in program delivery, and reduced effectiveness in achieving health outcomes.

4. **Integration with Health Systems:** For poverty reduction programs to have a meaningful impact on health, they must be integrated with the broader health system. However, there is often a lack of coordination between social welfare programs and healthcare services, leading to missed opportunities for synergy and comprehensive support for beneficiaries.

The Way Forward: Enhancing the Impact of Poverty Reduction Programs on Health

To enhance the impact of poverty reduction programs on health in Nigeria, several strategies can be pursued [17 - 19]:

1. **Expand Coverage and Reach:** Efforts should be made to expand the coverage of poverty reduction programs, particularly in underserved and rural areas. This includes scaling up successful programs like CBHI and CCT and ensuring that they reach the most vulnerable populations.
2. **Ensure Sustainability:** To ensure the sustainability of poverty reduction programs, it is essential to diversify funding sources, including partnerships with international donors, private sector involvement, and innovative financing mechanisms. Additionally, building the capacity of local governments and communities to manage and sustain these programs is crucial.
3. **Strengthen Implementation and Monitoring:** Improving the implementation and monitoring of poverty reduction programs requires greater transparency, accountability, and efficiency. This can be achieved through the use of technology for monitoring and evaluation, as well as by strengthening anti-corruption measures and ensuring that resources are used effectively.
4. **Integrate with Health Systems:** Integrating poverty reduction programs with the health system can enhance their impact on health outcomes. This includes linking CCT programs with maternal and child health services, ensuring that beneficiaries of economic empowerment programs have access to healthcare, and coordinating efforts between social welfare and health ministries.
5. **Promote Community Participation:** Engaging communities in the design, implementation, and evaluation of poverty reduction programs can lead to more effective and culturally appropriate interventions. Community participation ensures that programs are tailored to the specific needs of the population and that beneficiaries have a sense of ownership and commitment to the program's success.

CONCLUSION

Poverty reduction programs play a vital role in improving public health outcomes in Nigeria. By addressing the socioeconomic determinants of health, these programs contribute to better access to healthcare, improved nutrition, reduced mortality rates, and enhanced mental health. However, to maximise their impact, it is essential to overcome challenges related to coverage, sustainability, implementation, and integration with the health system. Through targeted strategies and a commitment to continuous improvement, poverty reduction programs can significantly contribute to the health and well-being of Nigeria's population.

SOCIAL PROTECTION SYSTEMS FOR HEALTH

Social protection systems are fundamental to reducing poverty, inequality, and vulnerability by providing support to individuals and households, especially during times of need. When designed effectively, these systems can significantly improve health outcomes by ensuring that all citizens, regardless of their socio-economic status, have access to essential healthcare services. This section delves into the role of social protection systems in health, focusing on their design, implementation, and impact on public health in Nigeria and other developing nations [20 - 22].

Understanding Social Protection Systems

Social protection encompasses a wide range of policies and programs aimed at reducing poverty and vulnerability by promoting efficient labour markets, diminishing people's exposure to risks, and enhancing their capacity to manage economic and social risks, such as unemployment, exclusion, sickness, disability, and old age. Social protection systems typically include the following components [20]:

1. **Social Insurance:** This involves contributions from employers, employees, and sometimes the state, to protect against specific risks, such as unemployment, sickness, and old age. Examples include health insurance, unemployment insurance, and pension schemes.
2. **Social Assistance:** These are non-contributory transfers provided to individuals or households in need, such as cash transfers, food assistance, and subsidies for basic services like healthcare and education.
3. **Labour Market Programs:** These include measures to promote employment, protect workers, and ensure adequate wages and working conditions. Programs

may include job creation schemes, skills development initiatives, and wage subsidies.

4. **Universal Health Coverage (UHC):** UHC is a critical component of social protection, aiming to ensure that all individuals and communities receive the health services they need without suffering financial hardship. UHC encompasses the entire spectrum of essential health services, from health promotion to prevention, treatment, rehabilitation, and palliative care.

The Role of Social Protection in Health

Social protection systems are vital for ensuring access to healthcare and improving health outcomes, particularly for the most vulnerable populations. Key roles of social protection in health include [21]:

1. **Financial Risk Protection:** Social protection systems provide financial risk protection by covering the cost of healthcare, thus preventing individuals from falling into poverty due to high medical expenses. This is particularly important in countries where out-of-pocket spending on health is high. By reducing financial barriers, social protection systems enable more people to access timely and appropriate healthcare, which can prevent the escalation of minor health issues into major illnesses.
2. **Increased Access to Healthcare:** Social protection mechanisms, such as health insurance and cash transfers, increase access to healthcare services for marginalised and vulnerable populations. For example, in Nigeria, the National Health Insurance Authority (NHIA) aims to provide access to healthcare for all citizens, particularly those in the informal sector. By subsidising healthcare costs, these programs ensure that more people can seek medical care when needed.
3. **Promotion of Preventive Care:** Social protection systems often include components that encourage preventive care and healthy behaviours. For instance, Conditional Cash Transfer (CCT) programs may require beneficiaries to attend regular health check-ups, vaccinate their children, or participate in health education sessions. These conditions promote preventive care and early detection of diseases, which are crucial for improving overall health outcomes.
4. **Support for Vulnerable Groups:** Social protection systems are designed to provide targeted support to vulnerable groups, such as the elderly, disabled, pregnant women, and children. In many developing countries, these groups are at higher risk of poor health outcomes due to limited access to healthcare and other essential services. Social protection programs, such as maternity benefits, disability pensions, and child grants, provide critical support to these populations, ensuring that they have access to the care and services they need.

Social Protection Systems in Nigeria

Nigeria has made significant strides in developing social protection systems that contribute to health. However, challenges remain in achieving comprehensive coverage and ensuring the effectiveness of these systems. Key social protection programs in Nigeria that impact health include [22]:

1. **National Health Insurance Authority (NHIA):** Established in 2005, NHIA aims to provide universal health coverage to all Nigerians, with a particular focus on formal sector workers. However, coverage remains low, particularly among informal sector workers and rural populations. Efforts are ongoing to expand coverage and improve the scheme's effectiveness in reducing financial barriers to healthcare.
2. **Conditional Cash Transfer (CCT) Program:** The CCT program, part of the National Social Investment Program (NSIP), provides financial support to poor and vulnerable households, with conditions related to health and education. For example, beneficiaries are required to ensure that their children receive vaccinations and attend school regularly. The program has shown positive impacts on health, particularly in improving child health and nutrition.
3. **Maternity Benefits and Child Grants:** Some states in Nigeria have introduced maternity benefits and child grants as part of their social protection efforts. These programs aim to reduce maternal and child mortality by providing financial support to pregnant women and young mothers, enabling them to access necessary healthcare services.

Challenges in Implementing Social Protection for Health

Despite the potential of social protection systems to improve health outcomes, several challenges hinder their effectiveness in Nigeria [21, 22]:

1. **Limited Coverage:** A significant portion of the population, particularly those in the informal sector and rural areas, remains uncovered by social protection systems. Expanding coverage to these populations is critical for ensuring that all Nigerians have access to essential healthcare services.
2. **Funding and Sustainability:** Social protection programs are often underfunded and reliant on government budgets, which can be inconsistent. Economic downturns, budget constraints, and political instability can threaten the sustainability of these programs, limiting their long-term impact on health.
3. **Fragmentation and Coordination:** Social protection programs in Nigeria are often fragmented, with multiple agencies and levels of government involved in their implementation. This can lead to inefficiencies, duplication of efforts, and

gaps in coverage. Improved coordination between programs and alignment with broader health system goals are necessary to maximise their impact.

4. **Implementation and Monitoring:** Effective implementation and monitoring of social protection programs are crucial for their success. However, challenges related to capacity, transparency, and accountability can undermine program effectiveness. Strengthening monitoring and evaluation systems, as well as ensuring that resources are used effectively, is essential for achieving the desired health outcomes.

Strengthening Social Protection Systems for Health

To enhance the impact of social protection systems on health in Nigeria, several strategies can be pursued [21, 22]:

1. **Expand Coverage and Reach:** Efforts should be made to extend social protection coverage to all citizens, particularly those in the informal sector and rural areas. This includes scaling up programs like NHIA and ensuring that social protection systems are inclusive and accessible to all.
2. **Ensure Adequate Funding and Sustainability:** Diversifying funding sources, including public-private partnerships and international support, can help ensure the sustainability of social protection programs. Additionally, integrating social protection systems into broader development strategies can enhance their long-term viability.
3. **Improve Coordination and Integration:** Better coordination between social protection programs and the health system is essential for maximising their impact. This includes aligning social protection goals with health system priorities and ensuring that programs are complementary rather than duplicative.
4. **Strengthen Implementation and Monitoring:** Enhancing the capacity of institutions responsible for implementing and monitoring social protection programs is crucial for their success. This includes investing in training, improving data collection and analysis, and ensuring transparency and accountability in program management.
5. **Promote Equity and Inclusion:** Social protection systems must be designed to address the needs of the most vulnerable populations. This includes ensuring that programs are equitable and inclusive, with a focus on reaching those who are most at risk of poor health outcomes.

CONCLUSION

Social protection systems are a vital tool for improving health outcomes in Nigeria and other developing nations. By providing financial risk protection, increasing access to healthcare, promoting preventive care, and supporting vulnerable populations, these systems play a critical role in addressing the socio-economic determinants of health. However, to fully realise their potential, it is essential to overcome challenges related to coverage, funding, coordination, and implementation. With the right strategies and a commitment to equity and sustainability, social protection systems can make a significant contribution to the health and well-being of all Nigerians.

EMPOWERING COMMUNITIES THROUGH ECONOMIC DEVELOPMENT

Economic development plays a pivotal role in transforming public health, particularly in developing nations where poverty is a major barrier to accessing healthcare and achieving better health outcomes. Empowering communities through economic development not only improves the standard of living but also creates a foundation for sustainable health improvements. This section explores the critical intersection of economic development and public health, emphasising strategies for empowering communities to drive their own health and economic prosperity [23 - 26].

The Link Between Economic Development and Health

Economic development and health are intricately linked, with each influencing the other. Improved economic conditions lead to better access to healthcare, nutrition, education, and other social services, which in turn enhance public health outcomes. Conversely, a healthier population contributes to economic growth through increased productivity, reduced healthcare costs, and a more vibrant workforce. Key aspects of this relationship include [23]:

1. **Income and Health:** Higher income levels enable individuals and families to afford better healthcare, nutritious food, and safe living conditions. Economic development initiatives that increase household income can directly reduce health inequalities and improve overall health outcomes.
2. **Education and Employment:** Education is a key determinant of health, as it equips individuals with the knowledge and skills needed to make informed health decisions. Economic development strategies that focus on improving education and creating employment opportunities can have a profound impact on public health by reducing poverty and enhancing access to healthcare.
3. **Infrastructure and Services:** Economic development often involves investment in infrastructure, such as roads, water supply, sanitation, and healthcare facilities. These investments are crucial for improving public health, particularly in rural and underserved areas. Improved infrastructure enhances

access to healthcare services, reduces the spread of diseases, and improves the overall quality of life.

Strategies for Economic Empowerment and Health Improvement

Empowering communities through economic development requires a multi-faceted approach that addresses the underlying causes of poverty and promotes sustainable growth. The following strategies are key to achieving this goal [24]:

1. **Microfinance and Entrepreneurship:** Microfinance programs provide small loans and financial services to individuals and small businesses, particularly in rural and low-income communities. By enabling people to start or expand businesses, microfinance can boost household income, create jobs, and reduce poverty. These economic gains translate into better access to healthcare and improved health outcomes.
2. **Skills Development and Vocational Training:** Investing in skills development and vocational training equips individuals with the knowledge and abilities needed to secure employment or start their own businesses. These programs are particularly effective in empowering women and youth, often marginalised in the labour market. By improving employment prospects, skills development initiatives contribute to economic stability and better health for communities.
3. **Agricultural Development and Food Security:** In many developing nations, agriculture is the backbone of the economy and a primary source of livelihood for rural communities. Enhancing agricultural productivity through improved farming techniques, access to markets, and support for smallholder farmers can significantly boost household income and food security. Adequate nutrition is essential for good health, and economic empowerment in agriculture can lead to substantial health improvements.
4. **Community-Based Cooperatives:** Cooperatives are community-driven organisations that pool resources and share profits among members. They can be particularly effective in promoting economic development in rural areas by providing access to credit, markets, and other resources. Cooperatives often focus on sectors like agriculture, crafts, and small-scale manufacturing, where they can have a significant impact on poverty reduction and community health.
5. **Public-Private Partnerships (PPPs):** Collaborations between the public and private sectors can leverage resources, expertise, and innovation to drive economic development and improve public health. PPPs can support infrastructure development, healthcare delivery, and the creation of sustainable economic opportunities in underserved communities. By aligning the interests of both sectors, PPPs can contribute to long-term economic and health benefits.

Case Studies: Successes in Economic Empowerment and Health

Examining real-world examples of successful economic empowerment initiatives provides valuable insights into the potential for improving public health through economic development. The following case studies highlight innovative approaches that have led to significant health and economic gains [24 - 26]:

1. **Grameen Bank in Bangladesh:** The Grameen Bank is a pioneering microfinance institution that provides small loans to the rural poor, particularly women, to start businesses and improve their livelihoods. The success of Grameen Bank has led to widespread economic empowerment and significant improvements in health, including better access to healthcare, education, and nutrition.
2. **BRAC's Integrated Development Program:** BRAC, a global development organisation based in Bangladesh, implements an integrated approach to economic empowerment and health improvement. Its programs combine microfinance, education, healthcare, and livelihood support to lift people out of poverty. BRAC's holistic model has been replicated in several countries and has demonstrated the potential of integrated development programs to achieve sustainable health and economic outcomes.
3. **Kenya's M-Pesa and Financial Inclusion:** M-Pesa, a mobile money platform in Kenya, has revolutionised financial inclusion by providing millions of people with access to banking services through their mobile phones. This has empowered individuals and businesses, particularly in rural areas, to engage in economic activities, save money, and access healthcare services more easily. The success of M-Pesa has led to improved economic stability and better health outcomes for many Kenyans.

Challenges and Opportunities in Economic Empowerment

While economic empowerment offers significant potential for improving public health, several challenges must be addressed to achieve sustainable outcomes [24 - 26]:

1. **Inequality and Exclusion:** Economic development efforts often fail to reach the most marginalised populations, exacerbating inequalities and leaving vulnerable groups behind. Ensuring that economic empowerment initiatives are inclusive and equitable is essential for achieving broad-based health improvements.
2. **Sustainability and Resilience:** Economic empowerment programs must be designed to be sustainable and resilient to economic shocks, such as market

fluctuations, natural disasters, and political instability. Building local capacity, diversifying income sources, and promoting community ownership are key strategies for enhancing the sustainability of these programs.

3. **Integration with Health Systems:** Economic empowerment initiatives should be integrated with health systems to maximise their impact on public health. This requires collaboration between different sectors, including health, education, agriculture, and finance, to ensure that economic development efforts are aligned with health goals.
4. **Monitoring and Evaluation:** Robust monitoring and evaluation mechanisms are necessary to assess the impact of economic empowerment programs on health and make data-driven decisions. Continuous learning and adaptation are essential for improving program effectiveness and achieving desired outcomes.

CONCLUSION

In Nigeria and other developing countries, poverty is the central structural determinant of population health. Achieving a measurable reduction in mortality, malnutrition, and disease burden depends on integrating social protection, place-sensitive health services, and community-level livelihood support under a data-driven governance framework. Targeted cash transfers, community nutrition programs, and empowerment of women and rural communities should be the bedrock to converting poverty-reduction budgets into lasting health gains. Empowering communities through economic development is a powerful strategy for improving public health in Nigeria and other developing nations. By addressing the root causes of poverty and creating opportunities for sustainable economic growth, these initiatives can lead to significant health improvements and reduce health disparities. However, to achieve lasting impact, economic empowerment programs must be inclusive, sustainable, and integrated with broader health systems. By fostering collaboration across sectors and prioritising the needs of the most vulnerable, we can create a pathway to better health and economic prosperity for all.

REFERENCES

[1] The World Bank Group. (2025). Mortality rate, under-5 (per 1,000 live births) – Nigeria. Available from: https://data.worldbank.org/indicator/SH.DYN.MORT?locations=NG&utm

[2] The World Bank Group. (2024). Gini Index – Nigeria. Available from: https://data.worldbank.org/indicator/SI.POV.GINI?locations=NG&utm

[3] Osimen GU, Etoroma OM, Pokubo I, Adi I. N-Power program and youth empowerment in Nigeria. Cogent Soc Sci 2025; 11(1): 2466786. [http://dx.doi.org/10.1080/23311886.2025.2466786]

[4] Ibok OW, Okon IE, Akpan OP, Isip IF. Impact of conditional cash transfer on households food security in Akwa Ibom State, Nigeria. PLoS One 2025; 20(6): e0325594. [http://dx.doi.org/10.1371/journal.pone.0325594] [PMID: 40531883]

[5] Evaluations – Conditional Cash Transfers. Available from: https://www.worldbank.org/en/programs/sief-trust-fund/brief/evaluations-conditional-cash-transfers?utm

[6] UNICEF. (2025). Nutrition - Nigeria. Available from: https://www.unicef.org/nigeria/nutrition?utm

[7] Global Nutrition Report 2025, Nigeria. The burden of malnutrition at a glance: Available from: https://globalnutritionreport.org/resources/nutrition-profiles/africa/western-africa/nigeria/

[8] World Health Organisation. (2010). Equity, Social Determinants and Public Health Programmes. Edited by Erik Blas and Anand Sivasankara Kurup. Geneva: WHO Press.

[9] Commission on Social Determinants of Health. (2008). Closing the Gap in a Generation: Health Equity through Action on the Social Determinants of Health. Geneva: WHO.

[10] Lichterman BL. Pathologies of Power: Health, Human Rights, and the New War on the Poor. BMJ 2003; 327(7425): 1232.

[11] Wagstaff A, Doorslaer E. Catastrophe and impoverishment in paying for health care: with applications to Vietnam 1993–1998. Health Econ 2003; 12(11): 921-33. [http://dx.doi.org/10.1002/hec.776] [PMID: 14601155]

[12] Peters DH, Garg A, Bloom G, Walker DG, Brieger WR, Hafizur Rahman M. Poverty and access to health care in developing countries. Ann N Y Acad Sci 2008; 1136(1): 161-71. [http://dx.doi.org/10.1196/annals.1425.011] [PMID: 17954679]

[13] Xu K, Evans DB, Carrin G, Aguilar-Rivera AM, Musgrove P, Evans T. Protecting households from catastrophic health spending. Health Aff (Millwood) 2007; 26(4): 972-83. [http://dx.doi.org/10.1377/hlthaff.26.4.972] [PMID: 17630440]

[14] Black RE, Allen LH, Bhutta ZA, *et al.* Maternal and child undernutrition: global and regional exposures and health consequences. Lancet 2008; 371(9608): 243-60. [http://dx.doi.org/10.1016/S0140-6736(07)61690-0] [PMID: 18207566]

[15] World Health Organization (2021) Levels and Trends in Child Malnutrition UNICEF/ WHO/World Bank Group Joint Child Malnutrition Estimates Key Findings of the 2021 Edition. Available form: https://www.who.int/publications/i/item/9789240025257

[16] Pinstrup-Andersen P. Food and Agricultural Policy for a Globalizing World: Preparing for the Future. Am J Agric Econ 2002; 84(5): 1201-14. [http://dx.doi.org/10.1111/1467-8276.00381]

[17] Rawlings LB, Rubio GM. Evaluating the impact of conditional cash transfer programs. World Bank Res Obs 2005; 20(1): 29-55. [http://dx.doi.org/10.1093/wbro/lki001]

[18] Narayan D, Pritchett L. Cents and Sociability: Household Income and Social Capital in Rural Tanzania. Econ Dev Cult Change 1999; 47(4): 871-97. [http://dx.doi.org/10.1086/452436]

[19] Chronic Poverty Research Centre (2008) The Chronic Poverty Report (2008-09). Escaping Poverty Traps. Belmont Press Ltd., Northampton.

[20] Palacios R, Sluchynsky O. Social pensions Part I : their role in the overall pension system. Social Protection Discussion Papers and Notes 36237, The World Bank, 2006.

[21] ILO. (2017). World Social Protection Report 2017-19: Universal Social Protection to Achieve the Sustainable Development Goals. Geneva: ILO.

[22] Barrientos A, Hulme D. Social Protection for the Poor and Poorest in Developing Countries: Reflections on a Quiet Revolution. Oxf Dev Stud 2009; 37(4): 439-56. [http://dx.doi.org/10.1080/13600810903305257]

[23] Sen A. Development as Freedom. Oxford University Press 1999.

[24] Alsop R, Bertelsen M, Holland J. Empowerment in Practice: From Analysis to Implementation. Washington, DC: The World Bank 2006.

[25] Banuth RM, Simone P, Salles M. The Impact of Cash Transfers on Local Economies. Econ Dev Cult Change 2015; 11(1): 707-34.

[26] Saleh J-EA. Resilient Communities: Navigating Public Health Challenges in Developing Nations. Bentham Science Publishers 2025.
[http://dx.doi.org/10.2174/97898153056091250101]

CHAPTER 3

Strengthening Fragile Health Systems

Abstract: This chapter delves into the essential components that constitute a robust health system, emphasising the need for comprehensive reforms in developing nations, particularly Nigeria. It begins by outlining the critical elements of a well-functioning health system, including governance, health financing, workforce, essential medicines, information systems, and service delivery. The chapter then explores the significant infrastructure gaps that hinder healthcare delivery and discusses the opportunities for improvement through investments and public-private partnerships. A detailed analysis of supply chain management highlights the challenges and strategies for ensuring a consistent supply of essential medicines. The importance of health information systems for data-driven decision-making is underscored, followed by an examination of the financing mechanisms needed to sustain health systems. The chapter concludes with a discussion on building resilience in health systems, drawing lessons from past crises to enhance their capacity to respond to future challenges. Overall, this chapter provides a roadmap for policymakers and healthcare providers to strengthen health systems, ensuring they are capable of delivering quality care to all individuals, even in the face of adversity.

Keywords: Developing nations, Essential medicines, Governance, Health systems, Health infrastructure, Health information systems, Health financing, Nigeria, Public-private partnerships, Resilience, Supply chain management.

INTRODUCTION

Health systems form the backbone of any nation's ability to deliver essential services, respond to public health emergencies, and ensure the well-being of its population. In many developing countries, including Nigeria, health systems are often fragile, characterised by weak infrastructure, inadequate financing, poor governance, and limited access to essential medicines and technologies. These vulnerabilities have been further exposed during global health crises, such as the COVID-19 pandemic, highlighting the urgent need for reforms. This chapter explores the various components of a robust health system, identifies existing gaps, and discusses opportunities for strengthening these systems to build resilience and ensure sustainable health outcomes.

Jalal-Eddeen Abubakar Saleh

COMPONENTS OF A ROBUST HEALTH SYSTEM

A robust health system is the cornerstone of any nation's ability to deliver quality healthcare, respond to public health emergencies, and improve the overall well-being of its population. In developing nations, where health systems are often fragile and under-resourced, understanding the key components of a robust health system is critical for guiding efforts to strengthen these systems and achieve sustainable health outcomes. This section explores the fundamental components that constitute a robust health system, drawing on global best practices and lessons learned from both successful and struggling health systems [1 - 3].

Fig. (**1**) and Table **1** present the WHO's six building blocks of a functional health system, contextualised with practical examples from Nigeria. The six components, service delivery, health workforce, information systems, essential medicines, financing, and governance, are critical for sustainable public health. The table helps readers understand how each element interrelates to support the broader system; for instance, efficient health information systems underpin evidence-based policymaking, while an adequate health workforce ensures service accessibility. Through localised examples such as the DHIS2 data platform, the Basic Health Care Provision Fund, and national drug policy initiatives, the table illustrates the current strengths and gaps in Nigeria's health system. By breaking down complex structural concepts into digestible segments, the table enables readers, especially policy practitioners and health planners, to identify which areas require investment and reform to strengthen resilience and ensure equitable health outcomes.

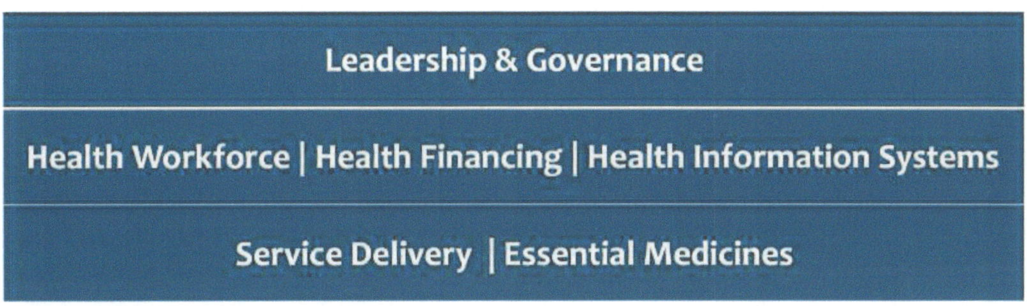

Fig. (1). Health system building blocks.

Table 1. Health system building blocks.

Building Block	Description	Example in Nigeria
Service Delivery	Quality and availability of health services	Immunization campaigns
Health Workforce	Availability and competence of staff	Community health workers

(Table 1) cont.....

Building Block	Description	Example in Nigeria
Health Information Systems	Data collection and use	DHIS2 platform
Essential Medicines	Availability of necessary drugs and equipment	National Drug Policy
Health Financing	Adequate and equitable funding	Basic Health Care Provision Fund
Leadership/Governance	Policy and oversight	National Health Policy

Health Service Delivery

At the heart of any health system is the delivery of health services that are accessible, equitable, and of high quality. Effective health service delivery requires the following elements [1]:

- **Availability of Services:** A strong health system guarantees that essential health services, including preventive, curative, rehabilitative, and palliative care, are accessible to all parts of the population. This encompasses a wide range of services from primary care to specialised medical services, tailored to meet the diverse needs of the community.
- **Accessibility and Equity:** Services must be physically and financially accessible to all, regardless of geographic location, socio-economic status, or cultural background. A strong health system actively addresses barriers to access, such as distance, cost, and discrimination, to ensure that no one is left behind.
- **Quality of Care:** The quality of health services is a critical determinant of health outcomes. A robust health system emphasises the continuous improvement of service quality through the implementation of evidence-based practices, adherence to clinical guidelines, regular training of healthcare providers, and the integration of patient safety measures.
- **Continuity of Care:** Ensuring that patients receive coordinated and uninterrupted care across different levels of the health system, from primary care to tertiary services, is essential for achieving positive health outcomes. This requires effective referral systems, patient tracking, and integration of services across different care settings.

Health Workforce

The health workforce is the backbone of any health system, and its strength is a key determinant of the system's overall performance. Critical aspects of a strong health workforce include [2]:

- **Adequate Staffing:** A robust health system must have a sufficient number of healthcare workers, including doctors, nurses, midwives, community health workers, and allied health professionals, to meet the population's needs. Addressing workforce shortages and ensuring an equitable distribution of health workers, particularly in rural and underserved areas, is crucial.
- **Competency and Training:** The competency of the health workforce is essential for delivering high-quality care. This requires continuous education and training, certification processes, and opportunities for professional development to ensure that health workers are equipped with the latest knowledge and skills.
- **Motivation and Retention:** Health systems must prioritize the well-being and motivation of their workforce. This involves providing adequate compensation, creating a supportive work environment, ensuring job security, and offering career advancement opportunities. Retention strategies are particularly important in regions where health workers are often lured away by better opportunities elsewhere.
- **Leadership and Governance:** Effective leadership and governance within the health workforce are essential for guiding the system's strategic direction, fostering teamwork, and ensuring accountability. Strong leadership at all levels, from health facility managers to national health authorities, is critical for the success of health workforce initiatives.

Health Information Systems

A robust health system relies on accurate, timely, and comprehensive health information to guide decision-making, monitor progress, and respond to emerging challenges. Key components of an effective health information system include [3]:

- **Data Collection and Management:** Reliable data collection processes are essential for capturing health-related information at all levels of the system. This includes data on health outcomes, service delivery, resource allocation, and population health indicators. Health systems must invest in infrastructure and technology to support efficient data collection and management.
- **Data Quality and Accuracy:** Ensuring the accuracy, completeness, and reliability of health data is critical for informed decision-making. This requires the implementation of standardised data collection methods, regular data quality assessments, and continuous capacity building for health information personnel.
- **Data Use and Dissemination:** A strong health information system not only collects data but also ensures that it is effectively used for policy formulation, program planning, and resource allocation. Data should be easily accessible to stakeholders at all levels, including policymakers, healthcare providers, and the

public. Regular dissemination of health information through reports, dashboards, and other communication channels is essential for transparency and accountability.

- **Surveillance and Early Warning Systems:** Robust health information systems include surveillance mechanisms to detect and respond to health threats, such as disease outbreaks and natural disasters. Early warning systems are critical for enabling timely interventions and mitigating the impact of public health emergencies.

Medical Products, Vaccines, and Technologies

The availability of essential medical products, vaccines, and technologies is a key pillar of a robust health system. These components ensure that health services can be delivered effectively and that populations are protected from diseases. Key aspects include [2, 3]:

- **Supply Chain Management:** An efficient supply chain system is essential for ensuring the continuous availability of medical products and vaccines. This includes procurement, storage, distribution, and inventory management processes that minimize stockouts, reduce waste, and ensure that products reach those who need them.
- **Quality Assurance:** Ensuring the quality, safety, and efficacy of medical products and vaccines is critical for maintaining public trust and achieving desired health outcomes. This requires rigorous regulatory oversight, adherence to international standards, and regular quality control measures.
- **Access to Technologies:** Access to appropriate health technologies, including diagnostic tools, medical devices, and information technologies, is vital for effective healthcare delivery. Health systems must invest in the development, procurement, and maintenance of these technologies to enhance service delivery and improve health outcomes.
- **Innovation and Adaptation:** Health systems must be adaptable and open to innovation to address emerging health challenges and take advantage of new technologies. This includes fostering research and development, promoting the adoption of new medical technologies, and ensuring that health workers are trained in their use.

Health Financing

Sustainable health financing is a cornerstone of a robust health system, ensuring that adequate resources are available to deliver quality healthcare to all. Key components of health financing include [1 - 3]:

- **Revenue Generation:** A robust health system requires diverse and sustainable revenue sources to fund its operations. This can include government funding, health insurance schemes, donor contributions, and out-of-pocket payments. Expanding revenue generation mechanisms, such as through taxation and innovative financing models, is crucial for achieving universal health coverage.
- **Equitable Resource Allocation:** Resources must be allocated equitably across the health system to ensure that all population groups, particularly the most vulnerable, have access to necessary services. This requires transparent budgeting processes, priority setting based on health needs, and mechanisms to track and evaluate resource allocation.
- **Financial Protection:** A key goal of health financing is to protect individuals from financial hardship due to healthcare costs. This involves implementing financial protection mechanisms, such as health insurance schemes and social safety nets, to reduce out-of-pocket payments and ensure that healthcare is affordable for all.
- **Efficiency and Accountability:** Efficient use of financial resources is essential for maximising the impact of health expenditures. Health systems must implement measures to reduce waste, prevent corruption, and ensure that funds are used effectively. Strong financial management systems, regular audits, and accountability mechanisms are critical for achieving this.

Leadership and Governance

Effective leadership and governance are essential for guiding the health system's strategic direction, ensuring accountability, and fostering collaboration across different sectors. Key aspects include [1 - 3]:

- **Policy Formulation and Implementation:** Robust health systems have clear policies and strategies that are based on evidence and aligned with national health goals. Effective policy formulation involves stakeholder engagement, cross-sector collaboration, and continuous monitoring and evaluation to ensure that policies are implemented as intended.
- **Regulation and Oversight:** Strong regulatory frameworks are necessary to ensure the quality, safety, and equity of health services. This includes the regulation of healthcare providers, medical products, and health facilities, as well as the enforcement of standards and guidelines to protect public health.
- **Community Engagement and Participation:** Engaging communities in the governance of the health system is critical for ensuring that services are responsive to the needs of the population. This involves promoting community participation in decision-making processes, fostering transparency, and empowering local leaders to take ownership of health initiatives.

- **Crisis Management and Resilience:** A robust health system must be resilient to shocks and able to respond effectively to public health emergencies. This requires strong crisis management structures, emergency preparedness plans, and the capacity to mobilize resources quickly in response to emerging threats.

CONCLUSION

The components of a robust health system are interconnected and mutually reinforcing, creating a framework that supports the delivery of quality healthcare, promotes equity, and enhances the overall health of the population. In developing nations, where health systems are often fragile and under-resourced, strengthening these components is essential for achieving sustainable health outcomes and addressing the complex challenges of public health. By investing in health service delivery, workforce development, health information systems, medical products and technologies, health financing, and leadership and governance, we can build resilient health systems that are capable of meeting the needs of all citizens and contributing to the broader goals of national development and prosperity.

INFRASTRUCTURE GAPS AND OPPORTUNITIES

The strength of a health system is inextricably linked to the quality and availability of its infrastructure. In many developing nations, including Nigeria, significant infrastructure gaps undermine the ability of health systems to deliver quality care, respond to emergencies, and improve population health outcomes. This section explores the critical infrastructure challenges faced by fragile health systems and identifies opportunities for investment and innovation to bridge these gaps [4 - 6].

Current Infrastructure Gaps

The challenges of inadequate health infrastructure in developing nations manifest in several ways, each impacting the efficiency and effectiveness of the health system [4, 5]. The Primary Health Centre State of Power Report 2024-2025 for six states (Cross River, Anambra, Benue, Osun, Sokoto, Taraba) reveals critical deficiencies in the PHCs. These gaps include power instability, infrastructure deficits, personnel shortages hindering accessible and affordable healthcare quality services, and a lack of clean water sources, functional sanitation, and adequate waste disposal systems. Strengthening these systems is essential for building resilient communities and supporting Nigeria's economic stability. The report, which examines the state of power supply in 345 PHCs across six states, revealed that 66% of PHCs lack a reliable power source, 45% connected to the national grid, 26% adopted solar energy, and 25% rely on generators. This electricity gap significantly impacts vaccine storage, emergency services, and patient care, resulting in avoidable delays, inefficiencies, and increased mortality rates in rural communities [4 - 7].

- **Health Facility Distribution:** There is often an uneven distribution of health facilities, with urban areas typically better served than rural regions. This geographic disparity leaves large portions of the population without easy access to healthcare services, exacerbating health inequities.
- **Condition of Health Facilities:** Many existing health facilities are in poor condition, with outdated or poorly maintained infrastructure. This includes crumbling buildings, a lack of basic amenities like clean water and electricity, and insufficient space to accommodate patients and healthcare workers.
- **Lack of Essential Medical Equipment:** Health facilities in fragile systems frequently lack essential medical equipment, such as diagnostic tools, surgical instruments, and life-saving devices. This limits the range of services that can be offered and compromises the quality of care.
- **Inadequate Transportation Networks:** Poor transportation infrastructure, including roads and public transit systems, makes it difficult for patients to reach health facilities, especially in rural areas. It also hampers the distribution of medical supplies, vaccines, and emergency response teams.
- **Information and Communication Technology (ICT) Deficiencies:** The lack of robust ICT infrastructure hampers the development of health information systems, telemedicine services, and efficient communication between health facilities. This leads to delays in data collection, reporting, and decision-making, weakening the overall health system.
- **Power Supply Issues:** Reliable electricity is a critical need for health facilities, yet many facilities in developing countries experience frequent power outages or lack access to electricity altogether. This affects the operation of medical equipment, storage of vaccines and medicines, and overall patient care.

Impact of Infrastructure Gaps on Health Outcomes

The infrastructure gaps outlined above have a direct and detrimental impact on health outcomes. Some of the most significant effects include [4, 5]:

- **Delayed and Inadequate Care:** Infrastructure deficiencies often result in delays in treatment, compromised quality of care, and reduced patient satisfaction. This can lead to worsened health outcomes, particularly for conditions requiring timely intervention, such as trauma, obstetric emergencies, and infectious diseases.
- **Increased Morbidity and Mortality:** The lack of essential infrastructure contributes to higher morbidity and mortality rates, particularly among

vulnerable populations such as pregnant women, children, and the elderly. For instance, inadequate maternal health facilities are a leading cause of high maternal mortality rates in many developing countries.

- **Health Inequities:** The uneven distribution of health infrastructure exacerbates health inequities, as those living in underserved areas are less likely to receive timely and appropriate care. This deepens the divide between urban and rural populations and between wealthy and poor communities.
- **Reduced System Resilience:** Fragile health systems with weak infrastructure are less resilient to shocks, such as natural disasters, disease outbreaks, or conflicts. Inadequate infrastructure hampers the system's ability to respond quickly and effectively to emergencies, leading to preventable deaths and prolonged crises.

Opportunities for Infrastructure Development

Addressing the infrastructure gaps in fragile health systems requires strategic investments, innovative approaches, and strong partnerships. Several opportunities exist to strengthen health infrastructure [4, 5]:

- **Investment in Health Facility Upgrades:** Governments, donors, and private sector partners can prioritise investments in upgrading and expanding health facilities, particularly in underserved areas. This includes building new facilities, renovating existing ones, and ensuring that all facilities meet basic standards for safety, hygiene, and patient care.
- **Public-Private Partnerships (PPPs):** Leveraging public-private partnerships can mobilise additional resources for infrastructure development. PPPs can be used to finance the construction of new health facilities, improve the supply chain for medical equipment, and enhance ICT infrastructure.
- **Telemedicine and Mobile Health (mHealth) Solutions:** Expanding telemedicine and mHealth initiatives can help bridge the gap between healthcare providers and patients in remote areas. These technologies enable remote consultations, monitoring, and diagnosis, reducing the need for physical infrastructure and expanding access to care.
- **Renewable Energy Solutions:** Investing in renewable energy sources, such as solar power, can provide reliable electricity to health facilities, particularly in areas with unreliable power grids. This not only ensures the continuous operation of medical equipment but also supports sustainable development goals.
- **Strengthening Transportation Networks:** Improving transportation infrastructure, including roads, bridges, and public transport, is essential for enhancing access to health services. Investments in transportation also facilitate

the efficient distribution of medical supplies and the rapid deployment of emergency response teams.

- **Digital Health Infrastructure:** Building robust digital health infrastructure, including health information systems, electronic medical records, and data-sharing platforms, is critical for improving the efficiency and effectiveness of health services. Digital tools can streamline administrative processes, enhance patient care, and support evidence-based decision-making.

Strategic Approaches to Infrastructure Development

To effectively address infrastructure gaps and seize the development opportunities, health systems must adopt strategic approaches [4 - 6]:

- **Needs Assessment and Planning:** Comprehensive needs assessments should guide infrastructure development efforts. These assessments should consider current gaps, population needs, and future health demands to ensure that investments are targeted and effective.
- **Integrated Infrastructure Development:** Infrastructure development should be integrated with broader health system strengthening efforts, including workforce development, supply chain management, and health financing. This ensures that new or improved infrastructure contributes to overall system resilience and sustainability.
- **Community Involvement and Ownership:** Engaging communities in the planning and implementation of infrastructure projects can enhance their relevance, acceptability, and sustainability. Community involvement ensures that infrastructure developments are responsive to local needs and are maintained over the long term.
- **Monitoring and Evaluation:** Continuous monitoring and evaluation of infrastructure projects are essential for ensuring that they achieve their intended outcomes. This includes tracking progress, assessing impact, and making necessary adjustments to improve effectiveness.

CONCLUSION

Addressing the infrastructure gaps in fragile health systems is a critical step toward achieving universal health coverage and improving health outcomes in developing nations. By investing in health facility upgrades, leveraging technology, and adopting strategic approaches to infrastructure development, we can build a resilient health system that is capable of meeting the needs of all citizens. Strengthening health infrastructure not only enhances the delivery of quality care but also contributes to broader social and economic development, paving the way for a healthier and more prosperous future.

SUPPLY CHAIN MANAGEMENT AND ESSENTIAL MEDICINES

The availability of essential medicines is a fundamental component of a functional health system, particularly in developing nations where health challenges are often exacerbated by supply chain inefficiencies. Effective supply chain management ensures that essential medicines are consistently available, affordable, and accessible to all who need them. This section explores the critical role of supply chain management in strengthening health systems, with a focus on the challenges and opportunities related to essential medicines in Nigeria and other developing nations [8 - 10].

The Role of Supply Chain Management in Health Systems

Supply chain management in healthcare encompasses a series of processes that involve the planning, procurement, storage, distribution, and delivery of medical products, including essential medicines, to health facilities and ultimately to patients. The efficiency and reliability of these processes directly impact the quality of care provided and the health outcomes of the population. Key functions of supply chain management in health systems include [8]:

- **Procurement:** Ensuring that essential medicines are procured on time, at the right quantity, and at a competitive price is crucial. Procurement processes must adhere to international standards and regulations to guarantee the quality and safety of medicines.
- **Inventory Management:** Effective inventory management is necessary to maintain an optimal stock of medicines, avoiding both shortages and overstock situations. This involves regular monitoring of stock levels, accurate forecasting of demand, and the use of data-driven decision-making tools.
- **Warehousing and Storage:** Medicines must be stored in appropriate conditions to preserve their efficacy and prevent degradation. This requires investment in proper warehousing infrastructure, temperature control systems, and rigorous adherence to storage protocols.
- **Distribution:** The timely and efficient distribution of medicines from central warehouses to health facilities is critical. This process must account for the geographic and logistical challenges that are often present in developing nations, such as poor road networks and limited transportation options.
- **Quality Assurance:** Throughout the supply chain, rigorous quality assurance measures must be implemented to ensure that medicines remain safe and effective until they reach the patient. This includes monitoring for counterfeit products, maintaining cold chain logistics for temperature-sensitive medicines, and conducting regular quality inspections.

Challenges in Supply Chain Management for Essential Medicines

Developing nations, including Nigeria, face a multitude of challenges in managing the supply chain for essential medicines. Table **2** shows Health Supply-Chain Challenges and Digital/Logistics Mitigation Strategies in Nigeria. These challenges often lead to frequent stockouts, wastage, and inequitable access to medicines, particularly in rural and underserved areas [8 - 10]:

Table 2. Health Supply-Chain Challenges and Digital/Logistics Mitigation Strategies in Nigeria.

Supply-Chain Challenges	Mitigation / Digital and Logistical Innovations
Frequent stockouts of essential medicines and diagnostics at Primary Health Centres (PHCs) due to poor forecasting, weak last-mile distribution, and equipment failure.	Deployment of Logistics Management Information Systems (LMIS) to track stock levels and anticipate shortages; integration of data from health facilities to improve forecasting accuracy.
Cold-chain breakdowns, especially in remote or rural areas, lead to vaccine wastage and compromised immunization integrity.	Use of mobile-based cold-chain monitoring systems and real-time temperature tracking devices (*e.g.*, remote temperature loggers, solar-powered cold rooms) to maintain vaccine potency and reduce wastage.
Procurement and shipment delays at the federal and state levels are caused by bureaucratic bottlenecks, lengthy approval processes, and poor coordination.	Digital procurement platforms and automated approval workflows (piloted in some states) to enhance transparency, speed up supply processes, and reduce administrative delays.
Inadequate visibility of supply chain performance across multiple levels (federal–state–LGA), resulting in poor accountability and inefficiencies.	Integrated supply-chain dashboards and eHealth analytics tools providing real-time visibility of stock movements and logistics performance indicators.
Inefficient redistribution of medical commodities leads to simultaneous stockouts and overstocks in different facilities.	Digital mapping and telemedicine-assisted supply redirection systems, enabling facilities to identify surplus and shortage points and coordinate redistribution within zones.

- **Inadequate Infrastructure:** Poor transportation networks, lack of reliable electricity, and insufficient storage facilities undermine the efficiency of the supply chain. These infrastructure deficits contribute to delays in the distribution of medicines and increase the risk of spoilage, especially for temperature-sensitive products like vaccines.
- **Weak Procurement Practices:** Inefficient procurement processes, including delays in tendering, lack of transparency, and corruption, result in the inconsistent availability of essential medicines. Weak procurement practices also lead to higher costs, making it difficult to sustain adequate supplies within limited budgets.
- **Poor Data Management:** Inaccurate or incomplete data on medicine consumption, stock levels, and demand forecasting hinders effective supply

chain management. Without reliable data, it is challenging to anticipate needs, plan procurement, and manage inventories, leading to either shortages or excesses.

- **Limited Human Resources:** The lack of trained personnel in supply chain management is a critical issue in many developing nations. Health facilities often struggle to maintain skilled staff who can effectively manage the logistics of medicine supply, from procurement to distribution.
- **Financial Constraints:** Insufficient funding for the health sector, particularly for the procurement and distribution of medicines, exacerbates supply chain challenges. Financial constraints limit the ability to maintain adequate stock levels, invest in infrastructure, and implement quality assurance measures.
- **Counterfeit Medicines:** The prevalence of counterfeit medicines in developing nations poses a significant threat to public health. Weak regulatory frameworks, coupled with porous borders and inadequate enforcement, allow counterfeit products to infiltrate the supply chain, undermining the safety and efficacy of medicines.

Opportunities for Improving Supply Chain Management

Addressing the challenges in supply chain management requires a multifaceted approach that involves investment, capacity building, and innovation. Several opportunities exist to strengthen supply chain management for essential medicines [8, 9]:

- **Investment in Infrastructure:** Improving transportation networks, warehousing facilities, and cold chain logistics are critical investments that can enhance the efficiency and reliability of medicine distribution. Public-private partnerships can play a key role in mobilising the resources needed for these infrastructure improvements.
- **Strengthening Procurement Systems:** Implementing transparent, efficient, and competitive procurement processes is essential for ensuring the timely and cost-effective acquisition of essential medicines. This includes adopting international procurement standards, utilising digital procurement platforms, and enhancing oversight to reduce corruption.
- **Leveraging Technology:** The use of digital tools and technologies can significantly improve supply chain management. For example, electronic inventory management systems, real-time tracking of shipments, and data analytics for demand forecasting can enhance the accuracy and efficiency of the supply chain.
- **Capacity Building and Training:** Investing in the training and development of supply chain management professionals is crucial. Health systems should focus on building the skills of personnel involved in procurement, logistics, and

inventory management through continuous education and specialised training programs.

- **Enhancing Data Management:** Strengthening health information systems to provide accurate and timely data on medicine supply and consumption is essential for effective decision-making. Integrating data across different levels of the health system and utilising data analytics can improve forecasting, reduce wastage, and ensure that medicines are available when and where they are needed.
- **Regulatory Strengthening:** Strengthening regulatory frameworks and enforcement mechanisms is necessary to combat the proliferation of counterfeit medicines. This includes enhancing the capacity of national regulatory authorities, improving border controls, and promoting public awareness about the dangers of counterfeit products.
- **Promoting Regional Collaboration:** Regional collaboration among neighbouring countries can help address supply chain challenges by pooling resources, harmonising procurement practices, and facilitating the cross-border movement of medicines. Regional initiatives can also support the sharing of best practices and the development of joint strategies to combat counterfeit medicines.

Strategic Approaches to Supply Chain Management

To effectively improve supply chain management and ensure the availability of essential medicines, health systems must adopt strategic approaches that are tailored to their specific contexts [8 - 10]:

- **Integrated Supply Chain Planning:** Supply chain management should be integrated into broader health system strengthening efforts, with a focus on aligning supply chain activities with national health priorities. This includes coordinating with other health programs, such as immunization and maternal health, to ensure a seamless supply of medicines.
- **Focus on Equity:** Ensuring equitable access to essential medicines should be a central goal of supply chain management. This involves prioritizing the distribution of medicines to underserved and hard-to-reach areas, reducing disparities in access, and addressing the specific needs of vulnerable populations.
- **Monitoring and Evaluation:** Continuous monitoring and evaluation of supply chain performance are essential for identifying bottlenecks, assessing the impact of interventions, and making data-driven improvements. This includes setting performance indicators, conducting regular audits, and involving stakeholders in the evaluation process.

- **Sustainability and Resilience:** Building a sustainable and resilient supply chain requires long-term planning and investment. Health systems should focus on creating supply chains that can withstand shocks, such as pandemics or natural disasters, and that are adaptable to changing health needs and market dynamics.

CONCLUSION

Effective supply chain management is a critical determinant of the availability and accessibility of essential medicines, which are foundational to any robust health system. By addressing the challenges and seizing the opportunities for improvement, developing nations can ensure that their populations have reliable access to the medicines they need to lead healthy lives. Strengthening supply chain management not only enhances the performance of the health system but also contributes to the broader goals of achieving universal health coverage, reducing health inequities, and improving public health outcomes.

HEALTH INFORMATION SYSTEMS: DATA FOR DECISION-MAKING

A well-functioning Health Information System (HIS) is the backbone of an effective health system. It provides the data needed to monitor health trends, manage resources, evaluate programs, and make informed decisions that ultimately improve health outcomes. In fragile health systems, such as those found in Nigeria and other developing nations, strengthening health information systems is essential for overcoming challenges and advancing public health goals. This section delves into the importance of HIS, the challenges faced, and the strategies needed to leverage data for effective decision-making [11 - 13].

The Role of Health Information Systems in Strengthening Health Systems

Health Information Systems are integral to every aspect of the health system, serving as the primary source of data for decision-making at all levels. HIS encompasses a wide range of data collection, storage, analysis, and dissemination processes that provide critical information to health practitioners, policymakers, and stakeholders. The key roles of HIS in strengthening health systems include [11]:

- **Monitoring and Surveillance:** HIS allows for the continuous monitoring of health indicators, such as disease incidence, mortality rates, and immunisation coverage. This data is vital for detecting and responding to health emergencies, outbreaks, and emerging health threats on time.
- **Resource Management:** Effective HIS supports the management of health resources, including human resources, medical supplies, and financial allocations. By providing accurate data on resource availability and utilisation,

HIS helps ensure that resources are allocated efficiently and that gaps are identified and addressed.

- **Program Evaluation:** HIS enables the evaluation of health programs and interventions by tracking progress toward health goals, measuring impact, and identifying areas for improvement. This evidence-based approach is crucial for refining programs and ensuring that they deliver the desired health outcomes.
- **Policy Development:** Reliable data from HIS informs the development of health policies and strategies. Policymakers rely on data to understand health trends, prioritize interventions, and allocate resources in ways that maximize public health impact.
- **Patient Care and Clinical Decision-Making:** HIS supports clinical decision-making by providing healthcare providers with access to patient records, treatment histories, and diagnostic data. This information is essential for delivering personalised care, improving patient outcomes, and reducing medical errors.
- **Public Health Research:** HIS provides a rich source of data for public health research, enabling the study of health trends, risk factors, and the effectiveness of interventions. Research findings based on HIS data contribute to the global body of knowledge and inform best practices in public health.

Challenges in Health Information Systems

Despite the critical role of HIS, many developing nations face significant challenges in establishing and maintaining effective systems. These challenges can undermine the quality, reliability, and use of health data, leading to gaps in decision-making and weakened health systems. Key challenges include [12]:

- **Fragmented and Siloed Systems:** In many developing nations, HIS are often fragmented, with multiple systems operating independently across different health programs or regions. This lack of integration leads to duplication of efforts, inconsistent data, and difficulties in sharing and analysing information.
- **Inadequate Infrastructure:** The lack of reliable infrastructure, including electricity, internet connectivity, and hardware, hampers the effective functioning of HIS. In rural areas, these infrastructure challenges are particularly pronounced, limiting the ability to collect, store, and transmit health data.
- **Limited Human Resources:** A shortage of trained personnel in data management, analysis, and information technology is a significant barrier to the effective operation of HIS. Many health facilities lack the staff needed to manage HIS effectively, leading to delays in data entry, errors, and underutilization of available data.
- **Poor Data Quality:** The quality of data collected through HIS is often compromised by factors such as incomplete reporting, errors in data entry, and

inconsistent use of data collection tools. Poor data quality reduces the reliability of HIS and undermines confidence in the data for decision-making.
- **Financial Constraints:** Insufficient funding for HIS development and maintenance is a major challenge. Without adequate financial resources, health systems struggle to invest in the necessary infrastructure, technology, and training to support robust HIS.
- **Resistance to Change:** In some cases, resistance to adopting new technologies or data-driven decision-making processes can hinder the effective implementation of HIS. This resistance may stem from a lack of understanding of the benefits of HIS, fear of increased workload, or concerns about data privacy and security.

Strategies for Strengthening Health Information Systems

To address these challenges and leverage the full potential of HIS, health systems must adopt strategic approaches that prioritise integration, capacity building, and data utilisation. Key strategies include [12]:

- **System Integration and Interoperability:** Developing an integrated HIS that allows for the seamless exchange of data across different health programs and regions is essential. Interoperable systems enable health facilities to share data in real-time, reducing duplication and improving the quality of data available for decision-making.
- **Investment in Infrastructure:** Strengthening the infrastructure that supports HIS is critical for its success. This includes investing in reliable electricity, internet connectivity, and modern hardware, particularly in rural and underserved areas. Mobile health technologies can also play a role in extending the reach of HIS to remote locations.
- **Capacity Building and Training:** Developing the skills of health workers and data managers is essential for the effective operation of HIS. Training programs should focus on data collection, analysis, and the use of HIS tools, as well as fostering a culture of data-driven decision-making within the health system.
- **Enhancing Data Quality:** Improving data quality requires the standardisation of data collection tools and processes, regular data quality audits, and the implementation of feedback mechanisms to address errors and inconsistencies. Clear guidelines and protocols should be established to ensure that data is collected, entered, and reported accurately.
- **Promoting Data Use for Decision-Making:** To maximise the impact of HIS, it is essential to promote the use of data for decision-making at all levels of the health system. This involves creating platforms for data sharing, developing user-friendly data dashboards, and providing training on data interpretation and application.

- **Ensuring Data Privacy and Security:** Protecting the privacy and security of health data is crucial for maintaining trust in HIS. Health systems must implement robust data protection measures, including encryption, access controls, and data anonymisation, to safeguard sensitive information.

The Role of Technology in Advancing Health Information Systems

Technology plays a transformative role in advancing HIS by enabling more efficient data collection, storage, analysis, and dissemination. Emerging technologies offer new opportunities to overcome traditional barriers and enhance the functionality of HIS. Key technological innovations include [12, 13]:

- **Electronic Health Records (EHRs):** The adoption of EHRs allows for the digitisation of patient records, facilitating easier access to medical histories, reducing paperwork, and improving the continuity of care. EHRs also enable the integration of patient data across different levels of the health system.
- **Mobile Health (mHealth) Solutions:** mHealth technologies, such as mobile apps and SMS-based reporting, can extend the reach of HIS to remote and underserved areas. These solutions facilitate real-time data collection and reporting, enhancing the timeliness and accuracy of health data.
- **Geographic Information Systems (GIS):** GIS technology allows for the spatial analysis of health data, providing insights into geographic patterns of disease, access to health services, and resource distribution. This information is valuable for targeted interventions and resource allocation.
- **Big Data and Analytics:** The use of big data analytics in HIS can unlock new insights from large and complex datasets. Advanced analytics enable the identification of trends, prediction of health outcomes, and optimization of resource use, supporting more informed decision-making.
- **Cloud Computing:** Cloud-based HIS solutions offer scalability, cost-effectiveness, and improved accessibility of health data. Cloud computing enables health systems to store large volumes of data securely and access it from multiple locations, facilitating data sharing and collaboration.

CONCLUSION

The successful implementation of robust Health Information Systems is essential for transforming fragile health systems in developing nations. By addressing challenges and leveraging technological advancements, health systems can harness the power of data to drive decision-making, improve health outcomes, and achieve universal health coverage. A data-driven health system is not only more efficient and effective but also more resilient, capable of responding to emerging health threats and adapting to changing needs. Strengthening HIS is, therefore, a critical step toward building a healthier and more equitable future for all.

FINANCING HEALTH SYSTEMS: PUBLIC AND PRIVATE CONTRIBUTIONS

The financing of health systems is a critical component in building and sustaining robust health systems, particularly in developing nations such as Nigeria. Effective financing strategies are essential to ensure that health systems are adequately resourced, equitable, and capable of delivering high-quality services to the population. This section explores the roles of both public and private contributions in financing health systems, the challenges faced in this area, and potential strategies for improving health financing to achieve better health outcomes [14 - 16].

The Importance of Health Financing

Health financing involves the collection, pooling, and allocation of financial resources to ensure that the health system can function effectively and meet the needs of the population. In the 2024 fiscal year, the Federal Government allocated N1.336 trillion to the health sector, representing 4.6% of the total federal budget [17]. In the analysed budget documents, it was revealed that in 2024, the health sector allocation has risen to 5.15%. Out of this, about 57.5% was for personnel, and 41% for capital (infrastructure) projects [18]. However, despite these increases, the allocation remains well below the 15% target established in the Abuja Declaration. Adequate financing is necessary to [14]:

- **Ensure Universal Health Coverage (UHC):** UHC aims to provide all individuals with access to necessary health services without financial hardship. Effective health financing mechanisms are critical to achieving UHC, as they determine the availability, accessibility, and affordability of health services.
- **Sustain Health Infrastructure and Services:** Health systems require continuous funding to maintain infrastructure, procure medical supplies, pay healthcare workers, and deliver essential services. Stable financing ensures that health facilities can operate efficiently and consistently.
- **Promote Equity:** Health financing mechanisms play a key role in reducing health disparities by ensuring that resources are distributed equitably across different regions and population groups. This is particularly important in developing nations, where health inequities are often pronounced.
- **Respond to Health Crises:** Adequate and flexible financing allows health systems to respond swiftly to emergencies, such as disease outbreaks, natural

disasters, or economic shocks. A well-financed health system is more resilient and better equipped to manage crises.
- **Foster Innovation and Improvement:** Continuous investment in health systems is necessary to foster innovation, improve the quality of care, and adapt to changing health needs. Financing supports research, the adoption of new technologies, and the development of more effective health interventions.

Public Contributions to Health Financing

Public financing, primarily through government revenue, plays a central role in health system funding. In many developing nations, including Nigeria, the government is the primary source of health financing, responsible for funding public health programs, subsidising healthcare services, and investing in health infrastructure. Key aspects of public contributions to health financing include [15]:

- **Tax-Based Financing:** Many health systems rely on tax revenues to fund health services. This includes general taxes, such as income tax, Value-Added Tax (VAT), and corporate tax, which are pooled to finance health expenditures. Tax-based financing is a progressive approach that can promote equity, as wealthier individuals contribute more to the system.
- **Social Health Insurance (SHI):** SHI schemes involve mandatory contributions from employees, employers, and sometimes the government to a health insurance fund that covers healthcare costs for beneficiaries. SHI can provide a sustainable source of financing and reduce out-of-pocket expenses for individuals, though it requires effective management and broad coverage to be successful.
- **Government Budget Allocations:** Governments allocate a portion of the national budget to health services, which are used to fund public health facilities, procure medicines, and support health programs. Adequate budgetary allocations are essential for maintaining and expanding health services, though many developing nations face challenges in meeting recommended health spending targets.
- **External Aid and Donor Funding:** In many developing nations, external aid from international donors, non-governmental organizations (NGOs), and multilateral agencies plays a significant role in health financing. Donor funding supports various health initiatives, including disease control programs, immunization campaigns, and maternal health services. However, reliance on external aid can lead to sustainability issues, particularly if funding is unpredictable or tied to specific projects.
- **Subsidies and Free Health Services:** To promote equity and access, governments often subsidise health services or provide them free of charge,

particularly for vulnerable populations such as children, pregnant women, and the elderly. These subsidies reduce financial barriers to care but require substantial public funding to be sustainable.

Private Contributions to Health Financing

Private contributions to health financing come from individuals, households, private health insurance, and private sector investments. In many developing nations, the private sector plays a crucial role in supplementing public financing and expanding access to healthcare services. Key aspects of private contributions to health financing include [15, 16]:

- **Out-of-Pocket Payments (OOPs):** OOPs refer to direct payments made by individuals or households for healthcare services at the point of care. In many developing nations, OOPs represent a significant share of health financing. However, high OOPs can lead to financial hardship and deter individuals from seeking necessary care, undermining efforts to achieve UHC.
- **Private Health Insurance:** Private health insurance provides coverage for healthcare costs, typically in exchange for regular premium payments. In some contexts, private insurance complements public financing by offering coverage for services not included in public health schemes or by reducing the burden on public facilities. However, private insurance can also exacerbate health inequities if it is only accessible to wealthier individuals.
- **Corporate Contributions and Philanthropy:** Corporations and philanthropic organizations contribute to health financing through donations, corporate social responsibility (CSR) initiatives, and direct investments in health programs. These contributions can support specific health initiatives, such as building health infrastructure or funding disease prevention programs, and play a crucial role in supplementing public resources.
- **Private Sector Investments:** The private sector is increasingly involved in health service delivery, from operating private hospitals and clinics to manufacturing pharmaceuticals and medical devices. Private sector investments can expand access to health services, introduce innovations, and increase the overall efficiency of the health system. However, the privatisation of health services raises concerns about affordability and equity.

Challenges in Health Financing

Despite the importance of both public and private contributions to health financing, many developing nations face significant challenges in securing adequate and sustainable funding for their health systems. These challenges include [15, 16]:

- **Insufficient Public Funding:** Many governments in developing nations struggle to allocate sufficient resources to the health sector, often due to limited fiscal capacity, competing priorities, and economic constraints. As a result, public health facilities may be underfunded, leading to shortages of medical supplies, inadequate infrastructure, and low healthcare worker salaries.
- **High Out-of-Pocket Expenditures:** In the absence of robust public financing and social health insurance systems, many individuals in developing nations are forced to pay for healthcare out of pocket. High OOPs can lead to financial hardship, deter individuals from seeking care, and exacerbate health inequities.
- **Reliance on External Aid:** While donor funding is crucial for many health programs, reliance on external aid can create vulnerabilities, particularly if funding is unpredictable or donor priorities do not align with national health needs. Furthermore, over-reliance on external aid can undermine the sustainability of health systems if domestic financing mechanisms are not adequately developed.
- **Fragmentation of Health Financing:** In many developing nations, health financing is often fragmented, with multiple sources of funding and disparate programs operating independently. This fragmentation can lead to inefficiencies, duplication of efforts, and difficulties in coordinating and managing resources effectively.
- **Weak Financial Management Systems:** Effective health financing requires strong financial management systems to ensure that resources are allocated efficiently, accounted for accurately, and used effectively. Weak financial management systems, including poor budgeting, accounting, and auditing practices, can lead to misallocation of resources, corruption, and wastage.

Strategies for Strengthening Health Financing

To address the challenges in health financing and ensure the sustainability and effectiveness of health systems, a multifaceted approach is required. Key strategies include [15, 16]:

- **Increasing Public Funding:** Governments need to prioritise health in their budgets and increase public funding for the health sector. This may involve expanding the tax base, improving tax collection, and reallocating resources from other sectors to health. Increasing public funding is essential to reduce reliance on OOPs and external aid, and to ensure the sustainability of health services.
- **Expanding Social Health Insurance:** Expanding social health insurance coverage can provide a sustainable source of financing for health services and reduce the burden of OOPs on individuals. Governments should focus on deve-

loping inclusive and equitable SHI schemes that cover a broad range of services and are accessible to all population groups.

- **Enhancing Financial Management:** Strengthening financial management systems is crucial for ensuring that health resources are used efficiently and transparently. This includes improving budgeting and accounting practices, conducting regular audits, and enhancing oversight and accountability mechanisms.
- **Leveraging Private Sector Contributions:** Engaging the private sector in health financing can help to mobilize additional resources and expand access to healthcare services. Governments should foster public-private partnerships, encourage private sector investments in health infrastructure and services, and promote CSR initiatives that support health programs.
- **Reducing Reliance on External Aid:** While external aid remains important, developing nations should work toward reducing their reliance on donor funding by strengthening domestic financing mechanisms. This includes increasing public funding, expanding SHI, and fostering private sector contributions. Governments should also work to align donor funding with national health priorities and ensure that aid is used effectively to complement domestic resources.
- **Promoting Equity in Health Financing:** Ensuring that health financing mechanisms promote equity is essential for achieving UHC and reducing health disparities. This includes designing progressive tax systems, subsidizing healthcare for vulnerable populations, and implementing targeted interventions to address the needs of underserved communities.

CONCLUSION

Sustainable and equitable health financing is the cornerstone of a strong and resilient health system. By effectively mobilizing and managing both public and private contributions, developing nations can ensure that their health systems are adequately resourced to meet the needs of their populations. Achieving this requires a comprehensive approach that addresses the challenges in health financing, promotes equity, and fosters collaboration between the public and private sectors. Ultimately, sustainable health financing is key.

BUILDING RESILIENCE IN HEALTH SYSTEMS: LESSONS FROM CRISES

The COVID-19 pandemic, Ebola outbreaks, and other health emergencies in recent decades have starkly highlighted the vulnerabilities in health systems, particularly in developing nations like Nigeria. These crises have exposed the fragility of health infrastructure, the inadequacies in service delivery, and the gaps in preparedness and response. However, they have also provided valuable lessons on how to build resilience in health systems, making them more capable of withstanding shocks, adapting to changing circumstances, and continuing to deliver essential services under stress. This section explores the concept of health system resilience, examines the lessons learned from past crises, and discusses strategies for enhancing resilience to protect public health in the face of future challenges [19 - 21].

Understanding Health System Resilience

Health system resilience refers to the ability of a health system to prepare for, respond to, and recover from crises while maintaining core functions and services. A resilient health system is not only able to absorb shocks but also adapt and transform in response to changing conditions, emerging threats, and new opportunities. The key characteristics of a resilient health system include [19]:

- **Robustness:** The capacity to withstand shocks without collapsing. This involves having strong infrastructure, sufficient resources, and effective systems in place that can continue functioning during a crisis.
- **Redundancy:** The existence of backup systems, resources, and personnel that can be activated when primary systems are overwhelmed or fail. Redundancy ensures that health services can continue even when certain components of the system are compromised.
- **Flexibility:** The ability to adapt to new circumstances, including shifting health needs, evolving threats, and changes in the availability of resources. Flexible health systems can modify their operations, reallocate resources, and implement new strategies as needed.
- **Preparedness:** The extent to which a health system is ready to respond to emergencies, including having contingency plans, trained personnel, and essential supplies in place before a crisis occurs.
- **Learning and Adaptation:** The capacity to learn from past experiences, identify weaknesses, and implement changes that improve the system's ability to handle future crises. This involves continuous monitoring, evaluation, and the incorporation of lessons learned into policy and practice.

Lessons from Past Crises

Various health crises over the years have provided valuable lessons that can inform efforts to build more resilient health systems. Some of the key lessons learned include [20]:

- **The Importance of Early Detection and Surveillance:** The COVID-19 pandemic and Ebola outbreaks have underscored the critical need for strong disease surveillance systems that can detect emerging threats early. Early detection allows for prompt response, reducing the spread of diseases and minimising their impact on health systems and populations.
- **The Role of Community Engagement:** Community involvement is essential for effective crisis response. During the Ebola outbreaks in West Africa, communities that were actively engaged in public health efforts, such as contact tracing, public education, and the enforcement of quarantine measures, experienced better outcomes. Engaging communities in preparedness and response efforts helps build trust, ensures compliance with public health measures, and enhances the effectiveness of interventions.
- **The Need for Flexible and Adaptive Health Systems:** Crises often require health systems to adapt quickly to changing circumstances, such as surges in patient numbers, disruptions in supply chains, and shifts in health needs. Health systems that are flexible and can reallocate resources, repurpose facilities, and implement new protocols are better able to manage the demands of a crisis.
- **Strengthening Health Workforce Capacity:** Crises place immense pressure on health workers, who are often the frontline responders. Ensuring that health systems have a well-trained, adequately staffed, and supported workforce is crucial for resilience. This includes not only clinical staff but also public health professionals, logisticians, and support personnel who play critical roles in crisis response.
- **Supply Chain Resilience:** The COVID-19 pandemic highlighted the vulnerabilities in global and national supply chains for essential medical supplies, such as personal protective equipment (PPE), medicines, and vaccines. Ensuring that health systems have resilient supply chains, capable of withstanding disruptions, scaling up production, and ensuring timely delivery of supplies, is critical for crisis preparedness and response.
- **The Value of Multisectoral Collaboration:** Crises often require coordinated efforts across multiple sectors, including health, finance, education, and security. The response to the COVID-19 pandemic demonstrated the importance of multisectoral collaboration in mobilising resources, implementing public health measures, and addressing the broader social and economic impacts of the crisis.
- **Investing in Health Information Systems:** Reliable data is essential for effective crisis management. Health information systems that provide timely, accurate, and actionable data enable health authorities to make informed decisions, allocate resources effectively, and monitor the impact of interventions. The use of digital technologies and data analytics can enhance the capacity of health systems to respond to crises.

Strategies for Building Resilience in Health Systems

Building resilience in health systems requires a proactive and comprehensive approach that addresses the vulnerabilities exposed by past crises while preparing for future challenges. Key strategies for enhancing health system resilience include [21, 22]:

- **Strengthening Surveillance and Early Warning Systems:** Investing in robust disease surveillance systems is critical for the early detection of emerging health threats. This includes enhancing laboratory capacity, improving data collection and analysis, and establishing early warning systems that can trigger timely responses to potential crises.
- **Enhancing Health Workforce Resilience:** Developing a resilient health workforce involves ensuring that health workers are adequately trained, supported, and protected. This includes investing in workforce development, providing mental health support, ensuring adequate supplies of PPE, and implementing policies that protect health workers during crises.
- **Improving Supply Chain Management:** Building resilient supply chains requires diversifying suppliers, maintaining strategic stockpiles of essential supplies, and investing in logistics infrastructure. Health systems should also develop contingency plans for supply chain disruptions and establish mechanisms for rapid procurement and distribution of medical supplies during emergencies.
- **Fostering Community Resilience:** Engaging communities in health system resilience efforts is essential for building trust and ensuring the effectiveness of public health interventions. This includes involving communities in preparedness planning, providing public health education, and empowering local leaders to take an active role in crisis response.
- **Investing in Health Infrastructure:** Resilient health systems require strong infrastructure that can withstand the pressures of a crisis. This includes ensuring that health facilities are well-maintained, equipped with necessary medical supplies, and supported by reliable utilities such as electricity, water, and telecommunications.
- **Promoting Multisectoral Collaboration:** Building resilience requires collaboration across different sectors and levels of government. Health systems should establish partnerships with other sectors, such as finance, education, and social services, to address the broader determinants of health and ensure a coordinated response to crises.
- **Leveraging Technology and Innovation:** Digital technologies, such as telemedicine, mobile health (mHealth) solutions, and health information systems, can enhance the resilience of health systems by improving access to

care, streamlining data collection, and enabling remote monitoring of health indicators. Health systems should invest in these technologies and explore innovative solutions to enhance crisis preparedness and response.

- **Implementing Continuous Learning and Adaptation:** Resilient health systems are those that continuously learn from past experiences and adapt to changing circumstances. This involves conducting after-action reviews following crises, identifying areas for improvement, and integrating lessons learned into health policies and practices. Continuous learning and adaptation help ensure that health systems are better prepared for future challenges.

CONCLUSION

Building resilience in health systems is an ongoing process that requires sustained commitment, investment, and collaboration. The lessons learned from past crises provide valuable insights into the vulnerabilities of health systems and highlight the need for proactive measures to enhance resilience. By strengthening surveillance systems, investing in health infrastructure, supporting the health workforce, and fostering community engagement, developing nations like Nigeria can build health systems that are more capable of withstanding shocks and continuing to deliver essential services in times of crisis. A resilient health system is not only better equipped to manage emergencies but also more capable of achieving long-term health goals, improving health equity, and ensuring the well-being of the population.

REFERENCES

[1] World Health Organisation. (2007). Everybody's Business: Strengthening Health Systems to Improve Health Outcomes: WHO's Framework for Action. Geneva. Available from: https://www.who.int/healthsystems/strategy/everybodys_business.pdf

[2] Frenk J. The global health system: strengthening national health systems as the next step for global progress. PLoS Med 2010; 7(1): e1000089. [http://dx.doi.org/10.1371/journal.pmed.1000089] [PMID: 20069038]

[3] Kruk ME, Myers M, Varpilah ST, Dahn BT. What is a resilient health system? Lessons from Ebola. Lancet 2015; 385(9980): 1910-2. [http://dx.doi.org/10.1016/S0140-6736(15)60755-3] [PMID: 25987159]

[4] Malkin RA. Design of health care technologies for the developing world. Annu Rev Biomed Eng 2007; 9(1): 567-87. [http://dx.doi.org/10.1146/annurev.bioeng.9.060906.151913] [PMID: 17430083]

[5] Bhutta ZA, Lassi ZS, Pariyo G, Huicho L. Global Experience of Community Health Workers for Delivery of Health Related Millennium Development Goals: A Systematic Review, Country Case Studies, and Recommendations for Integration into National Health Systems. Geneva: WHO 2010. Available from: https://www.who.int/workforcealliance/knowledge/publications/alliance/Global_CHW_web.pdf

[6] McPake B, Hanson K. Managing the public–private mix to achieve universal health coverage. Lancet 2016; 388(10044): 622-30. [http://dx.doi.org/10.1016/S0140-6736(16)00344-5] [PMID: 27358252]

[7] Nairametrics. (2024). FG allocates N1.3 trillion, 4.6% of its 2024 fiscal year budget, to Nigeria's health sector. Available from: https://nairametrics.com/2024/02/01/fg-allocates-n1-3-trillion-4-6- of-its-2024-fiscal-year-budget-to-nigerias-health-sector/?utm

[8] Yadav P. Health Product Supply Chains in Developing Countries: Diagnosis of the Root Causes of Underperformance and an Agenda for Reform. Health Syst Reform 2015; 1(2): 142-54. [http://dx.doi.org/10.4161/23288604.2014.968005] [PMID: 31546312]

[9] USAID. The Logistics Handbook: A Practical Guide for the Supply Chain Management of Health Commodities, 2011.

[10] MSH. MDS-3: Managing Access to Medicines and Health Technologies. Arlington, VA: MSH 2012.

[11] Lippeveld T, Sauerborn R, Bodart C. Design and Implementation of Health Information Systems. Geneva: WHO 2000. Available from: https://apps.who.int/iris/handle/10665/42289

[12] MEASURE Evaluation. Strengthening Health Information Systems in Low- and Middle-Income Countries: A Model to Frame What We Know and What We Need to Learn. Chapel Hill, NC: MEASURE Evaluation 2017.

[13] AbouZahr C, Boerma T. Health information systems: the foundations of public health. Bull World Health Organ 2005; 83(8): 578-83. Available from: https://www.scielosp.org/j/bwho/a/mQtDmBjbRvjNVCpGJSY9vML/?lang=en [PMID: 16184276]

[14] World Health Organisation. Health Systems Financing: The Path to Universal Coverage. World Health Report 2010. Geneva: WHO, 2010. Available from: https://www.who.int/whr/2010/en/

[15] McIntyre D, Kutzin J. Health Financing Country Diagnostic: A Foundation for National Strategy Development. Health Financing Guidance No. 1. WHO, Geneva, 2016. Available from: https://apps.who.int/iris/bitstream/handle/ 10665/204283/9789241510110_eng.pdf

[16] Moreno-Serra R, Smith PC. Does progress towards universal health coverage improve population health? Lancet 2012; 380(9845): 917-23. [http://dx.doi.org/10.1016/S0140-6736(12)61039-3] [PMID: 22959388]

[17] BUDGIT. (2024). Recalibrating Government Agencies for Resource Efficiency and Economic Growth. A review of Nigeria's 2024 Federal Government Budget of Renewed Hope. Available from: https://budgit.org/wp-content/uploads/2024/05/2024-FG-Budget-Analysis-2.pdf?utm

[18] Orodata Science. (2025). Primary Health Centre State of Power Report 2024-2025. (2025). Available from: https://www.orodata.org/download/primary-health-center-state-of-power-report-2024-2025/

[19] Nuzzo JB, Meyer D, Snyder M, *et al.* What makes health systems resilient against infectious disease outbreaks and natural hazards? Results from a scoping review. BMC Public Health 2019; 19(1): 1310. [http://dx.doi.org/10.1186/s12889-019-7707-z] [PMID: 31623594]

[20] Kieny MP, Dovlo D. Beyond Ebola: a new agenda for resilient health systems. Lancet 2015; 385(9963): 91-2. [http://dx.doi.org/10.1016/S0140-6736(14)62479-X] [PMID: 25706456]

[21] Blanchet K, Nam SL, Ramalingam B, Pozo-Martin F. Governance and Capacity to Manage Resilience of Health Systems: Towards a New Conceptual Framework. Int J Health Policy Manag 2017; 6(8): 431-5. [http://dx.doi.org/10.15171/ijhpm.2017.36] [PMID: 28812842]

[22] Saleh J-EA. Resilient Communities: Navigating Public Health Challenges in Developing Nations. Bentham Science Publishers 2025. [http://dx.doi.org/10.2174/97898153056091250101]

CHAPTER 4

Education as a Catalyst for Health Improvement

Abstract: This chapter explores the pivotal role of education as a driving force in improving public health. The chapter highlights the interconnectedness between education and health outcomes, emphasizing how health literacy serves as the foundation for public health. It examines the impact of basic education on health, the importance of integrating health education into school curricula, and the role of adult education in community health. Additionally, the chapter discusses the influence of media on health promotion and presents case studies of successful health education initiatives. By demonstrating the transformative power of education, this chapter advocates for increased investment in educational programs as a critical strategy for enhancing public health.

Keywords: School curricula, Adult education, Basic education, Community health, Health literacy, Health outcomes, Health education initiatives, Media in health promotion, Public health.

INTRODUCTION

Education is universally recognised as a critical driver of individual and societal progress. Beyond its intrinsic value, education serves as a powerful tool for improving public health outcomes. This chapter delves into the multifaceted relationship between education and health, illustrating how education serves as a catalyst for health improvement at both the individual and community levels. From basic health literacy to the integration of health education into school curricula, education empowers people to make informed health decisions, promotes healthier behaviours, and fosters environments that support better health outcomes.

HEALTH LITERACY: THE FOUNDATION OF PUBLIC HEALTH

Health literacy is increasingly recognised as a cornerstone of public health, particularly in developing nations like Nigeria, where the burden of disease remains high and access to healthcare services is often limited. Health literacy, broadly defined, is the degree to which individuals can obtain, process, and understand basic health information and services needed to make appropriate health decisions. It encompasses not only the ability to read and comprehend health-related materials but also the capacity to navigate complex healthcare systems, communicate effectively with healthcare providers, and apply health knowledge in everyday life [1 - 3].

The Importance of Health Literacy

Health literacy is fundamental to achieving positive health outcomes and improving public health. It serves as the foundation upon which individuals and communities can build healthy behaviours, access healthcare services, and engage in preventive health practices. The importance of health literacy can be understood through several key dimensions [1]:

- **Empowerment and Autonomy:** Health literacy empowers individuals by providing them with the knowledge and skills needed to make informed decisions about their health. This includes understanding medical instructions, recognising symptoms of illness, knowing when to seek care, and adhering to prescribed treatments. Empowered individuals are more likely to take control of their health, leading to better health outcomes and reduced healthcare costs.
- **Disease Prevention and Health Promotion:** Individuals with high health literacy are more likely to engage in preventive health behaviors, such as getting vaccinated, practicing safe hygiene, and adopting healthy lifestyles. Health literacy also plays a critical role in disease prevention by enabling individuals to understand risk factors, recognize early signs of illness, and seek timely medical care. By promoting healthy behaviors, health literacy contributes to the overall well-being of communities and reduces the burden of disease.
- **Access to Healthcare Services:** Health literacy is essential for navigating the healthcare system. Individuals with adequate health literacy can more effectively communicate with healthcare providers, understand their rights and responsibilities, and access the services they need. This is particularly important in contexts where healthcare systems are complex and resources are limited. Health literacy helps individuals overcome barriers to care, such as language, cultural differences, and a lack of familiarity with healthcare processes.
- **Health Equity:** Health literacy is closely linked to health equity. Populations with low health literacy are often the most vulnerable, including those with low socio-economic status, limited education, and marginalized communities. These populations are at greater risk of poor health outcomes due to limited access to health information and services. Improving health literacy can help address health disparities by ensuring that all individuals, regardless of their background, have the knowledge and skills needed to make informed health decisions.

- **Cost-Effectiveness:** Health literacy is also associated with cost savings in healthcare. Individuals with high health literacy are less likely to require emergency services, be hospitalized for preventable conditions, or experience medication errors. By improving health literacy, health systems can reduce the financial burden of preventable diseases and improve the efficiency of healthcare delivery.

Challenges in Achieving Health Literacy

Despite its importance, achieving high levels of health literacy remains a significant challenge, particularly in developing nations like Nigeria. Several factors contribute to low health literacy [2]:

- **Educational Barriers:** In many developing countries, access to quality education is limited, particularly in rural and underserved areas. Low levels of general literacy, especially among women and marginalized groups, contribute to low health literacy. Educational systems that do not prioritize health education further exacerbate this issue.
- **Cultural and Linguistic Diversity:** Nigeria is a linguistically and culturally diverse nation, with over 500 languages spoken across the country. This diversity presents challenges in delivering health information that is accessible and understandable to all populations. Health messages that are not culturally sensitive or delivered in a language that individuals can comprehend are less likely to be effective.
- **Complexity of Health Information:** Health information is often complex and difficult to understand, particularly for individuals with low literacy levels. Medical terminology, complicated instructions, and the use of technical language can create barriers to comprehension. Health literacy efforts must focus on simplifying and clarifying health information to make it more accessible.
- **Misinformation and Health Mistrust:** The spread of misinformation, particularly through social media and informal networks, poses a significant challenge to health literacy. Misinformation can lead to harmful health behaviors, such as vaccine hesitancy, and undermine public health efforts. Additionally, mistrust in the healthcare system, fueled by historical and ongoing inequalities, can prevent individuals from seeking accurate health information and care.
- **Resource Constraints:** In many developing nations, health systems are under-resourced and overburdened. Limited funding for health education programs, a shortage of trained health educators, and inadequate infrastructure for delivering health information contribute to low health literacy. Resource constraints also

limit the ability to reach remote and underserved populations with effective health literacy interventions.

Strategies for Improving Health Literacy

Improving health literacy requires a multifaceted approach that addresses the barriers to understanding and accessing health information. Effective strategies for enhancing health literacy in developing nations include [3]:

- **Integrating Health Education into School Curricula:** Schools are critical settings for health education. By integrating health education into school curricula from an early age, students can develop the knowledge and skills needed to make informed health decisions throughout their lives. Health education should cover a range of topics, including nutrition, hygiene, sexual and reproductive health, and the prevention of infectious and non-communicable diseases.
- **Promoting Community-Based Health Education:** Community-based approaches are essential for reaching populations with low health literacy. Community health workers, local leaders, and peer educators can play a key role in delivering health information that is culturally relevant and accessible. Community-based programs can also foster trust and encourage active participation in health-promoting activities.
- **Utilizing Digital Health Technologies:** Digital health technologies offer new opportunities for improving health literacy, particularly in contexts where access to healthcare is limited. Mobile health (mHealth) platforms, social media, and online resources can provide individuals with accurate and timely health information. However, digital health initiatives must be designed with the target population in mind, ensuring that content is accessible, easy to understand, and culturally appropriate.
- **Simplifying Health Communication:** Health communication should be clear, simple, and tailored to the literacy levels of the target audience. This includes using plain language, avoiding medical jargon, and incorporating visual aids, such as infographics and videos, to enhance understanding. Health messages should also be delivered in local languages and through channels that are trusted by the community.
- **Addressing Misinformation and Building Trust:** Combating misinformation requires proactive efforts to provide accurate health information and engage communities in dialogue. Health authorities should work with trusted community leaders and influencers to disseminate accurate information and counteract myths and misconceptions. Building trust in the healthcare system is also critical, particularly in communities that have historically been marginalized or underserved.

- **Strengthening Health System Support for Health Literacy:** Health systems should prioritize health literacy as a key component of public health strategies. This includes investing in health education programs, training healthcare providers in effective communication skills, and creating supportive environments that encourage patients to ask questions and seek information. Health literacy should also be integrated into national health policies and programs, with dedicated funding and resources allocated to its promotion.

CONCLUSION

Health literacy is not just a personal skill; it is a public health imperative that underpins the success of health systems and the well-being of populations. In developing nations like Nigeria, where health challenges are compounded by socio-economic disparities, low literacy levels, and limited access to healthcare, improving health literacy is essential for achieving better health outcomes and reducing health inequities. By investing in health education, simplifying health communication, and engaging communities in health promotion efforts, we can build a more health-literate society that is empowered to take charge of its health and well-being. In this way, health literacy serves as the foundation of public health, enabling individuals and communities to lead healthier, more informed lives.

THE IMPACT OF BASIC EDUCATION ON HEALTH OUTCOMES

Education is a powerful social determinant of health, with profound implications for individual well-being and population health outcomes. Basic education, which encompasses primary and secondary schooling, is particularly crucial as it lays the foundation for lifelong learning, shapes health behaviours, and influences access to health-related resources and opportunities. In the context of developing nations like Nigeria, where disparities in education and health are stark, the relationship between basic education and health outcomes is of paramount importance. This section explores how basic education impacts health, the mechanisms through which education influences health outcomes, and the broader implications for public health policy [4 - 6].

The Relationship Between Education and Health

The link between education and health is well-established, with extensive research demonstrating that higher levels of education are associated with better health outcomes. Individuals with basic education tend to live longer, healthier lives and are less likely to suffer from chronic diseases, malnutrition, and mental health issues. This relationship is multifaceted and can be understood through several key mechanisms [4]:

- **Health Knowledge and Literacy:** Education provides individuals with the knowledge and skills needed to understand health information, make informed decisions, and engage in health-promoting behaviors. For example, individuals with basic education are more likely to understand the importance of vaccination, practice safe hygiene, and adopt healthy dietary habits. Health literacy, as discussed in the previous section, is a direct outcome of basic education and plays a critical role in shaping health outcomes.
- **Economic Empowerment:** Education is a key driver of economic mobility, providing individuals with the qualifications and skills needed to secure better-paying jobs and achieve financial stability. Economic empowerment, in turn, improves access to healthcare, nutritious food, and safe living conditions, all of which are essential for good health. Conversely, a lack of education often perpetuates cycles of poverty, which are closely linked to poor health outcomes.
- **Access to Health Services:** Individuals with basic education are more likely to utilize healthcare services, including preventive care, maternal and child health services, and treatment for illnesses. Education enhances the ability to navigate complex healthcare systems, understand medical instructions, and advocate for one's health needs. This is particularly important in contexts where access to healthcare is limited and health services are underutilized.
- **Social and Psychological Well-being:** Education contributes to social and psychological well-being by fostering a sense of self-efficacy, reducing stress, and promoting social connectedness. Educated individuals are more likely to engage in social networks and community activities, which can provide emotional support and reduce the risk of mental health issues. Education also plays a role in shaping positive health behaviors, such as avoiding risky behaviors (*e.g.*, smoking, substance abuse) and seeking help when needed.
- **Intergenerational Health Benefits:** The benefits of education extend beyond the individual to their families and communities. Educated parents are more likely to prioritize their children's health and education, leading to better health outcomes for the next generation. For example, mothers with basic education are more likely to seek prenatal care, practice breastfeeding, and ensure that their children receive immunizations. This intergenerational transmission of health knowledge and behaviors helps break the cycle of poor health and poverty.

The Impact of Basic Education on Specific Health Outcomes

Basic education has a significant impact on various specific health outcomes, particularly in developing nations. Some of the key health outcomes influenced by education include [5]:

- **Maternal and Child Health:** Education is one of the most important determinants of maternal and child health. Women with basic education are more likely to access prenatal care, give birth in healthcare facilities, and practice proper infant feeding. This, in turn, reduces maternal and child mortality rates, improves birth outcomes, and enhances child development. Education also empowers women to make informed decisions about family planning, leading to healthier spacing of pregnancies and reduced fertility rates.

- **Infectious Disease Prevention:** Basic education plays a critical role in preventing the spread of infectious diseases, such as HIV/AIDS, malaria, and tuberculosis. Educated individuals are more likely to understand and adopt preventive measures, such as using insecticide-treated nets, practicing safe sex, and seeking early treatment for symptoms of infection. Education also contributes to greater awareness of vaccination programs and adherence to treatment regimens, which are essential for controlling infectious diseases.
- **Nutrition and Food Security:** Education is closely linked to improved nutrition and food security. Individuals with basic education are more likely to understand the importance of a balanced diet, recognize signs of malnutrition, and make informed food choices. Education also contributes to better household food management, including budgeting, food preparation, and storage. In regions where malnutrition is prevalent, such as parts of Nigeria, basic education can have a profound impact on reducing undernutrition and improving dietary diversity.
- **Chronic Disease Management:** As the burden of non-communicable diseases (NCDs) rises in developing nations, education becomes increasingly important for the prevention and management of chronic conditions such as diabetes, hypertension, and cardiovascular disease. Individuals with basic education are more likely to engage in regular physical activity, avoid tobacco and excessive alcohol use, and adhere to prescribed treatments for chronic conditions. Education also enhances the ability to recognize early signs of chronic disease and seek timely medical care.
- **Mental Health:** Education contributes to better mental health outcomes by promoting social and emotional well-being, reducing stress, and increasing access to mental health services. Educated individuals are more likely to seek help for mental health issues, adhere to treatment plans, and engage in coping strategies that reduce the risk of depression and anxiety. Education also reduces stigma associated with mental illness, encouraging more open discussions and support for those affected.

The Role of Education Policy in Health Improvement

Given the strong link between education and health, education policy has a crucial role to play in public health improvement. Governments and policymakers must prioritize investments in basic education, particularly in regions where educational attainment is low and health outcomes are poor. Key policy recommendations include [6]:

- **Expanding Access to Quality Education:** Ensuring universal access to quality basic education is essential for improving health outcomes. This includes addressing barriers to education, such as poverty, gender discrimination, and geographic disparities. Policies should focus on increasing school enrollment, reducing dropout rates, and ensuring that all children, regardless of their background, have access to a quality education.
- **Integrating Health Education into School Curricula:** Schools are critical settings for health education. Integrating comprehensive health education into school curricula can equip students with the knowledge and skills needed to make informed health decisions. Health education should cover topics such as nutrition, hygiene, sexual and reproductive health, disease prevention, and mental health. Schools should also promote healthy behaviors through physical education, school feeding programs, and access to health services.
- **Promoting Gender Equality in Education:** Gender disparities in education have significant implications for health outcomes. Girls who receive a basic education are more likely to delay marriage and childbirth, have fewer children, and access healthcare services. Promoting gender equality in education, including efforts to keep girls in school, is essential for improving maternal and child health and achieving broader public health goals.
- **Supporting Lifelong Learning and Adult Education:** While basic education is critical, opportunities for lifelong learning and adult education are also important for health improvement. Adult education programs can provide individuals with the knowledge and skills needed to manage their health, particularly for those who missed out on formal schooling. These programs can also address specific health issues, such as chronic disease management, nutrition, and reproductive health.
- **Leveraging Partnerships for Health and Education:** Achieving the full potential of education to improve health outcomes requires collaboration across sectors. Governments, non-governmental organizations, and the private sector should work together to promote education and health through coordinated programs and initiatives. This includes partnerships to improve school infrastructure, provide health services in schools, and support community-based education and health initiatives.

CONCLUSION

Basic education is a powerful catalyst for improving health outcomes in developing nations like Nigeria. By providing individuals with the knowledge, skills, and economic opportunities needed to make informed health decisions, education has the potential to transform public health and reduce health disparities. As we continue to confront the challenges of poverty, disease, and inequity, investing in basic education must remain a top priority for policymakers, educators, and public health professionals. Through a sustained commitment to education, we can empower individuals and communities to achieve better health, greater well-being, and a brighter future for all.

INTEGRATING HEALTH EDUCATION INTO SCHOOL CURRICULA

Integrating health education into school curricula is a crucial strategy for promoting public health, particularly in developing nations where the burden of disease is high and access to healthcare is limited. Schools are key environments where young people acquire the knowledge, skills, and attitudes necessary to lead healthy lives. By embedding health education into the formal education system, we can equip students with the tools they need to make informed decisions about their health, prevent illness, and contribute to the overall well-being of their communities [7 - 9].

The Rationale for Health Education in Schools

The inclusion of health education in school curricula is driven by several compelling reasons [7]:

- **Early Intervention:** Schools provide a unique opportunity to reach children and adolescents during their formative years, when they are developing habits and behaviours that will last a lifetime. By introducing health education early, we can influence behaviours before they become entrenched, reducing the risk of chronic diseases, substance abuse, and other health issues later in life.
- **Widespread Reach:** In many developing nations, schools are among the few institutions that reach a broad segment of the population, including those in rural and underserved areas. By integrating health education into school curricula, we can ensure that all children, regardless of their background, receive essential health information and skills.
- **Linking Education and Health Outcomes:** There is a strong correlation between education and health outcomes. Students who receive comprehensive health education are more likely to engage in health-promoting behaviors, such as regular physical activity, healthy eating, and safe sexual practices. By fostering a culture of health within schools, we can improve not only individual health outcomes but also the health of entire communities.
- **Promoting Health Equity:** Health education in schools can help address health disparities by providing all students with equal access to information and resources that promote health. This is particularly important in contexts where

access to healthcare is limited and where socio-economic factors create barriers to health. By empowering students with knowledge, we can reduce inequities and improve health outcomes across different population groups.

Key Components of a Comprehensive Health Education Curriculum

A comprehensive health education curriculum should be holistic, addressing a wide range of health topics and skills. The following components are essential for a robust health education program [8]:

- **Physical Health:** Education about physical health should cover topics such as nutrition, physical activity, hygiene, and the prevention of communicable and non-communicable diseases. Students should learn about the importance of a balanced diet, regular exercise, and personal hygiene practices in maintaining good health. Additionally, education on infectious diseases, including HIV/AIDS, malaria, and tuberculosis, is crucial in regions where these diseases are prevalent.
- **Mental and Emotional Health:** Mental health is an integral part of overall well-being. A comprehensive curriculum should include education on mental and emotional health, addressing topics such as stress management, coping skills, and the importance of seeking help for mental health issues. Teaching students about mental health can reduce stigma, promote emotional resilience, and encourage positive mental health practices.
- **Sexual and Reproductive Health:** Sexual and reproductive health education is essential for empowering young people to make informed decisions about their bodies and relationships. This component should include information on puberty, reproductive anatomy, contraception, sexually transmitted infections (STIs), and the prevention of unintended pregnancies. Culturally sensitive and age-appropriate education on sexual and reproductive health can reduce the rates of teenage pregnancy, STIs, and HIV transmission.
- **Substance Abuse Prevention:** Education on the risks associated with tobacco, alcohol, and drug use is critical for preventing substance abuse among young people. A comprehensive curriculum should include information on the physical, mental, and social consequences of substance use, as well as strategies for resisting peer pressure and making healthy choices.
- **Safety and Injury Prevention:** Teaching students about safety and injury prevention can help reduce the risk of accidents and injuries. This includes education on road safety, water safety, first aid, and the prevention of violence and abuse. Students should also learn about the importance of creating safe environments at home, school, and in the community.
- **Health Advocacy and Decision-Making Skills:** Health education should equip students with the skills needed to advocate for their health and make informed

decisions. This includes critical thinking, problem-solving, communication, and the ability to access and evaluate health information. By developing these skills, students can become active participants in their health and well-being, both individually and collectively.

Strategies for Effective Integration of Health Education

Integrating health education into school curricula requires careful planning and implementation. The following strategies can enhance the effectiveness of health education programs [9]:

- **Curriculum Development and Alignment:** Health education should be integrated into existing school curricula, aligned with national education standards, and tailored to the local context. Collaboration between education and health ministries, curriculum developers, and educators is essential for creating a curriculum that meets the needs of students and communities. The curriculum should be age-appropriate, culturally relevant, and inclusive of diverse perspectives.
- **Teacher Training and Support:** Teachers play a critical role in delivering health education. To ensure effective implementation, teachers need to be trained in health education content and pedagogical methods. Professional development programs should provide teachers with the knowledge, skills, and resources needed to teach health topics confidently and effectively. Ongoing support, including access to teaching materials and collaboration with health professionals, can further enhance teacher capacity.
- **Interactive and Engaging Teaching Methods:** Health education is most effective when it is interactive and engages students in active learning. Teaching methods should include discussions, group activities, role-playing, and hands-on experiences that allow students to apply what they have learned. Incorporating technology, such as multimedia presentations and online resources, can also enhance student engagement and learning outcomes.
- **Community and Parental Involvement:** Engaging the broader community and parents in health education initiatives can reinforce the messages taught in schools and create a supportive environment for health promotion. Schools should involve parents and community leaders in health education activities, such as workshops, health fairs, and information sessions. Collaboration with community organizations and healthcare providers can also strengthen the delivery of health education and provide students with additional resources and support.
- **Monitoring and Evaluation:** To ensure the effectiveness of health education programs, it is important to monitor and evaluate their impact on student knowledge, attitudes, and behaviors. Schools should collect data on health

outcomes, such as changes in health behaviors, academic performance, and attendance rates, to assess the success of the curriculum. Feedback from students, teachers, and parents can also provide valuable insights for continuous improvement.

Challenges and Considerations

While integrating health education into school curricula offers significant benefits, it also presents challenges that must be addressed [8, 9]:

- **Cultural Sensitivity:** Health education programs must be culturally sensitive and respect the values and beliefs of the communities they serve. Topics such as sexual and reproductive health can be particularly sensitive, and educators must navigate these issues carefully to avoid alienating students and their families. Engaging community leaders and involving parents in the development of health education programs can help ensure cultural appropriateness.
- **Resource Constraints:** In many developing nations, schools face resource constraints that can hinder the effective implementation of health education. Limited funding, inadequate facilities, and a shortage of trained teachers can all pose challenges. Governments and stakeholders must prioritize investments in education and health to overcome these barriers and ensure that all students have access to quality health education.
- **Addressing Health Disparities:** Health education programs must be designed to address the needs of all students, including those from marginalized and disadvantaged groups. This includes ensuring that health education is accessible to students with disabilities, those living in rural areas, and those from low-income families. Programs should be inclusive and equitable, providing all students with the opportunity to benefit from health education.
- **Sustainability:** For health education programs to have a lasting impact, they must be sustainable over the long term. This requires ongoing commitment from governments, educators, and communities, as well as continuous funding and support. Building capacity within the education system and creating partnerships with health organizations can help ensure the sustainability of health education initiatives.

CONCLUSION

Integrating health education into school curricula is a powerful strategy for improving public health and fostering a healthier future for young people. By providing students with the knowledge, skills, and attitudes necessary to make informed health decisions, schools can play a pivotal role in preventing disease, promoting well-being, and reducing health disparities. As we continue to face complex health challenges, the role of education in health promotion must be recognised and strengthened. Through collaborative efforts, we can ensure that health education becomes an integral part of the school experience, empowering the next generation to lead healthy, productive lives.

ADULT EDUCATION AND COMMUNITY HEALTH

Adult education plays a crucial role in enhancing community health, especially in regions where literacy rates are low and access to formal education is limited. By empowering adults with knowledge and skills, we can improve health outcomes not just for individuals but for entire communities. Adult education encompasses a wide range of learning activities, from basic literacy and numeracy to health-specific programs that address critical issues such as disease prevention, nutrition, and family planning [10 - 12].

The Importance of Adult Education in Public Health

The link between education and health is well-established, with numerous studies showing that higher levels of education are associated with better health outcomes. However, in many developing nations, a significant portion of the adult population may not have had the opportunity to complete formal education. Adult education programs provide a second chance for these individuals to acquire essential knowledge that can directly impact their health and well-being [10].

- **Health Literacy and Decision-Making:** Health literacy, the ability to understand and use health information, is fundamental to making informed health decisions. Adult education programs can improve health literacy by teaching participants how to access, interpret, and apply health information. This, in turn, enables individuals to make better choices regarding nutrition, hygiene, disease prevention, and the use of healthcare services.
- **Empowerment and Agency:** Education empowers individuals by increasing their sense of agency, the ability to take control of their lives and health. Adult education programs can help participants develop critical thinking and problem-solving skills, which are essential for navigating complex health issues. This empowerment extends beyond individual health, as educated adults are more likely to advocate for health improvements within their communities.
- **Intergenerational Impact:** The benefits of adult education extend beyond the individual, affecting entire families and communities. Educated adults are better equipped to support the health and education of their children, breaking the cycle of poverty and poor health. They are also more likely to engage in community health initiatives and contribute to the overall well-being of their communities.

Key Components of Effective Adult Education Programs

For adult education programs to have a meaningful impact on community health, they must be designed to meet the specific needs of the target population. The following components are essential for effective adult education initiatives [11]:

- **Literacy and Numeracy:** Basic literacy and numeracy are foundational skills that enable individuals to engage with more complex health information. Adult education programs should prioritize these skills, particularly in regions where literacy rates are low. Teaching adults to read and write empowers them to access health information independently, understand medical instructions, and communicate effectively with healthcare providers.
- **Health Education:** Health education should be a central component of adult education programs. Topics such as nutrition, hygiene, maternal and child health, disease prevention, and sexual and reproductive health should be covered. These programs should be tailored to the local context, addressing the specific health challenges and cultural norms of the community.
- **Life Skills Development:** In addition to health education, adult education programs should focus on developing life skills that contribute to overall well-being. This includes skills such as financial literacy, which can help individuals manage healthcare costs, and conflict resolution, which can reduce violence and improve mental health. Life skills education also enhances individuals' ability to participate in community health initiatives and engage with healthcare systems.
- **Community-Based Learning:** Adult education programs are most effective when they are community-based and participatory. This approach encourages collective learning and problem-solving, fostering a sense of community ownership over health outcomes. Programs that involve local leaders and integrate traditional knowledge can also enhance cultural relevance and acceptance.
- **Use of Technology:** Technology can be a powerful tool in adult education, particularly in reaching remote or underserved populations. Mobile phones, radio programs, and online platforms can be used to deliver health education and literacy training. These tools can also facilitate ongoing learning and support, allowing participants to continue their education beyond the classroom.

Challenges in Implementing Adult Education Programs

While the benefits of adult education for community health are clear, there are several challenges to implementing effective programs [12]:

- **Resource Constraints:** Many regions, particularly in developing nations, face significant resource constraints that limit the availability and quality of adult education programs. Funding, trained educators, and educational materials may be in short supply, making it difficult to reach all those in need.
- **Cultural Barriers:** Cultural norms and beliefs can pose challenges to adult education, particularly in areas where there is resistance to certain types of health education, such as sexual and reproductive health. Programs must be designed with cultural sensitivity in mind, engaging community leaders and adapting content to align with local values.
- **Logistical Challenges:** Reaching adult learners, particularly in rural or remote areas, can be logistically challenging. Transportation, communication, and infrastructure issues may hinder the delivery of education programs. Flexible and innovative delivery methods, such as mobile learning or community-based classes, are essential to overcoming these barriers.
- **Sustainability:** Ensuring the sustainability of adult education programs is a significant challenge. Programs require ongoing funding, resources, and support to continue delivering education and to adapt to changing community needs. Building local capacity and fostering partnerships with government agencies, NGOs, and the private sector can enhance sustainability.

Case Studies and Best Practices

Several successful adult education initiatives provide valuable lessons for improving community health:

- **The Literacy and Health Education Project in Bangladesh:** This project integrated literacy training with health education, focusing on maternal and child health. The program's success was attributed to its community-based approach, which involved local health workers and used culturally relevant materials. The project resulted in significant improvements in health literacy and health outcomes, particularly in reducing child mortality rates.
- **The REFLECT Approach in Uganda:** REFLECT (Regenerated Freirean Literacy through Empowering Community Techniques) combines literacy and numeracy training with participatory learning methods to address health and social issues. In Uganda, this approach has been used to improve health literacy and empower communities to take action on health challenges such as HIV/AIDS and malaria. The program's emphasis on community participation and empowerment has been key to its success.
- **Mobile Health Education in Kenya:** In Kenya, mobile phones have been used to deliver health education to adult learners in remote areas. Text messages, voice messages, and interactive platforms provide health information on topics such as HIV prevention, maternal health, and nutrition. The use of technology

has expanded the reach of health education and enabled continuous learning, even in challenging environments.

CONCLUSION

Adult education is a powerful tool for improving community health and fostering sustainable development. By equipping adults with the knowledge and skills they need to make informed health decisions, we can enhance individual and collective well-being. The integration of health education into adult learning programs not only improves health outcomes but also empowers communities to take charge of their health and development. As we look to the future, it is essential to invest in adult education as a key strategy for public health promotion. Governments, NGOs, and community organizations must collaborate to create accessible, culturally sensitive, and sustainable adult education programs that address the unique needs of each community. Through these efforts, we can build healthier, more resilient communities and contribute to the broader goal of health equity and social justice.

THE ROLE OF MEDIA IN HEALTH PROMOTION

The media has long been recognised as a powerful tool for shaping public opinion and behaviour, making it an essential component in the promotion of public health. In the context of Nigeria and other developing nations, where access to formal education and healthcare services may be limited, the media can serve as a critical channel for disseminating health information, raising awareness, and influencing health-related behaviours on a large scale. This section explores the various roles that media play in health promotion, the challenges faced, and the strategies for maximising its impact [13 - 15].

Media as a Vehicle for Health Education: Media outlets, ranging from traditional platforms such as radio, television, and print to digital media, play a pivotal role in health education. They can reach broad audiences, transcending geographical and socio-economic barriers, to deliver critical health information [13].

- **Raising Awareness:** One of the primary roles of the media is to raise awareness about health issues. Through news reports, documentaries, public service announcements, and health-focused programs, the media can inform the public about prevalent health concerns, such as infectious diseases, maternal and child health, and non-communicable diseases. In regions where health literacy is low, media campaigns can provide the basic information needed to prevent and manage health issues.

- **Behavioral Change Communication (BCC):** The media is instrumental in promoting behavioral change, which is essential for disease prevention and health promotion. Campaigns that focus on issues such as vaccination, sanitation, nutrition, and safe sexual practices can significantly influence public behavior. By presenting information in engaging and relatable formats, the media can motivate individuals to adopt healthier lifestyles.
- **Health Advocacy:** Media can also serve as a platform for health advocacy, highlighting issues that require public attention and policy intervention. Journalists and media outlets can hold governments and institutions accountable by exposing gaps in healthcare delivery, corruption, and inefficiencies. Additionally, they can advocate for policies that improve public health, such as anti-tobacco laws, road safety regulations, and access to healthcare.

The Impact of Traditional Media in Health Promotion

In many developing nations, traditional media, especially radio and television, remain the most accessible and influential forms of communication. These platforms have unique advantages in health promotion efforts [14]:

- **Radio:** Radio is particularly effective in reaching rural and remote communities, where literacy levels may be low, and access to other forms of media is limited. Radio programs can be broadcast in local languages, making health messages more accessible. Interactive radio shows that allow listeners to call in with questions can also foster community engagement and provide personalized health advice.
- **Television:** Television has the power to reach a wide audience and convey health messages visually, which can enhance understanding and retention. Health dramas, talk shows, and documentaries can make complex health issues more relatable by depicting real-life scenarios. Visual media can also be used to demonstrate practical health tips, such as how to properly wash hands or prepare nutritious meals.
- **Print Media:** Newspapers, magazines, and pamphlets can be effective tools for health education, particularly in urban areas where literacy rates are higher. Print media allows for detailed coverage of health topics, providing readers with in-depth information. Health columns and articles in widely-read publications can influence public discourse on health issues and encourage readers to take proactive steps in managing their health.

The Role of Digital Media in Modern Health Promotion

The advent of digital media has revolutionized health promotion, offering new opportunities for reaching and engaging with diverse audiences. In Nigeria and other developing nations, the proliferation of mobile phones and internet access has expanded the reach of digital health campaigns [15].

- **Social Media:** Platforms like Facebook, Twitter, Instagram, and WhatsApp are increasingly being used to disseminate health information and engage with the public. Social media campaigns can rapidly spread health messages, reach younger audiences, and foster community support for health initiatives. Health organizations can use these platforms to share information, respond to questions, and debunk health myths and misinformation.
- **Mobile Health (mHealth):** Mobile technology has become a critical tool for health promotion, particularly in areas with limited healthcare infrastructure. mHealth initiatives use mobile phones to deliver health information, reminders, and educational content *via* text messages, apps, and interactive voice response systems. These services can be tailored to individual needs, providing personalized advice on topics such as maternal health, chronic disease management, and immunization schedules.
- **Online Health Portals and E-Learning:** The internet provides a wealth of health resources, from educational websites to online support groups. Health portals can offer reliable, evidence-based information on a wide range of health topics, while e-learning platforms can provide training and education for healthcare workers and the general public. In regions with internet access, these resources can complement traditional health education efforts and provide continuous learning opportunities.

Challenges in Utilising Media for Health Promotion

While media hold great potential for health promotion, several challenges must be addressed to maximise its effectiveness [13 - 15]:

- **Misinformation and Health Myths:** One of the significant challenges in the digital age is the spread of misinformation and health myths, particularly on social media. False information can lead to harmful behaviours, such as vaccine hesitancy or the use of ineffective treatments. It is crucial for health organisations to actively monitor and counter misinformation by providing accurate and timely information.
- **Access and Equity:** Despite the growing reach of digital media, access to technology remains unequal, particularly in rural areas and among low-income populations. Ensuring that all segments of the population benefit from media-based health promotion requires addressing the digital divide and making traditional media more accessible and inclusive.

- **Cultural Sensitivity:** Health messages must be culturally sensitive and tailored to the specific needs and beliefs of the target audience. Generic messages may not resonate with all communities and could be met with resistance. Engaging local leaders and using culturally appropriate language and symbols can enhance the effectiveness of health promotion efforts.
- **Sustainability:** Sustaining media-based health promotion campaigns can be challenging, especially in resource-constrained settings. Long-term funding, partnerships with media organisations, and the integration of health promotion into regular programming are essential for maintaining the momentum of health campaigns.

Strategies for Enhancing the Impact of Media in Health Promotion

To overcome these challenges and maximise the impact of media in health promotion, several strategies can be employed [13 - 19]:

- **Partnerships and Collaboration:** Collaboration between health organisations, media outlets, and the private sector can enhance the reach and effectiveness of health campaigns. Public-private partnerships can provide the resources and expertise needed to develop and sustain impactful media initiatives.
- **Capacity Building:** Training journalists and media professionals in health reporting is crucial for ensuring accurate and responsible coverage of health issues. Workshops, seminars, and collaborations with health experts can equip media personnel with the knowledge and skills needed to convey complex health information effectively.
- **Community Engagement:** Engaging communities in the development and dissemination of health messages can increase their relevance and impact. Community radio stations, local influencers, and grassroots organisations can play a vital role in tailoring health messages to local contexts and ensuring they resonate with the target audience.
- **Monitoring and Evaluation:** Continuous monitoring and evaluation of media-based health promotion campaigns are essential for assessing their effectiveness and making necessary adjustments. Data on audience reach, engagement, and behavior change can provide valuable insights for improving future campaigns.

CONCLUSION

The media will continue to be a critical tool in promoting public health, particularly as technology evolves and access to information expands. In Nigeria and other developing nations, leveraging the full potential of both traditional and digital media is essential for addressing health challenges and improving health outcomes. As we move forward, it is important to invest in media-based health promotion, ensuring that it is inclusive, culturally sensitive, and sustainable. By harnessing the power of media, we can reach broader audiences, inspire positive health behaviors, and ultimately contribute to the goal of achieving health equity for all.

CASE STUDIES: SUCCESSFUL HEALTH EDUCATION INITIATIVES

Health education initiatives are crucial for improving public health outcomes, particularly in developing nations where access to healthcare services may be limited, and health literacy levels are often low. This section explores several successful health education initiatives that have been implemented in Nigeria and other developing nations, highlighting the strategies used, the challenges encountered, and the impact on public health [16 - 19].

The National Immunisation Days in Nigeria

One of the most notable health education initiatives in Nigeria has been the National Immunisation Days (NIDs) aimed at eradicating polio. This campaign, launched in the 1990s, has been instrumental in reducing the incidence of polio in the country.

- **Strategy:** The NIDs were designed as a nationwide campaign to immunise all children under five against polio. The initiative combined mass media campaigns with community mobilisation efforts. Radio, television, and print media were used to raise awareness about the importance of immunisation, while community health workers and volunteers went door-to-door to ensure that children in even the most remote areas received the vaccine.
- **Challenges:** The campaign faced significant challenges, including vaccine hesitancy due to misinformation, myths, religious beliefs, and cultural resistance in some communities. In response, the initiative incorporated local religious and community leaders into the campaign to build trust and counteract myths about the vaccine.
- **Impact:** The NIDs have been highly successful, with Nigeria being declared polio-free in 2020. The campaign not only contributed to the eradication of polio but also strengthened the overall immunization system in the country and raised public awareness about the importance of vaccination.

The Bangladesh Oral Rehydration Therapy (ORT) Campaign

The Oral Rehydration Therapy (ORT) campaign in Bangladesh is another classic example of a successful health education initiative. In the 1980s, Bangladesh was facing a severe challenge with high child mortality rates due to diarrhea. The ORT campaign was launched to address this issue.

- **Strategy:** The campaign focused on educating mothers about the preparation and use of oral rehydration solution (ORS) to treat diarrhea at home. The message was disseminated through a combination of mass media campaigns, including radio and television, and grassroots efforts involving community health workers who conducted home visits and demonstrations.
- **Challenges:** One of the major challenges was the initial skepticism about the efficacy of ORS. The campaign had to overcome deeply entrenched traditional practices and convince mothers that ORS was a simple yet effective solution. To do this, the campaign utilized testimonials from mothers who had successfully used ORS and integrated these messages into the broader media strategy.
- **Impact:** The ORT campaign is credited with saving millions of lives and dramatically reducing the child mortality rate in Bangladesh. By the late 1990s, the use of ORS was nearly universal in the country, and the initiative became a model for similar campaigns worldwide.

The Heartfile Health Financing Initiative in Pakistan

In Pakistan, the Heartfile Health Financing (HHF) initiative was developed to address the financial barriers to accessing healthcare, particularly for low-income populations. Although primarily a financing initiative, it also incorporated significant health education components.

- **Strategy:** The HHF initiative used a combination of technology and community outreach to educate the public about the availability of financial support for healthcare. The program leveraged SMS technology to reach low-income households with information about the program and how to access funds. Additionally, community health workers were trained to educate families about the importance of seeking timely healthcare and to assist them in navigating the financial support system.
- **Challenges:** One of the primary challenges was reaching the most vulnerable populations, who were often unaware of the available support. The initiative had to overcome barriers related to illiteracy, lack of access to mobile phones, and distrust of formal systems. To address these issues, the program employed a community-based approach, working closely with local leaders and health workers to build trust and ensure that the information reached those in need.
- **Impact:** The HHF initiative significantly increased access to healthcare for low-income families in Pakistan. It not only provided financial support but also empowered individuals with the knowledge to seek care when needed. The program's success has led to its expansion and adaptation in other regions of the country.

The Jamaica Healthy Lifestyle Project

The Jamaica Healthy Lifestyle Project is an example of a multi-faceted health education initiative aimed at reducing the burden of non-communicable diseases (NCDs) in the country.

- **Strategy:** The project combined mass media campaigns with community-based interventions to promote healthy lifestyles. It focused on educating the public about the risks of NCDs, such as heart disease, diabetes, and hypertension, and encouraged behaviors like healthy eating, regular physical activity, and smoking cessation. The initiative used television, radio, and print media to reach a broad audience, while also organizing community events, health fairs, and school-based programs.
- **Challenges:** The project faced challenges related to changing long-standing behaviors and cultural attitudes towards diet and physical activity. To address this, the campaign worked to create supportive environments that made healthy choices easier. For example, the project partnered with local food vendors to offer healthier options and collaborated with schools to integrate physical activity into the daily routine.
- **Impact:** The Jamaica Healthy Lifestyle Project succeeded in raising awareness about NCDs and promoting healthier behaviors. While the reduction in NCD prevalence takes time to fully manifest, the project has laid the groundwork for long-term change by increasing public knowledge and creating environments that support healthy living.

The Safe Motherhood Initiative in Nigeria

The Safe Motherhood Initiative in Nigeria was launched to address the high rates of maternal and infant mortality in the country. The initiative focused on improving maternal health through education and access to quality healthcare.

- **Strategy:** The initiative employed a multi-pronged approach, including media campaigns, community outreach, and healthcare provider training. It aimed to educate women, particularly in rural areas, about the importance of prenatal care, skilled birth attendance, and postpartum care. Radio programs, print materials, and community meetings were used to disseminate information, while partnerships with local NGOs and health facilities ensured that the necessary services were available.
- **Challenges:** Cultural practices and beliefs, particularly in rural areas, were significant barriers to the success of the initiative. Many women relied on traditional birth attendants and were hesitant to seek care at health facilities. To

overcome this, the initiative engaged community leaders and traditional birth attendants in the campaign, helping to bridge the gap between traditional practices and modern healthcare.

- **Impact:** The Safe Motherhood Initiative has contributed to a notable reduction in maternal and infant mortality rates in targeted areas. By improving access to maternal health services and increasing awareness about the importance of skilled care during pregnancy and childbirth, the initiative has had a lasting impact on maternal and child health in Nigeria.

CONCLUSION

The case studies presented in this section highlight the importance of culturally sensitive, community-based approaches to health education. Successful initiatives often combine mass media campaigns with grassroots efforts to reach and engage diverse populations. They also emphasise the need for partnerships, capacity building, and sustainability to ensure long-term impact. These initiatives demonstrate that health education can be a powerful tool in improving public health outcomes, particularly in developing nations. By learning from these successes, future health education campaigns can be designed to effectively address the unique challenges faced in different contexts and contribute to the broader goal of achieving health equity for all.

REFERENCES

[1] Nutbeam D. Health literacy as a public health goal: a challenge for contemporary health education and communication strategies into the 21st century. Health Promot Int 2000; 15(3): 259-67. [http://dx.doi.org/10.1093/heapro/15.3.259]

[2] Berkman ND, Sheridan SL, Donahue KE, Halpern DJ, Crotty K. Low health literacy and health outcomes: an updated systematic review. Ann Intern Med 2011; 155(2): 97-107. [http://dx.doi.org/10.7326/0003-4819-155-2-201107190-00005] [PMID: 21768583]

[3] Ratzan SC, Parker RM. Introduction. In: Selden CR, Zorn M, Ratzan SC, Parker RM, Eds. National Library of Medicine Current Bibliographies in Medicine: Health Literacy. National Institutes of Health, U.S. Department of Health and Human Services 2000; pp. v-vi.

[4] Gakidou E, Cowling K, Lozano R, Murray CJL. Increased educational attainment and its effect on child mortality in 175 countries between 1970 and 2009: a systematic analysis. Lancet 2010; 376(9745): 959-74. [http://dx.doi.org/10.1016/S0140-6736(10)61257-3] [PMID: 20851260]

[5] Feinstein L, Sabates R, Anderson TM, Sorhaindo A, Hammond C. OECD. 2006; pp. What are the effects of education on health? In: Desjardins R, Schuller T, Eds. Proceedings of the Copenhagen Symposium. 171-354.

[6] Cutler, D. M., & Lleras-Muney, A. (2006). Education and health: Evaluating theories and evidence. National Bureau of Economic Research Working Paper Series, No. 12352.

[7] World Health Organization. (1997). Promoting health through schools: The World Health Organization's global school health initiative. WHO Technical Report Series No. 870. Geneva: World Health Organization.

[8] St Leger L. Schools, health literacy and public health: possibilities and challenges. Health Promot Int

2001; 16(2): 197-205.
[http://dx.doi.org/10.1093/heapro/16.2.197] [PMID: 11356758]

[9] Deschesnes M, Martin C, Hill AJ. Comprehensive approaches to school health promotion: how to achieve broader implementation? Health Promot Int 2003; 18(4): 387-96.
[http://dx.doi.org/10.1093/heapro/dag410] [PMID: 14695370]

[10] Coady DP, Parker SW. Cost-effectiveness analysis of demand- and supply-side education interventions: The case of PROGRESA in Mexico. Rev Dev Econ 2004; 8(3): 440-51.
[http://dx.doi.org/10.1111/j.1467-9361.2004.00244.x]

[11] Nutbeam D. The evolving concept of health literacy. Soc Sci Med 2008; 67(12): 2072-8.
[http://dx.doi.org/10.1016/j.socscimed.2008.09.050]

[12] Freire P. Pedagogy of the Oppressed. New York: Continuum Books. 1970.

[13] Wakefield MA, Loken B, Hornik RC. Use of mass media campaigns to change health behaviour. Lancet 2010; 376(9748): 1261-71.
[http://dx.doi.org/10.1016/S0140-6736(10)60809-4] [PMID: 20933263]

[14] Noar SM. A 10-year retrospective of research in health mass media campaigns: where do we go from here? J Health Commun 2006; 11(1): 21-42.
[http://dx.doi.org/10.1080/10810730500461059] [PMID: 16546917]

[15] Thompson TL, Parrott R, Nussbaum JF, Eds. The Routledge Handbook of Health Communication. 2nd ed., Routledge 2011.
[http://dx.doi.org/10.4324/9780203846063]

[16] Kreuter MW, Oswald DL, Bull FC, Clark EM. Are tailored health education materials always more effective than non-tailored materials? Health Educ Res 2000; 15(3): 305-15.
[http://dx.doi.org/10.1093/her/15.3.305] [PMID: 10977378]

[17] Nutbeam D. Evaluating health promotion—progress, problems and solutions. Health Promot Int 1998; 13(1): 27-44.
[http://dx.doi.org/10.1093/heapro/13.1.27]

[18] Laverack G. Health Promotion Practice: Power and Empowerment. Sage 2004.

[19] Saleh J-EA. Resilient Communities: Navigating Public Health Challenges in Developing Nations. Bentham Science Publishers 2025.
[http://dx.doi.org/10.2174/97898153056091250101]

CHAPTER 5

Insecurity and Public Health: Navigating Conflict Zones

Abstract: This chapter delves into the profound impact of insecurity on public health, particularly in conflict zones. It explores the multifaceted health consequences of conflict and displacement, including the spread of diseases, mental health issues, and the collapse of healthcare infrastructure. The chapter highlights the challenges of delivering healthcare in such dangerous environments, where health workers face significant risks. It also emphasizes the importance of mental health and psychosocial support in crises and examines strategies to protect health workers and maintain health service continuity during crises. The chapter concludes by discussing post-conflict recovery and the rebuilding of health systems, offering insights into creating resilient healthcare frameworks that can withstand the pressures of insecurity.

Keywords: Conflict zones, Crisis management, Displacement, Insecurity, Healthcare delivery, Health system resilience, Health worker protection, Mental health, Psychosocial support, Public health, Post-conflict recovery.

INTRODUCTION

Insecurity, whether from armed conflict, terrorism, or civil unrest, profoundly affects public health, particularly in developing nations. The interplay between insecurity and public health is multifaceted, with direct impacts ranging from physical injuries to long-term psychological trauma, and indirect consequences such as the disruption of healthcare services, displacement of populations, and the breakdown of health systems. In Nigeria, as in many other developing countries, insecurity presents one of the most significant challenges to achieving universal health coverage and improving public health outcomes. This chapter explores the health consequences of conflict and displacement, examines the unique challenges of delivering healthcare in conflict zones, and discusses strategies for protecting health workers, ensuring continuity of services, and rebuilding health systems post-conflict.

Jalal-Eddeen Abubakar Saleh

THE HEALTH CONSEQUENCES OF CONFLICT AND DISPLACEMENT

Conflict and displacement have profound and far-reaching effects on public health, particularly in developing nations where health systems are already fragile. The breakdown of infrastructure, the disruption of services, and the displacement of populations create a cascade of health challenges that can persist long after the immediate violence has ended. This section explores the various health consequences of conflict and displacement, with a focus on the direct and indirect impacts on individuals and communities [1 - 4].

In Nigeria, there is a large geographically concentrated humanitarian crisis that drives both displacement and worsens health outcomes of the vulnerable population, particularly in the northern region. Based on the IOM's Displacement Tracking Matrix (Round 16, February 2025) figures, there are approximately 1.32 million internally displaced persons (IDPs) in north-west and north-central zones. The figure is more leveraging broader monitoring that includes northeast and other conflict-affected areas, revealing a national figure of between 3.0 - 3.6 million IDPs, a figure that aligns with the UNHCR reports. It is important to mention that conflict and displacement result in acute health consequences, with a surge in acute malnutrition and child mortality in affected states, vaccine-preventable diseases outbreaks, and poor access to reproductive, maternal, and child health services, to mention but a few [1].

Direct Health Impacts of Conflict

The direct health consequences of conflict are often the most visible and immediate, including [1]:

- **Injury and Trauma:** Armed conflict leads to high levels of physical injury and trauma, including gunshot wounds, shrapnel injuries, and fractures. In conflict zones, access to emergency medical care is often limited, exacerbating the severity of these injuries and increasing the likelihood of long-term disability or death.
- **Psychological Trauma:** Conflict exposes individuals, particularly children, to severe psychological stress. Witnessing violence, losing loved ones, and living in constant fear can result in mental health conditions such as post-traumatic stress disorder (PTSD), depression, and anxiety. The lack of mental health services in conflict zones means that these conditions often go untreated, leading to long-term psychological morbidity.
- **Sexual and Gender-Based Violence (SGBV):** Conflict often leads to an increase in sexual violence, including rape, forced prostitution, and sexual

slavery. Women and girls are particularly vulnerable, but men and boys can also be victims. The physical and psychological consequences of SGBV are severe, including trauma, Sexually Transmitted Infections (STIs), and unwanted pregnancies.

Indirect Health Impacts of Conflict

Beyond the immediate injuries and trauma, conflict also creates conditions that lead to a host of indirect health consequences [1, 2]:

- **Disruption of Health Services:** Conflict often destroys health infrastructure, including hospitals, clinics, and supply chains. Health workers may flee or be targeted, leading to a critical shortage of personnel. As a result, essential health services, such as immunizations, maternal care, and chronic disease management, are often interrupted, leading to preventable deaths and the resurgence of infectious diseases.
- **Malnutrition:** Conflict disrupts food production, supply chains, and markets, leading to food shortages and increased food prices. Displaced populations, in particular, may struggle to access sufficient and nutritious food. Malnutrition, especially among children, can lead to stunting, wasting, and increased vulnerability to infectious diseases.
- **Spread of Infectious Diseases:** Conflict exacerbates the spread of infectious diseases due to overcrowded living conditions, poor sanitation, and lack of access to clean water. Displaced populations living in camps or informal settlements are particularly at risk for outbreaks of diseases such as cholera, measles, and respiratory infections. Additionally, the breakdown of immunisation programs can lead to the resurgence of vaccine-preventable diseases.

Health Consequences of Displacement

Displacement, whether internal or across borders, brings its own set of health challenges. The forced movement of people from their homes disrupts their lives and places them in precarious situations where their health and well-being are compromised [1 - 3].

- **Living Conditions in Refugee Camps:** Refugee camps and internally displaced persons (IDP) settlements are often overcrowded and lack basic amenities such as clean water, sanitation, and adequate shelter. These conditions create a breeding ground for communicable diseases and exacerbate existing health conditions. The lack of privacy and security also increases the risk of sexual and gender-based violence.

- **Access to Healthcare:** Displaced populations often face significant barriers to accessing healthcare. These barriers include a lack of healthcare facilities in camps, discrimination, and legal restrictions in host countries. Additionally, displaced individuals may have lost their identification documents, making it difficult to access services that require proof of identity.
- **Chronic Diseases and Disability:** Displacement often interrupts the treatment of chronic diseases such as diabetes, hypertension, and HIV/AIDS. The stress of displacement and the lack of consistent care can lead to worsening health outcomes and complications. Similarly, individuals with disabilities may find it particularly challenging to access the care and support they need in displacement settings.
- **Mental Health:** The trauma of displacement, combined with the stress of living in precarious conditions, takes a significant toll on mental health. Displaced individuals may experience high levels of anxiety, depression, and PTSD. The lack of mental health services in displacement settings means that these conditions are often left untreated, leading to a deterioration in overall well-being.

Long-Term Health Impacts

The health consequences of conflict and displacement do not end when the violence subsides or when displaced populations return home. The long-term health impacts can persist for years, affecting individuals, families, and communities [1 - 4].

- **Rebuilding Health Systems:** In the aftermath of conflict, rebuilding health systems is a daunting task. Infrastructure needs to be repaired, health workers need to be trained and recruited, and essential services need to be restored. The long-term impact of the disruption of health services during the conflict often results in higher mortality and morbidity rates for years to come.
- **Intergenerational Health Effects:** The health consequences of conflict and displacement can be passed on to future generations. For example, malnutrition during pregnancy can lead to low birth weight and developmental issues in children, while the psychological trauma experienced by parents can affect their ability to care for their children.
- **Social Determinants of Health:** Conflict and displacement exacerbate poverty, unemployment, and social exclusion, all of which are key determinants of health. The long-term impact of these factors can lead to a cycle of poor health outcomes, perpetuating the effects of conflict on future generations.

CONCLUSION

Addressing the health consequences of conflict and displacement requires a comprehensive and multifaceted approach. This includes not only providing immediate medical care and humanitarian assistance but also investing in the rebuilding of health systems, supporting mental health services, and addressing the social determinants of health. It is also crucial to involve displaced populations in the planning and implementation of health interventions to ensure that their needs and concerns are adequately addressed. The international community, governments, and non-governmental organisations must work together to develop sustainable solutions that go beyond emergency response and focus on long-term recovery and resilience. By doing so, it is possible to mitigate the devastating health impacts of conflict and displacement and to build healthier, more resilient communities in the aftermath of crises.

DELIVERING HEALTHCARE IN CONFLICT ZONES

Delivering healthcare in conflict zones is one of the most complex and challenging tasks in global health. The volatile and often dangerous environment, coupled with the breakdown of infrastructure and social order, makes the provision of medical services extremely difficult. This section examines the key challenges and strategies involved in delivering healthcare in conflict zones, with a focus on the principles of humanitarian action, the roles of different actors, and the innovative approaches required to overcome barriers [5 - 8].

Challenges in Delivering Healthcare in Conflict Zones

Delivering healthcare in conflict zones presents numerous challenges, many of which are interconnected and exacerbate each other [5]:

- **Insecurity and Violence:** Healthcare providers in conflict zones often operate in environments where they face threats from armed groups, crossfire, and targeted attacks. The lack of security makes it difficult for healthcare workers to reach those in need, and can result in the closure of health facilities.
- **Infrastructure Destruction:** Conflict frequently results in the destruction of hospitals, clinics, and other health facilities, as well as damage to roads, bridges, and other critical infrastructure. This destruction severely limits the ability to provide healthcare services and to transport medical supplies.
- **Shortage of Healthcare Workers:** Conflict zones often experience a shortage of healthcare workers due to displacement, death, or the flight of personnel to safer areas. Those who remain are often overworked and under-resourced, facing immense pressure to meet the needs of the affected population.

- **Supply Chain Disruptions:** The supply chains for essential medicines, medical equipment, and other supplies are often severely disrupted in conflict zones. This can lead to shortages of life-saving medications, vaccines, and other critical resources.
- **Population Displacement:** Large-scale displacement of populations creates additional challenges, as healthcare providers must track and address the health needs of people on the move, often in remote or hard-to-reach areas.
- **Legal and Bureaucratic Barriers:** Humanitarian organisations operating in conflict zones may face legal and bureaucratic barriers, such as restrictions on movement, difficulties in obtaining permits, and issues related to the neutrality and independence of their operations.

Principles of Humanitarian Healthcare Delivery

Despite these challenges, healthcare delivery in conflict zones is guided by key humanitarian principles that ensure the provision of care to those most in need [5, 6]:

- **Neutrality:** Healthcare providers must remain neutral and impartial, providing care based on need rather than on any political, ethnic, or religious affiliations. This principle is crucial for gaining access to conflict zones and for ensuring the safety of healthcare workers.
- **Impartiality:** Care must be provided to all individuals, regardless of their role in the conflict or their background. This principle ensures that the most vulnerable populations receive the care they need.
- **Independence:** Humanitarian organisations must operate independently of political and military actors to maintain their neutrality and to ensure that their actions are guided solely by the needs of the population.
- **Do No Harm:** Healthcare providers must ensure that their actions do not exacerbate the situation or put patients and staff at further risk. This includes careful planning and coordination to avoid unintentionally aiding one side of the conflict or becoming a target.

The Role of Different Actors

The delivery of healthcare in conflict zones involves a diverse array of actors, each with a specific role to play [5 - 7]:

- **Local Healthcare Providers:** Local doctors, nurses, and other healthcare workers are often the first responders in conflict zones. Their knowledge of the local context and their commitment to their communities make them indispensable, even though they may face significant risks.

- **International Humanitarian Organizations:** Organizations such as the International Committee of the Red Cross (ICRC), Médecins Sans Frontières (MSF), and various UN agencies play a critical role in providing medical care, supplying resources, and advocating for access to affected populations.
- **Non-Governmental Organisations (NGOs):** Many NGOs work alongside local and international actors to deliver healthcare, provide training, and support health system resilience in conflict zones.
- **Governments and Armed Forces:** In some cases, governments and armed forces may be involved in the delivery of healthcare, particularly in areas under their control. However, this involvement can be contentious, particularly if it is perceived as compromising the neutrality of healthcare delivery.
- **Community Health Workers:** In areas where access is limited, community health workers play a vital role in delivering primary care, health education, and referrals. Their close ties to the community often allow them to operate in areas where others cannot.
- **5.2.4 Innovative Approaches to Overcoming Barriers:** Given the unique challenges of delivering healthcare in conflict zones, innovative approaches are often required to ensure that care reaches those in need [5 - 7]. It is critical to maintain health information systems to track disease outbreaks, monitor health trends, and coordinate care. Innovative technologies, such as mobile apps and satellite communications, can be used to collect and transmit data in real-time. The importance of partnerships among government actors, UN agencies, international NGOs (such as MSF and ICRC), and local civil society cannot be overemphasised. Similarly, negotiated access, community liaison, leveraging the military and intel for updates on the security situation, and joint logistics enable predictable service delivery even in volatile areas. These collaborations often involve shared costs, pooling of resources, and adherence to the operational norms and agreed standard operating procedures.
- **Mobile Clinics and Outreach Teams:** Mobile clinics are used to reach populations in remote or hard-to-access areas, particularly those who are displaced. These clinics can provide essential services, including maternal care, vaccinations, and treatment for common illnesses. These mobile medical teams, led by government health ministries and in partnership with the WHO and other NGOs, deliver vaccinations, antenatal care, outpatient treatment, nutrition screening (CMAM), and basic stabilisation at the IDP camps or remote settlements. Similarly, MSF, in partnership with the WHO, has widespread mobile teams in Borno State, delivering therapeutic feeding and vaccination in inaccessible locations where fixed facilities are not delivering services due to insecurity, often with a clear referral linkage, security planning, and building trust with local communities [2].

- **Telemedicine:** In some conflict zones, telemedicine has been used to connect healthcare providers with specialists in other locations, allowing for remote diagnosis, consultation, and training. This approach can help to overcome the shortage of skilled personnel and to provide care in otherwise inaccessible areas. The Telemedicine platforms and remote consultation tools bridge specialist care, providing clinical supervision and management of chronic diseases because of a lack of geographic access or insecurity. In Nigerian conflict-affected zones, pilot programs have shown feasibility in supervising CHWs, supporting mental health services, and continuity of care for chronic illnesses, notwithstanding challenges with internet connectivity, privacy safeguards, and stable electricity, which are critical requirements.
- **Task Shifting:** In situations where healthcare professionals are in short supply, task shifting, where non-specialists are trained to perform specific tasks, can help to expand the availability of services. For example, community health workers may be trained to administer basic medical care or to manage chronic diseases. Because of disruption in facility-based care, CHWs trained in integrated Community Case Management (iCCM) fill in those critical gaps, diagnosing and treating common illnesses, detecting and referring severe cases, conducting malnutrition and growth monitoring, and providing health promotion and prevention at homes and or the IDP camps.
- **Emergency Health Kits and Pre-positioning of Supplies:** Pre-packaged emergency health kits containing essential medicines, medical supplies, and equipment can be rapidly deployed to conflict zones. These kits are designed to support health facilities and mobile clinics in providing care to large numbers of people. Similarly, prepositioning essential supplies, including medicines, rapid diagnostics, ready-to-use therapeutic foods (RUTF), and WASH supplies in secure hubs, is key in contexts with episodic access. Deploying digital logistics management information systems (LMIS) is critical to allow tracking of stock, redistribution of supplies, and early warning of shortages once access is restored.

Case Studies and Lessons Learned

Several case studies illustrate both the challenges and the successes of delivering healthcare in conflict zones [5 - 8]:

- **Syria:** The ongoing conflict in Syria has seen the destruction of much of the country's health infrastructure. However, despite these challenges, local healthcare providers, supported by international organisations, have continued to deliver care, often under extreme conditions. Mobile clinics, underground hospitals, and cross-border aid have all played a role in sustaining healthcare services.

- **South Sudan:** In South Sudan, conflict and displacement have severely impacted health services, particularly in rural areas. NGOs and international organisations have worked to fill the gaps by deploying mobile clinics, training community health workers, and providing emergency health kits. Despite the challenges, these efforts have helped to prevent major outbreaks and to provide critical care to displaced populations.
- **Yemen:** The conflict in Yemen has created one of the world's worst humanitarian crises, with widespread food insecurity and a collapsing health system. International organizations have responded by supporting local health facilities, providing vaccinations, and establishing cholera treatment centers. The use of telemedicine and health information systems has been critical in coordinating these efforts.

CONCLUSION

Delivering healthcare in conflict zones is fraught with challenges, but it is also an essential component of humanitarian action. The ability to provide care in these settings not only saves lives but also helps to build resilience and to lay the foundation for recovery once the conflict ends. Moving forward, it is crucial to continue investing in innovative approaches, to support local healthcare providers, and to advocate for the protection of healthcare workers and facilities in conflict zones. The international community, governments, and humanitarian organizations must work together to ensure that healthcare remains a priority in conflict zones and that those affected by violence receive the care they need. By doing so, we can help to mitigate the devastating impact of conflict on health and to support the long-term recovery and stability of affected communities.

MENTAL HEALTH AND PSYCHOSOCIAL SUPPORT IN CRISIS SITUATIONS

Crises, whether caused by conflict, natural disasters, or other emergencies, often have profound and lasting impacts on mental health. The psychological toll on individuals and communities can be as devastating as the physical harm, yet mental health and psychosocial support (MHPS) are frequently under-prioritised in humanitarian responses. This section explores the importance of MHPSS in crises, the challenges in delivering these services, and the strategies that can be employed to support the mental well-being of affected populations [9 - 12].

In Nigeria's conflict-affected regions, MSF and UNICEF have reported high demand for mental health services. Program evaluations point to success when non-specialists are trained, community-based psychosocial activities are offered, and safe referral pathways exist. Remote (telehealth) mental health consultations have also emerged but are limited by connectivity and privacy constraints.

Conflict zones produce widespread psychological distress: trauma, grief, depression, anxiety, sleep disorders, and caregiver burden. Though beyond the scope of this book, it is worth mentioning the International guidance from the IASC (Inter-Agency Standing Committee) MHPSS Guidelines and WHO's frameworks, which emphasise *layered intervention models*:

1. **Community and population-level psychosocial support** (*e.g.*, safe spaces, peer support networks, psycho-education).
2. **Focused non-specialised services:** psychological first aid, basic counselling, training CHWs or PHC workers in mental health awareness.
3. **Specialised care:** for severe conditions, PTSD, and psychiatric disorders, through referral or remote specialist support.

The Psychological Impact of Crisis Situations

Crises such as armed conflicts, natural disasters, and displacement can lead to a wide range of mental health issues, including [9]:

- **Acute Stress Reactions:** Individuals in crises often experience intense stress, leading to symptoms such as anxiety, insomnia, irritability, and hypervigilance. These reactions, while normal in the immediate aftermath of a crisis, can become debilitating if they persist.
- **Post-Traumatic Stress Disorder (PTSD):** PTSD is a common consequence of exposure to traumatic events, such as witnessing violence or experiencing life-threatening situations. Symptoms include flashbacks, nightmares, severe anxiety, and avoidance behaviors.
- **Depression:** The loss, displacement, and uncertainty that accompany crises often lead to depression. This condition is characterized by persistent sadness, loss of interest in activities, feelings of hopelessness, and, in severe cases, suicidal thoughts.
- **Anxiety Disorders:** Chronic anxiety can develop in response to ongoing threats, such as living in a conflict zone or in displacement camps. This can manifest as generalized anxiety, panic attacks, or phobias.
- **Substance Abuse:** In some cases, individuals may turn to alcohol or drugs as a coping mechanism, leading to substance abuse issues that further compound their mental health challenges.
- **Social and Behavioral Disorders in Children:** Children are particularly vulnerable in crises. They may exhibit behavioral issues, such as aggression or withdrawal, and may struggle with developmental delays or learning difficulties.

Challenges in Providing Mental Health and Psychosocial Support

Several challenges complicate the delivery of MHPSS in crises [10]:

- **Stigma and Cultural Barriers:** Mental health issues are often stigmatized, leading individuals to avoid seeking help. Cultural perceptions of mental illness can also affect how people understand and respond to psychological distress, potentially hindering the effectiveness of interventions.
- **Resource Constraints:** Crises often lead to resource shortages, including a lack of trained mental health professionals, inadequate facilities, and insufficient supplies of psychotropic medications. This limits the ability to provide comprehensive MHPSS services.
- **Security Concerns:** In conflict zones, ongoing violence and insecurity can make it difficult for MHPSS providers to reach affected populations. This can leave those in need without access to essential mental health services.
- **Integration into Humanitarian Response:** MHPSS is sometimes treated as an afterthought in humanitarian responses, with physical health and basic needs taking priority. This can result in delayed or inadequate mental health support.
- **Long-Term Needs vs. Short-Term Funding:** Mental health issues often persist long after the initial crisis has passed, but funding for humanitarian interventions is typically short-term. This creates a gap in services during the critical post-crisis recovery period.

Principles of Effective Mental Health and Psychosocial Support

To effectively address the mental health needs of populations in crisis, MHPSS interventions should adhere to the following principles [11]:

- **Community-Based Approaches:** Engaging communities in the design and implementation of MHPSS programs is essential for ensuring that interventions are culturally appropriate and accessible. Community-based approaches also help to build resilience and support systems that can continue to function after external aid is withdrawn.
- **Multi-Tiered Support Systems:** MHPSS interventions should be organized into a multi-tiered system of care, ranging from basic psychosocial support to specialized mental health services. This ensures that all individuals, regardless of the severity of their needs, receive appropriate care.
- **Integration with Other Services:** MHPSS should be integrated into broader health and social services, including primary healthcare, education, and protection programs. This holistic approach addresses the interconnected nature of mental health and other aspects of well-being.

- **Capacity Building:** Training local healthcare providers, community leaders, and volunteers in MHPSS is critical for creating sustainable support systems. Capacity building efforts should focus on developing the skills needed to recognize and address mental health issues within the community.
- **Protecting Human Rights:** MHPSS interventions must respect the dignity and rights of all individuals. This includes ensuring informed consent, protecting confidentiality, and providing care that is free from coercion or discrimination.

Strategies for Delivering MHPSS in Crisis Situations

Several strategies have proven effective in delivering MHPSS in crises [12]:

- **Psychological First Aid (PFA):** PFA is an evidence-informed approach that involves providing immediate emotional and practical support to individuals in distress. It can be delivered by trained laypeople and focuses on listening, comforting, and helping individuals meet their basic needs.
- **Safe Spaces:** Establishing safe spaces, such as child-friendly areas or women's centers, provides a supportive environment where vulnerable individuals can access MHPSS services, receive care, and engage in social activities. These spaces are particularly important for children and women who may be at higher risk of violence or exploitation.
- **Group-Based Interventions:** Group-based interventions, such as support groups, can be an effective way to provide psychosocial support. These interventions allow individuals to share their experiences, build social connections, and learn coping strategies.
- **Culturally Adapted Therapies:** Adapting therapeutic approaches to fit the cultural context of the affected population is crucial for their effectiveness. This may involve using traditional healing practices, incorporating local languages, or involving community elders in the therapeutic process.
- **Use of Technology:** In some crisis situations, technology can play a role in delivering MHPSS. Mobile health (mHealth) applications, telephone hotlines, and online counseling services can help reach individuals who are isolated or unable to access in-person support.
- **Monitoring and Evaluation:** Continuous monitoring and evaluation of MHPSS programs are essential for assessing their impact and making necessary adjustments. This includes collecting data on mental health outcomes, service utilization, and patient satisfaction.

Case Studies: MHPSS in Action

Several case studies illustrate the implementation of MHPSS in crises [12]:

- **Rohingya Refugee Crisis (Bangladesh):** The influx of Rohingya refugees into Bangladesh created significant mental health challenges, particularly among survivors of violence. Humanitarian organizations responded by establishing PFA training for local volunteers, creating safe spaces for women and children, and integrating MHPSS into health services provided in refugee camps. These efforts have helped to address the immediate psychological needs of the refugees and to build community resilience.
- **Earthquake in Nepal (2015):** The 2015 earthquake in Nepal led to widespread trauma and mental health issues among the affected population. In response, local and international organizations launched MHPSS programs that included PFA, group counseling, and community-based psychosocial support. The programs were designed to be culturally sensitive and were integrated with efforts to rebuild the country's health infrastructure.
- **Syria Conflict:** The protracted conflict in Syria has resulted in widespread mental health issues, including PTSD and depression. MHPSS interventions in Syria have included mobile clinics, telemedicine, and the training of local mental health professionals. Despite the challenges posed by ongoing violence, these efforts have provided critical support to those affected by the conflict.

CONCLUSION

Mental health and psychosocial support are essential components of any comprehensive humanitarian response. While the challenges are significant, the strategies and principles outlined in this section demonstrate that it is possible to provide effective MHPSS even in the most difficult circumstances. By prioritizing mental health and ensuring that it is integrated into broader health and social services, we can help individuals and communities to heal from the psychological wounds of crisis and to build the resilience needed for recovery and future well-being. The international community, humanitarian organizations, and governments must continue to advocate for the inclusion of MHPSS in crisis response plans and to ensure that mental health is recognized as a fundamental aspect of human rights and dignity in crises.

PROTECTING HEALTH WORKERS IN INSECURE AREAS

Health workers are often on the front lines in insecure areas, delivering essential care in the most challenging and dangerous environments. Their work is critical to maintaining public health, especially in regions affected by conflict, natural disasters, or political instability. However, health workers in these areas face significant risks, including targeted violence, abduction, and exposure to infectious diseases. This section explores the challenges of protecting health workers in insecure areas, the strategies employed to ensure their safety, and the broader implications for global health [13 - 16].

In conflict zones, Health workers face direct threats ranging from attacks on facilities, sexual violence, intimidation, kidnappings, threats to personal safety, and harassment. Protecting them is critical.

- **International Legal Frameworks:** The Geneva Conventions (specifically Additional Protocols) and International Humanitarian Law establish medical neutrality and protection of health personnel and facilities. The ICRC's "Health Care in Danger" initiative and WHO's "Stopping Attacks on Health Care" campaign provide frameworks for addressing violations.
- **Operational Protection Measures:** These include the use of protected medical markings on facilities, staff safety training, incident reporting mechanisms, safe housing, and secure transport for personnel, community acceptance strategies (dialogues and trust building), and negotiation for corridor or access agreements with conflicting parties.
- **Policy References and Standards:** Nigeria is a signatory to international treaties respecting humanitarian law. Domestic policy, however, requires strengthening: formal inclusion of health worker protection in national emergency and security policies; reporting mechanisms; and ensuring health worker insurance or support in conflict settings.

THE RISKS FACED BY HEALTH WORKERS IN INSECURE AREAS

Health workers in insecure areas. Health workers in Nigeria's conflict-affected areas are exposed to a variety of risks that can have serious consequences for their safety and well-being because of threats that compromise their safety, well-being, and ability to deliver care [13]. These risks extend beyond physical harm to encompass psychological, social, and occupational dimensions. Table **1** below summarises the major crises affecting health workers, their health impacts, and the mitigation responses designed to protect them.

- **Targeted Attacks:** Health workers are often targeted by armed groups who view them as representatives of the government, international organisations, or rival factions. These attacks can include physical violence, bombings, and assassinations, leading to injury or death.

- **Abduction and Hostage-Taking:** In conflict zones, health workers may be abducted and held for ransom or used as bargaining chips by armed groups. These incidents can result in prolonged captivity, psychological trauma, and, in some cases, death.
- **Sexual Violence:** Female health workers are particularly vulnerable to sexual violence in insecure areas. Sexual assault and harassment can occur both in the workplace and while travelling to and from work, creating an additional layer of fear and stress.
- **Exposure to Infectious Diseases:** Health workers in crises are often at increased risk of exposure to infectious diseases, particularly in the absence of adequate protective equipment. This risk is heightened in regions experiencing epidemics or in areas with poor sanitation and hygiene conditions.
- **Psychological Stress:** The constant threat of violence, combined with the demands of providing care in extreme conditions, can lead to high levels of stress and burnout among health workers. This stress can be compounded by witnessing the suffering of patients and the loss of colleagues.

Table 1. Examples of crisis, health impact, response, and outcome.

Crisis	Health Impact	Response	Outcome
Targeted attacks on HCWs deliberately by armed groups, viewed as government or international representatives.	Physical injury, death, loss of skilled personnel, and disruption of essential health services.	Strengthening of security coordination with military and local authorities, use of risk mapping, and training on security protocols for frontline workers.	Improved field security awareness and reduced fatalities in high-risk deployments; however, access to volatile areas remains constrained.
Abduction, hostage-taking, and kidnapping of HCWs for ransom or political leverage.	Severe psychological trauma, prolonged captivity, and occasional fatalities result in the interruption of health interventions.	Crisis response frameworks established through the WHO and UN security systems; community engagement and negotiated access to ensure safer humanitarian operations.	Enhanced local trust and cooperation in volatile areas; reduced incidents where local mediators are involved.
Sexual violence, especially against female HCWs in the form of sexual assault and harassment, occurs in insecure or remote regions.	Physical and mental health trauma, stigmatization, and reduced female participation in field deployment.	Implementation of gender-sensitive security policies, confidential reporting systems, and psychosocial and legal support for survivors.	Increased reporting of incidents and awareness, yet persistent underreporting due to stigma and fear of reprisal.

(Table 1) cont.....

Crisis	Health Impact	Response	Outcome
Exposure to infectious diseases in high-risk areas during outbreaks (*e.g.*, cholera, Lassa fever, Ebola) occurs due to inadequate PPE and poor sanitation.	Illness, reduced workforce capacity, and transmission to patients and communities.	Provision of PPE, infection prevention and control (IPC) training, and deployment of rapid response teams in emergencies.	Reduced infection rates among responders; institutionalized IPC protocols within humanitarian operations.
Psychological stress and burnout occur because of persistent exposure to violence, insecurity, and suffering.	High stress, burnout, anxiety, depression, and decreased job performance or retention.	Mental health and psychosocial support (MHPSS) services for health workers; peer-support networks and debriefing sessions post-deployment.	Improved resilience and retention among health workers; growing integration of MHPSS in emergency response plans.

Challenges in Protecting Health Workers

Protecting health workers in insecure areas is a complex task that involves addressing several challenges [14]:

- **Lack of Security Infrastructure:** Many insecure areas lack the basic security infrastructure needed to protect health workers, such as secure facilities, safe transportation, and communication networks. This leaves health workers vulnerable to attacks and other risks.
- **Impunity and Lack of Accountability:** In many conflict zones, attacks on health workers go unpunished due to weak legal systems, lack of enforcement, or the absence of effective governance. This impunity encourages further violence and undermines efforts to protect health workers.
- **Resource Constraints:** Health systems in insecure areas often operate with limited resources, making it difficult to implement comprehensive security measures. This includes a lack of funding for security personnel, protective equipment, and training.
- **Humanitarian Access Restrictions:** Armed groups or governments may restrict humanitarian access to certain areas, making it difficult to provide protection and support to health workers. These restrictions can also limit the ability of international organizations to monitor and respond to threats.
- **Complexity of Conflicts:** The complex and fluid nature of many conflicts makes it difficult to predict and mitigate risks to health workers. Shifting frontlines, the involvement of multiple armed groups, and the breakdown of social order all contribute to an unpredictable and dangerous environment.

Strategies for Protecting Health Workers

A range of strategies can be employed to protect health workers in insecure areas [15]:

- **Negotiation and Engagement with Armed Groups:** Engaging with armed groups to secure agreements that protect health workers and respect the neutrality of healthcare facilities is a critical strategy. This requires skilled negotiators who can build trust and navigate the complexities of local power dynamics.

- **Strengthening Legal Protections:** Advocating for stronger legal protections for health workers at both the national and international levels is essential. This includes pushing for the enforcement of existing laws, as well as the adoption of new legislation that criminalizes attacks on health workers.
- **Capacity Building and Training:** Providing health workers with training in personal security, risk assessment, and emergency response can enhance their ability to protect themselves in insecure areas. Training should also include mental health support to help workers cope with the stresses of their environment.
- **Use of Technology:** Technology can play a crucial role in protecting health workers. This includes the use of mobile phones and satellite communication for emergency alerts, GPS tracking for safe travel routes, and telemedicine to reduce the need for health workers to travel to dangerous areas.
- **Safe Access Zones and Humanitarian Corridors:** Establishing safe access zones or humanitarian corridors, where health workers can operate without fear of attack, can provide critical protection. These zones should be negotiated with all relevant parties and monitored by neutral observers to ensure their integrity.
- **Community Engagement and Support:** Building strong relationships with local communities can enhance the protection of health workers. Communities that value and support their health workers are more likely to provide information about potential threats and to intervene to prevent violence.
- **International Advocacy and Solidarity:** International advocacy campaigns can raise awareness of the dangers faced by health workers and put pressure on governments and armed groups to respect their rights. Solidarity actions, such as public statements, petitions, and diplomatic interventions, can also help to protect health workers.

Case Studies: Protecting Health Workers in Practice

Several case studies illustrate the successful implementation of strategies to protect health workers [16]:

- **Syria Conflict:** In the Syrian conflict, health workers have been targeted by both government forces and armed opposition groups. In response, international organisations have provided training in security and emergency response, while advocacy efforts have focused on raising awareness of the attacks and pushing for accountability. Some organisations have also established underground clinics to protect health workers and patients from airstrikes.
- **Ebola Outbreak in West Africa (2014-2016):** During the Ebola outbreak, health workers were at high risk of infection and violence. Protective measures included the provision of personal protective equipment (PPE), training in infection control, and the establishment of secure treatment centres. Community engagement efforts were also critical in reducing resistance to health interventions and protecting health workers from attacks.
- **Afghanistan:** In Afghanistan, health workers have faced threats from the Taliban and other armed groups. To protect these workers, international and local organizations have engaged in negotiations with armed groups to ensure safe access to healthcare facilities. Additionally, mobile health clinics have been deployed to reduce the need for health workers to travel through dangerous areas.

The Role of the International Community

The international community has a critical role to play in protecting health workers in insecure areas. This includes [15, 16]:

- **Advocating for the Protection of Health Workers:** International organizations, governments, and NGOs must continue to advocate for the protection of health workers in conflict zones. This includes pressing for the implementation of international humanitarian law, which prohibits attacks on healthcare facilities and personnel.
- **Providing Resources and Support:** The international community should provide financial and technical support to help countries implement protective measures for health workers. This includes funding for security infrastructure, training programs, and emergency response systems.
- **Monitoring and Reporting Violations:** International organizations should monitor and report on attacks against health workers, documenting violations and advocating for accountability. This can help to deter future attacks and ensure that perpetrators are held responsible.

CONCLUSION

The protection of health workers in insecure areas is not only a matter of human rights but also a critical component of maintaining public health in crises. Without adequate protection, health workers cannot perform their essential duties, leading to a breakdown in healthcare services and exacerbating the suffering of affected populations. To ensure the safety of health workers, it is essential to adopt a multi-faceted approach that includes legal protections, capacity building, community engagement, and international advocacy. By prioritising the protection of health workers, we can help to safeguard the health of communities in insecure areas and uphold the principles of humanity and impartiality that are at the core of global health efforts.

STRATEGIES FOR HEALTH SERVICE CONTINUITY DURING CRISES

Ensuring the continuity of health services during crises is a critical challenge for health systems, particularly in regions affected by conflict, natural disasters, or other emergencies. In such situations, the demand for healthcare often increases sharply, while the capacity to deliver services may be severely compromised. This section explores the strategies that can be employed to maintain health service delivery during crises, drawing on lessons learned from past emergencies and best practices in crisis management [17 - 20].

Understanding the Impact of Crises on Health Services

Crises can disrupt health services in multiple ways [17]:

- **Destruction of Infrastructure:** Conflict, natural disasters, and other crises can damage or destroy health facilities, cutting off access to essential services. In some cases, entire hospitals and clinics may be rendered unusable, forcing patients and health workers to relocate.
- **Displacement of Populations:** Large-scale displacement of populations due to conflict or disasters can overwhelm existing health services in host communities or camps. The sudden influx of people often leads to shortages of medical supplies, overcrowded facilities, and increased transmission of communicable diseases.
- **Staff Shortages:** Health workers may flee crisis areas, be injured or killed, or be unable to reach their workplaces due to insecurity. This can lead to severe staff shortages, further straining the capacity to deliver services.
- **Supply Chain Disruptions:** Crises can disrupt supply chains, leading to shortages of essential medicines, medical supplies, and equipment. This can hinder the delivery of routine healthcare services as well as emergency care.
- **Increased Disease Burden:** Crises often lead to a surge in health problems, including trauma, infectious diseases, malnutrition, and mental health issues. The increased burden on health systems requires rapid adaptation to meet the new demands.

Building Resilient Health Systems

To ensure the continuity of health services during crises, health systems must be resilient and adaptable. Key components of a resilient health system include [18]:

- **Strong Governance and Leadership:** Effective leadership and governance are crucial for coordinating crisis response efforts and ensuring that health services continue to function. This includes clear decision-making structures, efficient communication channels, and the ability to mobilize resources quickly.
- **Flexible Service Delivery Models:** Health systems must be able to adapt their service delivery models to the changing needs and constraints of a crisis situation. This may involve decentralizing services, establishing mobile clinics, or leveraging telemedicine to reach affected populations.
- **Robust Supply Chains:** Ensuring the continuity of supply chains is essential for maintaining access to medicines, medical supplies, and equipment during crises. This requires pre-crisis planning, including the establishment of emergency stockpiles, diversified supply sources, and contingency plans for logistics.
- **Community Engagement and Participation:** Engaging communities in crisis response efforts can enhance the resilience of health services. Communities can play a key role in identifying needs, providing local support, and helping to ensure that services reach those most in need.
- **Integration of Mental Health and Psychosocial Support:** Crises often result in significant psychological stress for both affected populations and health workers. Integrating mental health and psychosocial support into health services is essential for addressing the mental health impacts of crises.

Pre-Crisis Planning and Preparedness

Effective crisis management begins with pre-crisis planning and preparedness. Strategies for ensuring health service continuity include [19]:

- **Risk Assessment and Mapping:** Conducting risk assessments and mapping potential hazards can help identify vulnerabilities and prioritize areas for intervention. This includes assessing the risks of natural disasters, conflict, disease outbreaks, and other potential crises.
- **Development of Emergency Response Plans:** Health systems should have comprehensive emergency response plans in place that outline the roles and responsibilities of different stakeholders, procedures for rapid deployment of resources, and strategies for maintaining essential services.
- **Training and Capacity Building:** Health workers and other stakeholders should be trained in emergency response protocols, including triage, mass

casualty management, and infection control. Regular drills and simulations can help ensure that staff are prepared to respond effectively during a crisis.

- **Establishment of Rapid Response Teams:** Rapid response teams, composed of trained health workers and support staff, can be deployed quickly to crisis areas to provide emergency care and support local health services. These teams should be equipped with the necessary supplies and have the flexibility to operate in different settings.
- **Pre-positioning of Supplies:** Pre-positioning essential medicines, medical supplies, and equipment in strategic locations can help ensure that health services continue during a crisis. This includes stockpiling items such as vaccines, antibiotics, surgical kits, and personal protective equipment.

Strategies for Health Service Delivery During Crises

Once a crisis occurs, health systems must implement strategies to maintain service delivery [20]:

- **Establishment of Field Hospitals and Mobile Clinics:** In areas where health facilities have been damaged or are inaccessible, field hospitals and mobile clinics can provide critical care. These temporary facilities should be equipped to handle a range of medical needs, including trauma care, maternal and child health services, and treatment for communicable diseases.
- **Decentralization of Services:** Decentralizing health services can help ensure that care is accessible to people in remote or hard-to-reach areas. This may involve supporting smaller, local health facilities or empowering community health workers to deliver care at the household level.
- **Utilization of Telemedicine:** Telemedicine can be a valuable tool for maintaining health service delivery during crises. By leveraging digital technologies, health workers can provide remote consultations, monitor patients, and coordinate care without the need for physical contact.
- **Integration of Humanitarian and Health Services:** In crisis situations, it is important to integrate health services with broader humanitarian efforts, such as food distribution, water and sanitation programs, and shelter provision. This ensures a holistic approach to meeting the needs of affected populations.
- **Public Health Surveillance and Early Warning Systems:** Maintaining robust public health surveillance and early warning systems during a crisis is essential for detecting and responding to disease outbreaks. This includes monitoring for signs of infectious diseases, malnutrition, and other health threats.

Case Studies: Health Service Continuity in Practice

Several case studies demonstrate successful strategies for maintaining health service continuity during crises [20]:

- **The Rohingya Refugee Crisis in Bangladesh:** The massive influx of Rohingya refugees into Bangladesh created significant challenges for health service delivery. The response involved the rapid establishment of mobile clinics, vaccination campaigns, and the integration of mental health services into primary care. Coordination between humanitarian organizations and the Bangladeshi government was key to ensuring the continuity of services.
- **The 2010 Haiti Earthquake:** The 2010 earthquake in Haiti caused widespread destruction of health infrastructure. In response, international organizations set up field hospitals, while local health workers were trained to provide care in temporary shelters. Pre-positioned emergency supplies and the rapid deployment of international medical teams played a critical role in maintaining health services.
- **The COVID-19 Pandemic:** The COVID-19 pandemic has highlighted the importance of resilient health systems. Countries that successfully maintained health services during the pandemic implemented strategies such as the expansion of telemedicine, the repurposing of health facilities for COVID-19 care, and the integration of public health measures into routine services.

The Role of International and Local Partnerships

Partnerships between international organizations, governments, NGOs, and local communities are essential for ensuring health service continuity during crises [19, 20]:

- **International Support and Collaboration:** International organizations can provide technical assistance, funding, and logistical support to strengthen health systems in crisis-affected areas. This includes deploying emergency medical teams, providing supplies, and supporting the coordination of humanitarian response efforts.
- **Local Ownership and Leadership:** Local health authorities and communities must play a central role in crisis response efforts. This includes leading the planning and implementation of health services, ensuring that interventions are culturally appropriate, and mobilizing local resources and support.
- **Public-Private Partnerships:** Public-private partnerships can enhance the resilience of health systems by leveraging the expertise, resources, and innovation of the private sector. This includes partnerships with pharmaceutical

companies, technology firms, and logistics providers to ensure the availability of medicines, medical supplies, and communication technologies.

CONCLUSION

Ensuring the continuity of health services during crises is a complex but essential task. By building resilient health systems, engaging in pre-crisis planning, and implementing adaptable service delivery models, it is possible to maintain critical healthcare services even in the most challenging circumstances. The lessons learned from past crises underscore the importance of preparedness, flexibility, and collaboration in safeguarding public health during emergencies. By prioritising these strategies, we can better protect the health of vulnerable populations and ensure that health systems are equipped to respond to the crises of the future.

POST-CONFLICT RECOVERY: REBUILDING HEALTH SYSTEMS

Rebuilding health systems in the aftermath of conflict is a critical but challenging process that requires careful planning, resource allocation, and community engagement. The devastation wrought by conflict often leaves health infrastructure in ruins, disrupts service delivery, and causes significant loss of health personnel. Post-conflict recovery provides an opportunity to not only restore health services but also to build a more resilient and equitable health system. This section explores the key strategies and considerations for rebuilding health systems in post-conflict settings [21 - 25].

Assessing the Damage: Initial Needs and Prioritisation

The first step in post-conflict recovery is to conduct a comprehensive assessment of the damage to the health system. This assessment should identify [21]:

- **Damage to Infrastructure:** Assess the extent of physical damage to health facilities, including hospitals, clinics, and laboratories. Determine which facilities can be repaired and which need to be rebuilt entirely.
- **Health Workforce:** Evaluate the status of the health workforce, including the number of healthcare providers who remain in the area, those who have been displaced or killed, and the overall capacity of the workforce to meet the health needs of the population.
- **Service Delivery:** Assess the availability and quality of essential health services, including maternal and child health, infectious disease control, and emergency care. Identify gaps in service delivery and prioritize the restoration of critical services.

- **Supply Chains:** Evaluate the state of medical supply chains, including the availability of medicines, vaccines, and medical equipment. Identify bottlenecks and disruptions that need to be addressed to ensure the consistent delivery of supplies.
- **Health Information Systems:** Determine the functionality of health information systems, including the ability to collect, analyze, and use data for decision-making. Identify gaps in data collection and reporting that need to be addressed to support recovery efforts.

The findings from this assessment should inform the prioritization of recovery efforts, focusing on the most urgent needs and the most vulnerable populations.

Restoring Health Infrastructure

Rebuilding health infrastructure is a key component of post-conflict recovery. This includes [22]:

- **Rehabilitation of Existing Facilities:** Where possible, health facilities that have been damaged but not destroyed should be rehabilitated. This may involve repairing structural damage, restoring utilities such as water and electricity, and replacing damaged equipment.
- **Construction of New Facilities:** In areas where health facilities have been completely destroyed, new facilities must be constructed. This provides an opportunity to build more resilient and better-equipped facilities that can withstand future shocks.
- **Mobile Health Units:** In the interim, mobile health units can be deployed to provide essential health services to populations in areas where health facilities are not yet operational. These units can be particularly important in reaching remote or hard-to-access areas.
- **Infrastructure Resilience:** In rebuilding health infrastructure, it is important to incorporate resilience measures, such as building to higher structural standards, ensuring that facilities are located in safer areas, and incorporating renewable energy sources to reduce reliance on vulnerable utility networks.

Rebuilding the Health Workforce

Rebuilding the health workforce is another critical aspect of post-conflict recovery. Key strategies include [23, 26]:

- **Recruitment and Training:** Efforts should be made to recruit and train new health workers, particularly from within the affected communities. This can help to fill gaps left by displaced or deceased health workers and ensure that the workforce is culturally and linguistically appropriate.

- **Retention Strategies:** Incentives such as competitive salaries, housing, and career development opportunities can help retain health workers in post-conflict areas. Ensuring the safety and security of health workers is also essential to prevent further loss of personnel.
- **Psychosocial Support:** Health workers who have experienced the trauma of conflict may require psychosocial support to cope with the emotional and psychological toll. Providing mental health services and peer support networks can help health workers recover and return to their duties.
- **Task Shifting:** In settings where there are severe shortages of highly trained health workers, task shifting, whereby certain tasks are delegated to less specialized health workers, can be an effective strategy for maintaining service delivery.

Strengthening Health Governance

Effective governance is crucial for the successful recovery and rebuilding of health systems. Post-conflict recovery efforts should focus on [24, 26]:

- **Restoring Health System Leadership:** Re-establishing health system leadership at the national and local levels is essential for coordinating recovery efforts, managing resources, and ensuring accountability.
- **Engaging Communities:** Community engagement is vital for rebuilding trust in the health system and ensuring that recovery efforts are aligned with the needs and priorities of the population. Involving community leaders and organizations in the planning and implementation of recovery efforts can enhance the effectiveness and sustainability of interventions.
- **Promoting Transparency and Accountability:** Transparency and accountability mechanisms should be strengthened to ensure that resources allocated for health system recovery are used efficiently and equitably. This includes establishing monitoring and evaluation systems to track progress and identify areas for improvement.
- **Decentralization:** Decentralizing health governance can empower local authorities and communities to take ownership of the recovery process. This can enhance the responsiveness of health services to local needs and improve the sustainability of interventions.

Revitalizing Health Financing

Health financing is a key determinant of the success of post-conflict recovery efforts. Strategies for revitalizing health financing include [25]:

- **Mobilizing Domestic Resources:** Post-conflict governments should prioritize the allocation of domestic resources to health system recovery. This may involve reallocating funds from other sectors, increasing tax revenues, or leveraging natural resource wealth to finance health services.
- **International Assistance:** International donors and development partners can play a critical role in supporting post-conflict health system recovery. This includes providing financial assistance, technical expertise, and capacity building to strengthen health systems.
- **Innovative Financing Mechanisms:** Innovative financing mechanisms, such as health bonds, insurance schemes, and public-private partnerships, can help to mobilize additional resources for health system recovery. These mechanisms should be designed to ensure sustainability and equity in access to health services.
- **Ensuring Equity in Resource Allocation:** Recovery efforts should prioritise the allocation of resources to the most vulnerable populations and the most severely affected areas. This can help to address pre-existing inequalities and promote social cohesion in post-conflict settings.

Integrating Health and Development

Post-conflict recovery presents an opportunity to integrate health and development efforts to address the social determinants of health and promote long-term development. Key strategies include [24 - 26]:

- **Rebuilding Livelihoods:** Efforts to rebuild livelihoods, including job creation, income generation, and vocational training, can have a positive impact on health outcomes by improving access to food, shelter, and healthcare.
- **Strengthening Education:** Restoring and strengthening education systems can contribute to improved health outcomes by increasing health literacy, reducing risky behaviours, and empowering individuals to make informed health decisions.
- **Improving Water, Sanitation, and Hygiene (WASH):** Rebuilding WASH infrastructure is essential for preventing the spread of communicable diseases and promoting overall health. This includes ensuring access to clean water, adequate sanitation, and hygiene education.
- **Promoting Peace and Social Cohesion:** Health system recovery can contribute to peacebuilding and social cohesion by providing equitable access to health services, addressing health disparities, and fostering trust between communities and the state.

Case Studies: Successful Post-Conflict Health System Recovery

Several countries have successfully rebuilt their health systems after conflict, providing valuable lessons for future recovery efforts [24 - 26]:

- **Rwanda:** Following the 1994 genocide, Rwanda undertook comprehensive health system reforms that focused on decentralization, community engagement, and equity. The country's innovative community-based health insurance scheme and performance-based financing model have contributed to significant improvements in health outcomes.
- **Sierra Leone:** After a decade-long civil war, Sierra Leone rebuilt its health system with support from international partners. Key strategies included the recruitment and training of health workers, the construction of new health facilities, and the establishment of a free healthcare initiative for pregnant women, lactating mothers, and children under five.
- **Liberia:** In the aftermath of the civil war, Liberia focused on restoring primary healthcare services, rebuilding health infrastructure, and addressing the mental health needs of the population. The country's National Health Policy and Plan prioritized equitable access to essential services and the integration of health and development efforts.

CONCLUSION

Rebuilding health systems in post-conflict settings is a complex and multifaceted process that requires sustained commitment, collaboration, and innovation. By focusing on restoring health infrastructure, rebuilding the health workforce, strengthening governance, revitalising health financing, and integrating health and development efforts, post-conflict societies can lay the foundation for a resilient and equitable health system.

The lessons learned from successful post-conflict recovery efforts underscore the importance of a holistic approach that addresses the immediate needs of the population while also promoting long-term development and social cohesion. As countries emerge from conflict, the rebuilding of health systems can catalyse broader recovery and development, helping to heal the wounds of conflict and build a healthier, more prosperous future for all.

REFERENCES

[1] World Health Organisation. Health emergency and disaster risk management framework. Geneva: WHO 2019.

[2] UNHCR. Global Trends: Forced Displacement in 2021. United Nations High Commissioner for Refugees 2022.

[3] Ghobarah HA, Huth P, Russett B. Civil wars kill and maim people—long after the shooting stops. Am Polit Sci Rev 2003; 97(2): 189-202. [http://dx.doi.org/10.1017/S0003055403000613]

[4] Spiegel PB, Le P, Ververs MT, Salama P. Occurrence and overlap of natural disasters, complex emergencies and epidemics during the past decade (1995–2004). Confl Health 2007; 1(1): 2. [http://dx.doi.org/10.1186/1752-1505-1-2] [PMID: 17411460]

[5] Roberts L, Lafta R, Garfield R, Khudhairi J, Burnham G. Mortality before and after the 2003 invasion of Iraq: cluster sample survey. Lancet 2004; 364(9448): 1857-64. [http://dx.doi.org/10.1016/S0140-6736(04)17441-2] [PMID: 15555665]

[6] MSF, (2016). Where is everyone? Responding to emergencies in the most difficult places. MSF Report.

[7] Ryan JR. Health care in failed and failing states. J R Soc Promot Health 2004; 124(6): 252-3. [http://dx.doi.org/10.1177/146642400412400607] [PMID: 15602988]

[8] Bogale B, Scambler S, Mohd Khairuddin AN, Gallagher JE. Health system strengthening in fragile and conflict-affected states: A review of systematic reviews. PLoS One 2024; 19(6): e0305234. [http://dx.doi.org/10.1371/journal.pone.0305234] [PMID: 38875266]

[9] World Health Organisation. Building back better: sustainable mental health care after emergencies. Geneva: WHO 2013.

[10] Inter-Agency Standing Committee (IASC). IASC Guidelines on Mental Health and Psychosocial Support in Emergency Settings. Geneva: IASC 2007.

[11] Silove D, Steel Z. Understanding community psychosocial needs after disasters: implications for mental health services. J Postgrad Med 2006; 52(2): 121-5. [PMID: 16679676]

[12] Miller KE, Rasmussen A. War exposure, daily stressors, and mental health in conflict and post-conflict settings: Bridging the divide between trauma-focused and psychosocial frameworks. Soc Sci Med 2010; 70(1): 7-16. [http://dx.doi.org/10.1016/j.socscimed.2009.09.029] [PMID: 19854552]

[13] Guisolan SC, Ambrogi M, Meeussen A, Althaus F, Eperon G. Health and security risks of humanitarian aid workers during field missions: Experience of the International Red Cross. Travel Med Infect Dis 2022; 46: 102275. [http://dx.doi.org/10.1016/j.tmaid.2022.102275] [PMID: 35131427]

[14] The International Committee of the Red Cross. Health care in danger: A sixteen-country study. Geneva: ICRC 2011.

[15] Garfield R, Neugut AI. The human consequences of war. In: Levy BS, Sidel VW, Eds. War and Public Health. Oxford University Press 1997; pp. 27-38.

[16] MSF. Protection of medical personnel: IHL and humanitarian action. Médecins Sans Frontières 2015.

[17] World Health Organisation. Health Emergency and Disaster Risk Management Framework WHO, 2019.

[18] OCHA. Humanitarian response plan: Addressing the humanitarian consequences of conflict and displacement. New York: OCHA 2016.

[19] Leaning J, Guha-Sapir D. Natural disasters, armed conflict, and public health. N Engl J Med 2013; 369(19): 1836-42. [http://dx.doi.org/10.1056/NEJMra1109877] [PMID: 24195550]

[20] Doarn CR, Merrell RC. Telemedicine and e-health in disaster response. Telemed J E Health 2014; 20(7): 605-6. [http://dx.doi.org/10.1089/tmj.2014.9983] [PMID: 24918269]

[21] World Bank. World Bank Engagement in Situations of Conflict: An Evaluation of FY10–20 Experience Independent Evaluation Group. Washington, DC: World Bank 2021.

[22] Elwan AE, Holtzman SB, Scott CS. Post-conflict reconstruction: the role of the World Bank. Washington, DC: World Bank Group 1998. Available from: http://documents.worldbank.org/curated/en/175771468198561613

[23] Newbrander W, Waldman R, Shepherd-Banigan M. Rebuilding and strengthening health systems and providing basic health services in fragile states. Disasters 2011; 35(4): 639-60. [http://dx.doi.org/10.1111/j.1467-7717.2011.01235.x] [PMID: 21913929]

[24] World Health Organisation. (2020). Health cluster guide: a practical handbook. Geneva. Licence: CC BY-NC-SA 3.0 IGO.

[25] Duffield M. Global governance and the new wars: The merging of development and security. London: Zed Books 2014. [http://dx.doi.org/10.5040/9781350220430]

[26] Saleh J-EA. Resilient Communities: Navigating Public Health Challenges in Developing Nations. Bentham Science Publishers 2025. [http://dx.doi.org/10.2174/97898153056091250101]

CHAPTER 6

The Human Resources Crisis: Building a Sustainable Health Workforce

Abstract: The health workforce is a critical pillar of any functional health system, especially in developing nations like Nigeria, where shortages, inequitable distribution, and brain drain are prevalent. Chapter 6 explores the multifaceted challenges of the human resources crisis in the health sector, focusing on the causes and consequences of workforce shortages, training and capacity-building efforts, and strategies to retain skilled health workers. It also examines the role of community health workers in bridging service delivery gaps and offers policy recommendations for strengthening the health workforce. The chapter underscores the need for a coordinated approach to build a sustainable and resilient health workforce, crucial for achieving universal health coverage and improving public health outcomes in Nigeria and beyond.

Keywords: Brain drain, Capacity building, Community health workers, Developing nations, Health system, Health workforce, Human resources, Nigeria, Retention strategies, Workforce distribution.

INTRODUCTION

The health workforce is the backbone of any healthcare system, playing a pivotal role in delivering essential health services and ensuring the overall functioning of the health sector. In many developing nations, including Nigeria, the health workforce faces a myriad of challenges that undermine its ability to meet the population's health needs. This chapter delves into the human resources crisis in the health sector, exploring the causes and consequences of workforce shortages, strategies for training and capacity building, and approaches to retain and equitably distribute health workers. The chapter also highlights the critical role of community health workers in bridging service delivery gaps and offers policy recommendations to build a sustainable health workforce.

THE HEALTH WORKFORCE SHORTAGE: CAUSES AND CONSEQUENCES

The shortage of health workers is one of the most critical challenges facing health systems, particularly in developing nations like Nigeria. This crisis not only

Jalal-Eddeen Abubakar Saleh

hampers the delivery of essential health services but also exacerbates existing health disparities, leaving the most vulnerable populations without access to care. The WHO benchmark of 4.45 health workers per 1,000 people is not an easy target for Nigeria and many sub-Saharan African countries. In Nigeria, according to the World Bank, there are approximately 1.682 nurses and midwives per 1,000 people in 2022, an indication of a deep and multi-layered human resources for health crisis [1]. The available NHWA (National Health Workforce Accounts) indicate severe shortages of medical doctors, nurses, and midwives in Nigeria. The projected workforce modelling suggests a needs-based shortfall in Africa of several million health workers by 2030, and regional analyses highlight that Nigeria will require large-scale production and retention to close its gap [2]. Understanding the causes of the health workforce shortage and its far-reaching consequences is essential for developing effective strategies to address this issue [1, 2].

CAUSES OF HEALTH WORKFORCE SHORTAGE

Several factors contribute to the health workforce shortage, each intersecting with broader socio-economic and political dynamics. Some of these include [1, 2]:

1. Insufficient Training Capacity:
   - **Educational Bottlenecks:** Many countries cannot train a sufficient number of health professionals. Medical, nursing, and allied health schools are often underfunded, poorly equipped, and suffer from a shortage of qualified instructors. This limits the number of new graduates entering the workforce each year.
   - **Curriculum Misalignment:** In some cases, health education curricula do not align with the needs of the health system, resulting in graduates who are not adequately prepared for the realities of clinical practice or public health challenges in their communities.
2. Migration of Health Workers:
   - **Brain Drain:** The migration of health workers to more developed countries in search of better working conditions, higher salaries, and professional opportunities significantly depletes the health workforce in developing nations. This "brain drain" leaves countries like Nigeria with a severe shortage of skilled professionals.
   - **Regional Disparities:** Within countries, health workers often migrate from rural to urban areas, exacerbating the shortage in already underserved regions. The lack of incentives to work in rural or remote areas further fuels this internal migration.

3. Poor Working Conditions:
   - **Inadequate Infrastructure:** Health workers in many developing countries face poor working conditions, including inadequate infrastructure, a lack of essential supplies, and unsafe environments. These conditions contribute to job dissatisfaction and high attrition rates.
   - **Low Compensation:** Many health workers are underpaid, with salaries that do not reflect the demands and risks of their work. Inconsistent or delayed payment of salaries further demoralizes the workforce and drives many to seek alternative employment or migrate abroad.
4. Policy and Governance Challenges:
   - **Weak Health Governance:** Ineffective health governance, including poor workforce planning, a lack of data on workforce needs, and insufficient investment in human resources, undermines efforts to build a sustainable health workforce.
   - **Inadequate Health Financing:** Limited financial resources allocated to health systems often result in insufficient funding for health worker recruitment, training, and retention. This financial constraint further exacerbates the workforce shortage.
5. Health System Strain:
   - **Epidemics and Crises:** Public health emergencies, such as the COVID-19 pandemic, Ebola outbreaks, or natural disasters, place additional strain on the health workforce. These crises can lead to overwork, burnout, and increased mortality among health workers, further depleting the workforce.
   - **Population Growth:** Rapid population growth in many developing countries increases the demand for health services, which outpaces the growth of the health workforce. This results in higher patient-to-provider ratios and overburdened health workers.

Consequences of Health Workforce Shortage

The shortage of health workers has profound and far-reaching consequences for public health, socio-economic development, and global health security. The following consequences are worth noting [1]:

1. Compromised Health Service Delivery:
   - **Reduced Access to Care:** A shortage of health workers leads to reduced access to healthcare, particularly in rural and underserved areas. This can result in delayed treatment, unmet health needs, and an increase in preventable morbidity and mortality.
   - **Overburdened Health Workers:** Health workers in areas with severe shortages often face overwhelming workloads, leading to burnout, decreased

quality of care, and higher rates of medical errors. This also contributes to a vicious cycle of attrition and further workforce depletion.

2. Worsening Health Outcomes:
   - **Maternal and Child Health:** The shortage of skilled birth attendants and other maternal health professionals contributes to high rates of maternal and infant mortality. Inadequate staffing in pediatric care also affects child health outcomes, leading to higher rates of malnutrition, infectious diseases, and child mortality.
   - **Chronic Disease Management:** The lack of trained health workers hinders the management of chronic diseases such as diabetes, hypertension, and cancer. Patients may go undiagnosed, receive suboptimal treatment, or fail to adhere to treatment regimens due to inadequate follow-up care.
3. Exacerbation of Health Inequities:
   - **Urban-Rural Divide:** The concentration of health workers in urban areas exacerbates health inequities between urban and rural populations. Rural communities, often with the highest burden of disease, are left with limited access to qualified healthcare providers.
   - **Socioeconomic Disparities:** The shortage of health workers disproportionately affects low-income populations, who may be unable to afford care from private providers or travel to urban centers for treatment. This deepens existing socio-economic disparities in health outcomes.
4. Economic Impact:
   - **Reduced Productivity:** Poor health outcomes due to inadequate healthcare negatively impact economic productivity. Illness and premature death among the working-age population reduce the labor force, hinder economic growth, and perpetuate the cycle of poverty.
   - **Increased Healthcare Costs:** The lack of timely and adequate care can lead to the progression of diseases to more severe stages, resulting in higher treatment costs for both individuals and health systems. This places additional financial strain on already under-resourced health systems.
5. Global Health Security Risks:
   - **Pandemic Preparedness and Response:** A depleted health workforce undermines a country's ability to detect, prevent, and respond to public health emergencies. This poses a significant risk to global health security, as diseases can spread more rapidly and uncontrollably from regions with weak health systems.
   - **Vaccine Delivery:** The shortage of health workers also affects the delivery of vaccination programs, leading to lower immunisation rates and increased vulnerability to vaccine-preventable diseases. This is particularly concerning in the context of global efforts to eradicate diseases like polio and control outbreaks of measles and other infectious diseases.

Addressing the Health Workforce Shortage

Addressing the health workforce shortage requires a multifaceted approach that includes [1, 3]:

- **Investing in Health Education:** Expanding the capacity of medical and nursing schools, improving curricula, and providing scholarships or financial incentives to encourage enrollment in health professions can help increase the number of qualified health workers.
- **Enhancing Retention Strategies:** Improving working conditions, offering competitive salaries, and providing opportunities for professional development can help retain health workers in the public sector and in underserved areas.
- **Strengthening Health Governance:** Developing and implementing robust health workforce policies, improving data collection and management, and ensuring adequate health financing are critical for building a sustainable health workforce.
- **Promoting International Cooperation:** Addressing the brain drain requires international cooperation to develop policies that balance the rights of health workers to migrate with the needs of countries experiencing severe workforce shortages. This could include bilateral agreements, ethical recruitment practices, and support for health workforce development in source countries.

CONCLUSION

The health workforce shortage is a pressing global challenge with significant implications for health outcomes, equity, and security. By addressing the root causes of this shortage and implementing targeted strategies to build and sustain a robust health workforce, countries can improve the health and well-being of their populations and contribute to global health stability.

TRAINING AND CAPACITY BUILDING FOR HEALTH WORKERS

The training and capacity building of health workers is a cornerstone in the development of a resilient and effective health system, particularly in developing nations like Nigeria. As healthcare demands grow and evolve, so too must the skills and competencies of those who provide care. This section explores the critical components of training and capacity building, identifies challenges, and offers strategies for ensuring that health workers are well-equipped to meet the needs of the populations they serve [4, 5].

Although strained, Nigeria has an extensive training ecosystem. The key institutions that contribute to the training and supply of the health care workforce include:

- **Medical schools:** There is a wide range across the country providing undergraduate training, including University College Hospital at Ibadan, Ahmadu Bello University at Zaria, and University of Lagos. Similarly, there is the National Postgraduate Medical College of Nigeria (NPMCN), which runs residency and specialist training. The Medical and Dental Council of Nigeria (MDCN) is the overall regulatory body for medical practice in Nigeria [6].
- **Nursing and midwifery schools:** There are various schools of nursing and midwifery across the thirty-six states and the FCT that train this cadre of health care workers. Similarly, the Nursing and Midwifery Council of Nigeria (NMCN) regulates the practice [7].

However, despite the widespread presence of these schools across the country, there are limited seats in these training institutions because of increasing demand. Similarly, there is the issue of inadequate funding for clinical rotations in the postgraduate training institutions, slowing the conversion of graduates into fully licensed specialists.

The Importance of Continuous Professional Development

Health is a dynamic field, with new diseases emerging, technologies advancing, and treatment protocols constantly evolving. Continuous Professional Development (CPD) is essential for health workers to remain proficient in their fields. CPD encompasses formal training, workshops, conferences, and self-directed learning, allowing health workers to update their knowledge and skills regularly. This ongoing education is not just a professional obligation but a critical factor in improving patient outcomes and ensuring that healthcare delivery remains relevant and effective. For Nigeria and similar developing nations, CPD can bridge the gap between existing healthcare practices and global best practices. It helps in fostering a culture of lifelong learning among health workers, ensuring they are not just reactive but proactive in managing health crises and improving overall health standards. Some of these include [4, 5].

1. **Adapting to the Evolving Nature of Health and Disease:** Healthcare is an ever-changing field, with the regular emergence of new diseases, shifting epidemiological patterns, and frequent changes in global health priorities. The COVID-19 pandemic, for instance, underscored how rapidly the healthcare landscape can change and the need for up-to-date knowledge and skills. CPD ensures that health workers stay informed about new health threats, evolving clinical guidelines, and advances in disease surveillance, enabling them to respond effectively and promptly in both routine and emergencies.
2. **Keeping Pace with Advancements in Technology and Treatment:** Technological innovation is rapidly transforming diagnostics, patient

monitoring, telemedicine, and treatment delivery. Health workers must continuously update their competencies to effectively utilize new equipment, digital platforms, and therapeutic interventions. CPD provides opportunities for hands-on training and exposure to new technologies, ensuring that healthcare professionals do not fall behind, especially in developing countries where technological lag can compromise care quality and patient safety.

3. **Enhancing Professional Competence and Service Quality:** CPD helps maintain and improve the core competencies required for quality care delivery. Regular workshops, training programs, and refresher courses reinforce best practices, clinical protocols, and ethical standards, reducing the risk of errors and malpractice. By engaging in CPD, health workers remain clinically sharp, confident in their decision-making, and better equipped to provide evidence-based, patient-centered care. This directly contributes to improved patient outcomes and more efficient use of health system resources.
4. **Bridging the Gap Between Local Practices and Global Standards:** In many low- and middle-income countries, including Nigeria, there is often a lag between local health practices and international best practices due to limited access to current information or training. CPD serves as a bridge, exposing health workers to updated global guidelines, treatment protocols, and research findings. This alignment fosters a more standardized and globally competitive healthcare workforce, reducing disparities in care quality between urban and rural or underserved areas.
5. **Fostering a Culture of Lifelong Learning:** Beyond knowledge and skills, CPD cultivates a mindset of curiosity, self-improvement, and responsibility among health workers. This culture of lifelong learning ensures that professionals are not only reactive to emerging challenges but also proactive in seeking knowledge, anticipating risks, and innovating in their practice. In a rapidly changing world, this adaptability is crucial for resilience and leadership within the health sector.
6. **Supporting Health System Strengthening and Preparedness:** CPD is an essential pillar of health system strengthening. Well-trained and up-to-date health workers form the backbone of a responsive, efficient, and prepared health system. In times of crisis, such as outbreaks, humanitarian emergencies, or natural disasters, health systems depend on frontline workers who are not only skilled but agile and current in their knowledge. Investing in CPD is, therefore, a strategic move toward building stronger and more resilient health systems.

Addressing the Skill Gaps

One of the major challenges in the Nigerian healthcare system is the significant skill gap among health workers. This gap is often a result of inadequate initial training, limited access to advanced training opportunities, and the lack of infrastructure to support ongoing education. Addressing these skill gaps requires a multi-faceted approach [4, 5]:

1. **Curriculum Reform:** The curricula for medical, nursing, and allied health training institutions must be continuously updated to include the latest medical knowledge, technology, and best practices. Emphasis should be placed on practical, hands-on training that prepares health workers for real-world challenges.
2. **Specialized Training Programs:** In addition to general medical education, there is a need for specialized training programs in areas such as emergency care, mental health, infectious disease management, and maternal and child health. These specialised programs can help address critical shortages in key areas of healthcare delivery.
3. **In-service Training:** For those already in the workforce, in-service training programs are crucial. These can be in the form of short courses, workshops, or on-the-job training sessions that focus on specific skills or new technologies. Partnerships with international organisations can help bring in expertise and resources for these programs.

Building Training Infrastructure

Effective capacity building is dependent on the availability of adequate training infrastructure. This includes not just physical infrastructure like classrooms, laboratories, and simulation centres, but also digital infrastructure that supports e-learning and telemedicine. Developing nations must invest in both these areas to ensure that training programs are accessible and of high quality [4, 5].

1. **Simulation Centres:** These provide health workers with hands-on experience in a controlled environment, allowing them to practice procedures and decision-making without risk to patients. Simulation-based training has been shown to significantly improve clinical skills and confidence.
2. **E-learning Platforms:** Given the geographical and resource constraints in many parts of Nigeria, e-learning offers a flexible and scalable solution for training health workers. Online courses, webinars, and virtual classrooms can provide access to high-quality training materials, expert lectures, and collaborative learning opportunities.
3. **Telemedicine for Capacity Building:** Telemedicine can be used not only for patient care but also as a tool for capacity building. Through telemedicine platforms, health workers in remote areas can receive mentorship, consultation, and training from experts based in urban centres or even abroad.

Retention and Motivation Through Capacity Building

Training and capacity building are also key to retaining health workers in the system. When health workers feel competent and valued, they are more likely to remain in their positions and be motivated to provide high-quality care. However, retention strategies must go beyond training to include career development opportunities, recognition programs, and incentives that acknowledge the contributions of health workers [4, 5].

1. **Career Development Pathways:** Creating clear pathways for career advancement can help retain health workers by providing them with a sense of purpose and direction in their careers. This might include opportunities for further education, specialisation, or leadership roles within the health system.
2. **Incentive Programs:** Financial and non-financial incentives, such as scholarships for advanced training, recognition awards, and professional development grants, can motivate health workers to continue improving their skills and stay within the public health sector.
3. **Supportive Work Environments:** Finally, a supportive work environment that values continuous learning and professional growth is essential. Health workers should have access to mentors, peer networks, and resources that support their ongoing development.

Challenges and Future Directions

While the benefits of training and capacity building are clear, several challenges must be addressed to make these efforts effective. These include [4, 5]:

1. **Resource Constraints:** Financial limitations often restrict the scope of training programs. Governments and organisations must prioritise funding for capacity building, recognising it as an investment in the future of public health.
2. **Geographic Disparities:** Access to training is often limited in rural or underserved areas. Efforts must be made to decentralise training programs and make them accessible to health workers across the country.
3. **Sustainability:** Training programs must be designed with sustainability in mind, ensuring that they can continue and expand even in the face of financial or logistical challenges. This might involve building local capacity to run training programs independently over time.

CONCLUSION

Training and capacity building for health workers are essential components of a sustainable health workforce. By investing in continuous professional development, addressing skill gaps, and building the necessary infrastructure, Nigeria can strengthen its health system and improve the quality of care provided to its citizens. The challenges are significant, but with a strategic approach, the health workforce can be equipped to meet the needs of the nation now and in the future.

RETENTION STRATEGIES: TACKLING THE BRAIN DRAIN

The migration of doctors and nurses out of Nigeria to other countries is a major driver of the HRH gap among this cadre. The phenomenon of brain drain, where skilled health workers leave their home countries in search of better opportunities abroad, poses a significant challenge to the sustainability of health systems in developing nations like Nigeria. The loss of trained professionals not only exacerbates the already critical shortages in the healthcare workforce but also undermines the capacity to deliver quality care to the population. This section explores the factors driving brain drain and outlines strategies to retain health workers and mitigate its impact on the health sector [8, 9].

In a study by the Africa CDC, over 13,000 Nigerian health workers left for the UK alone (2021–2022), with additional clinicians expressing intention to leave [10].

The drivers of the brain drain include poor remuneration and delayed salaries, unsafe or hostile workplace conditions, limited career progression, lack of training opportunities, and inadequate Continuing Professional Development (CPD), amongst others.

Understanding the Drivers of Brain Drain

Several factors contribute to the migration of health workers from Nigeria and other developing countries. These can be broadly categorised into push and pull factors [8]:

1. **Push Factors:**
    - **Poor Working Conditions:** Health workers often face inadequate facilities, insufficient medical supplies, and a lack of essential resources, making it difficult to provide quality care. The resulting frustration drives many to seek better working environments.
    - **Low Wages and Delayed Payments:** Many health workers are underpaid or experience significant delays in salary payments. In contrast, opportunities abroad often offer significantly higher salaries and more stable income.
    - **Insecurity:** In regions affected by conflict or high levels of crime, health

workers are at risk of violence, kidnapping, and harassment, further incentivizing them to leave.
   - **Limited Career Opportunities:** A lack of professional development opportunities, including training, promotions, and career advancement, leaves many health workers feeling stagnant in their roles.
2. **Pull Factors:**
   - **Higher Salaries:** Health workers are often attracted to higher-paying jobs abroad, particularly in countries with strong healthcare systems that value and invest in their workforce.
   - **Better Living Conditions:** The prospect of living in a more stable, secure, and prosperous environment is a strong motivator for migration.
   - **Advanced Training Opportunities:** Many health workers seek opportunities for specialisation and advanced training that are not available in their home countries.

Enhancing Working Conditions and Compensation

Improving working conditions is one of the most effective strategies for retaining health workers. This involves not only providing adequate medical supplies and infrastructure but also ensuring that health workers are compensated fairly and on time. Key measures include [8, 9]:

1. **Salary Increases and Timely Payments:** Ensuring that health workers receive competitive salaries and timely payments can significantly reduce the financial incentives to leave. Governments and health institutions should regularly review and adjust salaries to match inflation and the cost of living.
2. **Provision of Adequate Resources:** Health workers are more likely to stay when they can perform their duties effectively. This requires the availability of essential medical supplies, equipment, and drugs, as well as proper maintenance of health facilities.
3. **Improved Working Conditions:** Investing in safe, well-equipped, and supportive work environments is crucial. This includes measures to protect health workers from violence, ensuring adequate staffing levels to prevent burnout, and providing opportunities for breaks and time off.

Professional Development and Career Advancement

Creating opportunities for professional growth and career advancement can help retain health workers by providing them with a clear path for development and a sense of purpose in their careers. The strategies include [8, 9]:

1. **Continuing Education and Training Programs:** Providing access to ongoing training and education helps health workers stay updated with the latest medical knowledge and practices, which can enhance job satisfaction and reduce the desire to seek opportunities abroad.
2. **Career Pathways:** Establishing clear and transparent career pathways, with opportunities for promotion, specialisation, and leadership roles, can motivate health workers to stay within the system. This could include mentorship programs, scholarships for advanced degrees, and leadership training.
3. **Recognition and Reward Systems:** Implementing recognition programs that reward outstanding performance and dedication can boost morale and job satisfaction. This could include awards, public recognition, and financial bonuses for exceptional service.

Addressing Insecurity and Ensuring Safety

Insecurity is a significant factor driving health workers away from conflict-affected regions. Addressing this requires a multi-pronged approach, including [8, 9]:

1. **Security Measures:** Governments and health institutions must prioritise the safety of health workers by providing security in high-risk areas, including escort services, secure transportation, and fortified health facilities.
2. **Insurance and Risk Compensation:** Offering comprehensive insurance packages and risk compensation for health workers in insecure areas can provide a safety net and reduce the fear of working in such environments.
3. **Psychosocial Support:** Providing mental health support and counselling services for health workers exposed to violence and trauma is essential for their well-being and retention.

Policy and Governance Interventions

Government policies play a critical role in retaining health workers. Strong governance, transparent policies, and political commitment are necessary to address the root causes of brain drain effectively. Key policy interventions include [8, 9]:

1. **Health Worker Retention Policies:** Governments should develop and implement policies specifically aimed at retaining health workers. These policies should address compensation, working conditions, and career development, with a focus on making the health sector more attractive to workers.

2. **Bilateral Agreements:** Countries experiencing brain drain can negotiate bilateral agreements with nations that attract their health workers. These agreements can include provisions for the return of health workers after a set period, financial compensation for training, or support for health system development in the source country.
3. **National Health Workforce Plans:** Developing and implementing comprehensive health workforce plans can ensure a strategic approach to workforce development, retention, and distribution. These plans should be data-driven, taking into account current and projected health workforce needs.

Community Engagement and Social Support

Retaining health workers is not solely a matter of financial and professional incentives; social and community factors also play a role. Strategies to foster community engagement and support include [8, 9]:

1. **Community Involvement:** Encouraging communities to actively participate in health system strengthening can create a sense of ownership and support for health workers. Community-led initiatives, such as housing schemes or local recognition awards, can enhance the social standing of health workers and reduce their desire to migrate.
2. **Support Networks:** Establishing professional and social networks for health workers can provide emotional and professional support, helping them cope with the challenges of their work and reducing feelings of isolation.
3. **Family Support Programs:** Providing support for the families of health workers, such as housing, education, and healthcare, can reduce the pressure to seek better opportunities abroad.

Monitoring and Evaluation

Effective retention strategies require continuous monitoring and evaluation to assess their impact and make necessary adjustments. This involves [8, 9]:

1. **Data Collection:** Regularly collecting and analyzing data on health worker retention, migration patterns, and the effectiveness of retention strategies is essential for informed decision-making.
2. **Feedback Mechanisms:** Establishing feedback mechanisms where health workers can express their concerns, challenges, and suggestions can help identify areas for improvement in retention strategies.
3. **Impact Assessment:** Periodically assessing the impact of retention strategies on the overall health system, including patient outcomes and service delivery, is crucial for understanding their effectiveness and sustainability.

CONCLUSION

Tackling the brain drain requires a comprehensive approach that addresses the multifaceted drivers of migration while creating a more supportive and rewarding environment for health workers in Nigeria. By improving working conditions, offering professional development opportunities, ensuring security, and implementing strong policy measures, the country can retain its valuable health workforce and build a more sustainable health system. The challenges are significant, but with targeted interventions and a commitment to health worker retention, Nigeria can reduce the impact of brain drain and improve healthcare delivery for its population.

EQUITABLE DISTRIBUTION OF HEALTH WORKERS ACROSS REGIONS

The equitable distribution of health workers across regions is a critical challenge for developing nations, particularly in countries like Nigeria, where disparities between urban and rural areas significantly impact healthcare delivery. The concentration of health workers in urban centres often leaves rural and underserved regions with severe shortages, leading to disparities in health outcomes. This section examines the factors contributing to the uneven distribution of health workers and proposes strategies for achieving a more balanced allocation across regions [11, 12].

The Scope of the Problem

In Nigeria, the distribution of health workers is heavily skewed toward urban areas, where better infrastructure, higher salaries, and more career opportunities are available. This urban bias has led to a situation where rural areas, which often have the greatest need for healthcare services, are left with inadequate staffing. The consequences are dire, including higher mortality rates, lower life expectancy, and the persistence of preventable diseases in these regions. Several factors contribute to the inequitable distribution of health workers [11]:

1. **Urbanisation and Infrastructure:** Urban areas generally offer better living conditions, infrastructure, and access to education and healthcare for health workers and their families. Rural areas, in contrast, often lack basic amenities such as electricity, clean water, and schools, making them less attractive to health professionals.
2. **Financial Incentives:** Health workers in urban areas typically receive higher salaries and more consistent payments compared to their rural counterparts.

The lack of financial incentives for rural postings exacerbates the reluctance of health workers to serve in these areas.

3. **Career Development Opportunities:** Urban centres offer more opportunities for professional growth, including access to specialised training, workshops, and conferences. Health workers in rural areas often face professional isolation, with limited opportunities for career advancement.
4. **Safety and Security:** In regions affected by conflict or high levels of crime, health workers are understandably reluctant to work due to concerns for their personal safety. This further compounds the shortage of health workers in these high-need areas.

Strategies for Equitable Distribution

Addressing the inequitable distribution of health workers requires a comprehensive approach that includes both policy interventions and practical measures. Key strategies include [11, 12]:

1. **Incentive Programs for Rural Service:**
   - **Financial Incentives:** Offering financial incentives such as hardship allowances, rural service bonuses, and housing subsidies can make rural postings more attractive to health workers. These incentives should be substantial enough to offset the disadvantages of working in underserved areas.
   - **Loan Forgiveness and Scholarships:** Programs that offer loan forgiveness or scholarships in exchange for a commitment to work in rural areas for a certain period can attract young health workers to underserved regions.
2. **Improving Rural Infrastructure:**
   - **Facility Upgrades:** Investing in the infrastructure of rural health facilities, including the provision of essential medical equipment and supplies, can improve working conditions and make these postings more appealing.
   - **Community Support:** Engaging local communities in supporting health workers, such as through housing provision, community-led security initiatives, and social integration programs, can enhance the attractiveness of rural postings.
3. **Career Development and Support:**
   - **Rural Training Programs:** Establishing training programs and centers of excellence in rural areas can provide health workers with access to ongoing education and professional development without needing to relocate to urban centers.
   - **Mentorship and Peer Networks:** Creating mentorship programs and professional networks that connect rural health workers with their peers and

experts in urban areas can reduce feelings of isolation and provide support for career advancement.

4. **Policy and Governance Interventions:**
    - **Mandatory Rural Service:** Implementing mandatory rural service for new health graduates, particularly for those who received government-sponsored education, can help address immediate shortages in underserved areas. This approach must be accompanied by adequate support to ensure that it does not lead to dissatisfaction or burnout.
    - **Decentralized Health Workforce Planning:** Governments should adopt decentralized health workforce planning, allowing for more targeted recruitment and deployment of health workers based on the specific needs of each region.
5. **Technology and Telemedicine:**
    - **Telemedicine Initiatives:** Leveraging telemedicine can help bridge the gap in healthcare services between urban and rural areas. Through telemedicine, rural health workers can consult with specialists in urban centres, enhancing their capacity to provide quality care.
    - **E-Learning Platforms:** Providing access to e-learning platforms can enable rural health workers to participate in ongoing education and professional development, even from remote locations.

Monitoring and Evaluation

To ensure the success of strategies aimed at equitable distribution, it is essential to establish robust monitoring and evaluation mechanisms. These should include [11, 12]:

1. **Data Collection and Analysis:** Regularly collecting data on health worker distribution, turnover rates, and health outcomes in different regions can help identify disparities and measure the effectiveness of interventions.
2. **Feedback Mechanisms:** Implementing feedback mechanisms where health workers can report challenges, successes, and suggestions related to their postings can inform policy adjustments and improve retention in rural areas.
3. **Impact Assessments:** Periodically assessing the impact of distribution strategies on overall health system performance, including patient outcomes and access to care, is crucial for refining approaches and ensuring sustainability.

CONCLUSION

Achieving equitable distribution of health workers across regions is essential for building a sustainable health workforce and ensuring that all populations have access to quality healthcare. By addressing the factors that contribute to the urban bias in health worker distribution and implementing targeted strategies, Nigeria can reduce disparities and improve health outcomes in underserved regions. The challenge is significant, but with a coordinated approach that includes incentives, infrastructure development, and policy support, it is possible to create a more balanced and effective health workforce.

THE ROLE OF COMMUNITY HEALTH WORKERS IN BRIDGING GAPS

Community Health Workers (CHWs) play a crucial role in addressing the health workforce shortages in developing nations, particularly in underserved and remote areas. They act as a bridge between the formal healthcare system and communities, delivering essential health services, promoting health education, and improving access to care. In Nigeria, where the distribution of health workers is often uneven, CHWs have become indispensable in filling the gaps left by the shortage of formally trained health professionals. This section explores the importance of CHWs, their roles, challenges, and the strategies needed to maximise their impact [13, 14].

Understanding the Role of Community Health Workers

CHWs are often members of the communities they serve, which positions them uniquely to understand and address local health needs. Their roles are diverse and include the following [13]:

1. **Health Education and Promotion:** CHWs are vital in raising awareness about key health issues, including maternal and child health, nutrition, hygiene, and infectious diseases. They use culturally appropriate methods to educate communities, thereby promoting healthier behaviours and preventing illness.
2. **Basic Health Services:** CHWs provide essential health services such as immunisations, antenatal care, distribution of medications, and first aid. In areas where access to healthcare facilities is limited, they are often the first point of contact for patients.
3. **Disease Surveillance and Reporting:** By collecting and reporting data on health conditions, CHWs contribute to disease surveillance efforts. This is particularly important in detecting outbreaks of infectious diseases and responding promptly to public health emergencies.
4. **Linking Communities with Health Systems:** CHWs act as liaisons between communities and the formal healthcare system, facilitating referrals to higher levels of care and helping to navigate the healthcare system. This role is

especially important in ensuring that marginalised populations receive the care they need.

5. **Supporting Chronic Disease Management:** For patients with chronic conditions such as diabetes, hypertension, and HIV/AIDS, CHWs provide ongoing support, including monitoring, counselling, and ensuring adherence to treatment regimens.

The Impact of Community Health Workers on Health Outcomes

The deployment of CHWs has been associated with significant improvements in health outcomes, particularly in low-resource settings. Some of the key impacts include [13, 14]:

1. **Reduction in Maternal and Child Mortality:** CHWs have been instrumental in reducing maternal and child mortality by providing antenatal care, promoting safe delivery practices, and ensuring that children receive essential vaccinations.
2. **Improved Access to Care:** CHWs increase access to healthcare by bringing services directly to communities, particularly in remote and underserved areas. This has led to higher coverage of essential health services and improved health equity.
3. **Enhanced Disease Control:** Through their role in disease surveillance and health education, CHWs contribute to the control and prevention of infectious diseases such as malaria, tuberculosis, and HIV/AIDS.
4. **Empowerment of Communities:** By involving community members in health promotion and service delivery, CHWs empower communities to take an active role in managing their health, leading to more sustainable health outcomes.

Challenges Faced by Community Health Workers

Despite their critical role, CHWs face several challenges that can limit their effectiveness [13, 14]:

1. **Inadequate Training and Support:** Many CHWs receive minimal training and lack ongoing support, which can hinder their ability to provide high-quality care. The lack of supervision and opportunities for professional development further exacerbates this issue.
2. **Insufficient Compensation and Incentives:** CHWs are often volunteers or receive low compensation, which can lead to high turnover rates and reduced motivation. The lack of financial incentives can also deter qualified individuals from becoming CHWs.

3. **Limited Resources and Supplies:** CHWs frequently operate with limited resources, including basic medical supplies, transport, and communication tools. This limits their ability to deliver services effectively and respond to health emergencies.
4. **Recognition and Integration into the Health System:** In some settings, CHWs are not fully recognised or integrated into the formal health system, which can result in a lack of coordination and support from healthcare professionals. This limits their potential to contribute to broader health system goals.

Strategies for Enhancing the Role of Community Health Workers

To maximise the impact of CHWs and address the challenges they face, several strategies can be implemented [13, 14]:

1. **Comprehensive Training and Continuous Education:** Providing CHWs with comprehensive initial training and ongoing education is essential for ensuring that they have the skills and knowledge needed to perform their roles effectively. This training should cover a broad range of topics, including basic healthcare, disease prevention, communication skills, and data collection.
2. **Adequate Compensation and Incentive Structures:** Developing compensation packages and incentive structures for CHWs can improve retention and motivation. These could include regular stipends, performance-based bonuses, opportunities for career advancement, and non-financial incentives such as community recognition.
3. **Provision of Necessary Resources and Tools:** Ensuring that CHWs have access to the necessary resources, such as medical supplies, transport, and mobile communication tools, is critical for their effectiveness. Investments in these areas can enhance the ability of CHWs to deliver services and respond to health needs in real-time.
4. **Integration into the Health System:** CHWs should be formally recognized as an integral part of the health system, with clear roles and responsibilities. This integration can be achieved through policies that define their role, standardized training and certification, and mechanisms for coordination with other healthcare professionals.
5. **Supportive Supervision and Mentorship:** Implementing systems for regular supervision and mentorship can provide CHWs with the support they need to perform their roles effectively. This supervision should be constructive and focus on problem-solving, skill development, and emotional support.
6. **Community Engagement and Ownership:** Engaging communities in the selection, support, and oversight of CHWs can enhance their effectiveness and

ensure that they are responsive to local needs. Community ownership of CHW programs can also improve sustainability and accountability.

Monitoring and Evaluation of CHW Programs

To ensure the success and sustainability of CHW programs, it is essential to establish robust monitoring and evaluation (M&E) systems. These systems should be able to do the following [13, 14]:

1. **Track Performance and Impact:** Regularly monitor the performance of CHWs, including the quality of services provided and the impact on health outcomes. This can help identify areas for improvement and ensure that CHWs are meeting the needs of their communities.
2. **Collect and Use Data for Decision-Making:** CHWs should be involved in the collection of health data, which can be used to inform decision-making at the local and national levels. This data can also be used to evaluate the effectiveness of CHW programs and make adjustments as needed.
3. **Provide Feedback and Continuous Improvement:** Establishing feedback mechanisms where CHWs can share their experiences, challenges, and suggestions is crucial for continuous improvement. This feedback should be used to refine training programs, supervision practices, and resource allocation.

CONCLUSION

Community Health Workers are essential in bridging the gaps in healthcare delivery, particularly in underserved and remote areas. By providing essential health services, promoting health education, and linking communities with the formal healthcare system, CHWs play a vital role in improving health outcomes and achieving health equity. However, to maximise their impact, it is crucial to address the challenges they face through comprehensive training, adequate compensation, resource provision, and integration into the health system. With the right support, CHWs can continue to be a cornerstone of public health efforts in Nigeria and other developing nations, helping to build a more sustainable and equitable health workforce.

POLICY RECOMMENDATIONS FOR STRENGTHENING THE HEALTH WORKFORCE

The health workforce is the backbone of any healthcare system, and in developing nations like Nigeria, where health challenges are numerous and resources are limited, the need for a robust, well-distributed, and adequately supported health workforce is critical. Addressing the challenges of workforce shortages, uneven distribution, and inadequate training requires comprehensive and targeted policy interventions. This section outlines key policy recommendations to strengthen the health workforce and ensure that it is capable of meeting the country's public health needs [15 - 17].

Enhancing Workforce Planning and Management

Effective health workforce planning and management are foundational to building a sustainable health workforce. This involves not only forecasting future health workforce needs but also managing the current workforce to ensure that health workers are deployed where they are most needed [15].

1. **Establishing a Health Workforce Observatory:** The creation of a health workforce observatory can facilitate better data collection, analysis, and dissemination on workforce trends, distribution, and requirements. This observatory should work closely with health ministries, educational institutions, and professional bodies to ensure accurate and timely information is available for policy-making.
2. **Strengthening Workforce Planning Capacities:** Investing in the capacity of health ministries and related agencies to plan and manage the health workforce is essential. This includes training in workforce modelling, projection techniques, and the use of data in decision-making processes.
3. **Developing a National Health Workforce Strategy:** A comprehensive national health workforce strategy should be developed, addressing the specific needs of different regions and populations. This strategy should include goals for workforce expansion, distribution, training, and retention, with clear timelines and accountability mechanisms.

Investing in Education and Training

Ensuring that health workers have the necessary skills and competencies to deliver high-quality care is vital. This requires sustained investment in health education and training programs aimed at the following [15 - 17]:

1. **Expanding and Improving Training Institutions:** The government should invest in expanding and improving health training institutions, particularly in underserved regions. This includes upgrading facilities, hiring qualified instructors, and increasing the capacity of these institutions to admit and train more students.
2. **Aligning Curricula with Health System Needs:** Health training curricula should be regularly reviewed and updated to align with the current and future needs of the health system. This includes integrating primary healthcare, public health, and community-based care into all training programs.

3. **Enhancing Continuing Professional Development (CPD):** Policies should mandate and support ongoing professional development for health workers. CPD programs should be accessible, relevant, and tailored to the needs of different cadres of health workers, with a focus on improving practical skills and knowledge.

Promoting Equitable Distribution of Health Workers

Addressing the disparities in the distribution of health workers across regions is crucial for ensuring that all populations have access to healthcare. There are imbalances in the distribution of healthcare workers, adding to the challenges of the HRH. It is common knowledge that female health workers (nurses, midwives) are the backbone of primary health care, and yet they often face lower remuneration, limited leadership roles in the hierarchy, and higher attrition. In the states, there is variability in female workforce participation across cadres, with lower densities of skilled attendants in rural LGAs compared with urban centres [18, 19]. The following should be considered [15 - 17]:

1. **Implementing Incentive Programs for Rural Service:** The government should develop and implement incentive programs to attract and retain health workers in rural and underserved areas. These incentives could include financial bonuses, housing support, educational opportunities for workers and their families, and career advancement opportunities.
2. **Mandating Rural Service:** As part of the licensing process, health professionals could be required to serve in rural areas for a specified period. This approach should be accompanied by adequate support to ensure that the experience is positive and sustainable for the workers involved.
3. **Supporting Decentralised Workforce Planning:** Decentralising workforce planning to regional or district levels allows for more targeted and context-specific strategies to address local health workforce challenges. Regional health authorities should be empowered and resourced to plan and manage their workforce needs.
4. **Gender balance and rural–urban distribution:** Gender imbalances and rural-urban maldistribution of the health workforce compound shortages. Although the female healthcare workers remain the backbone of primary maternal and child health services, the women healthcare workforce often faces fewer leadership roles and higher attrition due to caregiving burdens. Similarly, the state health workforce profiles show variability in female workforce participation across cadres and notably lower densities of skilled attendants in rural LGAs compared with urban centres. In Bauchi State, for example, the workforce audits reveal many PHCs staffed primarily by lower-cadre CHEWs

and community-based personnel, with skilled birth attendants disproportionately concentrated in urban hospitals [19, 20].

Enhancing Retention and Reducing Brain Drain

Retaining skilled health workers is essential to maintaining a stable and effective health workforce. Reducing brain drain requires both domestic policy interventions and international cooperation. The policymakers should consider the following [15 - 17]:

1. **Improving Working Conditions:** Governments should prioritise improving the working conditions of health workers, including ensuring regular payment of salaries, providing adequate resources and equipment, and ensuring a safe and supportive working environment.
2. **Offering Career Development Opportunities:** Providing clear career paths and opportunities for advancement within the healthcare system can help retain skilled workers. This includes offering specialised training, leadership development programs, and opportunities for promotion.
3. **Negotiating Bilateral Agreements on Health Worker Migration:** To address brain drain, the government should negotiate bilateral agreements with countries that are major destinations for Nigerian health workers. These agreements should include provisions for mutual benefit, such as the return of health workers after a specified period or support for domestic health workforce development.

Leveraging Technology and Innovation

Technology and innovation can play a critical role in addressing health workforce challenges, particularly in improving training, service delivery, and management. This approach should be prioritised [15 - 17]:

1. **Expanding E-Learning and Telemedicine:** The government should support the expansion of e-learning platforms to provide ongoing education and training for health workers, particularly those in remote areas. Telemedicine initiatives should also be scaled up to connect rural health workers with specialists and resources in urban centres.
2. **Implementing Workforce Management Systems:** Digital workforce management systems can improve the efficiency of workforce planning, deployment, and monitoring. These systems should include real-time data on workforce distribution, workloads, and health outcomes, enabling more responsive and informed decision-making.

3. **Promoting Research and Innovation in Health Workforce Development:** Supporting research and innovation in health workforce development can lead to new approaches and solutions to workforce challenges. This could include partnerships with universities, research institutions, and private-sector innovators.

Strengthening Governance and Accountability

Strong governance and accountability mechanisms are essential for the successful implementation of health workforce policies. It is critical to consider the following [15 - 17]:

1. **Establishing Clear Accountability Structures:** Clear accountability structures should be established within health ministries and related agencies to ensure the effective implementation of workforce policies. This includes defining roles and responsibilities at all levels and setting up monitoring and evaluation systems.
2. **Engaging Stakeholders in Policy Development:** Engaging a broad range of stakeholders, including health professionals, professional associations, community representatives, and development partners, in the development and implementation of workforce policies can ensure that policies are relevant, feasible, and widely supported.
3. **Monitoring and Evaluation of Workforce Policies:** Regular monitoring and evaluation of workforce policies should be conducted to assess their effectiveness and impact. This should include the use of key performance indicators (KPIs) and feedback mechanisms to inform continuous improvement.

Policy Recommendations

Nigeria can build a sustainable health workforce that is well-distributed, adequately trained, and capable of meeting the health needs of its population. The success of these efforts will depend on strong political will, sustained investment, and collaboration across all sectors involved in health workforce development [18 - 20].

In moving from crisis to a sustainable workforce, the following pragmatic, measurable targets are recommended to align with global benchmarks and national feasibility:

1. Consider meeting up with the SDG workforce benchmark: set a national target to reach 4.45 doctors, nurses, and midwives per 1,000 population (44.5 per

10,000) as a medium-term objective (national roadmap to 2035), with interim milestones.
2. Expand pre-service capacity (medical, nursing, midwifery) by 50% within five years to increase training through accreditation-backed scale-up of training institutions and additional postgraduate residency slots (monitored by annual graduates).
3. Reduce migration and improve retention through improved financing and incentives by introducing measurable retention KPIs, improving remuneration, bonded service for public-funded trainees, support for CPD pathways, and rural hardship allowance. Monitor *via* registration and exit surveys.
4. Aim at equity targets by ensuring every LGA achieves a minimum skilled-birth-attendant-to-population ratio within seven years, and track disaggregated gender and rural/urban coverage annually using the HRH profiles.

CONCLUSION

Strengthening the health workforce in Nigeria requires a comprehensive and multifaceted approach that addresses the various challenges faced by the sector. The HRH crisis in Nigeria is both quantitative and qualitative. The policymakers should ensure that health care workers are fairly distributed and better supported, and must close the gap between training output and workforce retention.

By implementing these policy recommendations, Nigeria can build a sustainable health workforce that is well-distributed, adequately trained, and capable of meeting the health needs of its population. The success of these efforts will depend on strong political will, sustained investment, and collaboration across all sectors involved in health workforce development.

REFERENCES

[1] World Health Organisation. Global strategy on human resources for health: Workforce 2030. Geneva: WHO 2016.

[2] World Health Organisation. Global baseline on health workforce density: 4.45 doctors, nurses and midwives per 1,000 population. Geneva, 2019.

[3] Liu JX, Goryakin Y, Maeda A, Bruckner T, Scheffler R. Global Health Workforce Labor Market Projections for 2030. Hum Resour Health 2017; 15(1): 11. [http://dx.doi.org/10.1186/s12960-017-0187-2] [PMID: 28159017]

[4] Frenk J, Chen L, Bhutta ZA, *et al.* Health professionals for a new century: transforming education to strengthen health systems in an interdependent world. Lancet 2010; 376(9756): 1923-58. [http://dx.doi.org/10.1016/S0140-6736(10)61854-5] [PMID: 21112623]

[5] Omaswa F, Crisp N. African health leaders: making change and claiming the future. Oxford University Press 2014.

[6] National Postgraduate Medical College of Nigeria. Training capacity and annual residency intake report. Lagos 2023.

[7] Nursing and Midwifery Council of Nigeria. Annual report and registration statistics. Abuja 2022.

[8] Dovlo, D. (2003). The brain drain and retention of health professionals in Africa. A case study prepared for a regional training conference on improving tertiary education in Sub-Saharan Africa.

[9] World Health Organisation. Working together for health: World Health Report 2006. Geneva: World Health Organisation 2006.

[10] Africa CDC. Health workforce mobility and migration in Africa: trends and policy responses. Addis Ababa: Africa CDC 2022.

[11] Lehmann U, Sanders D. Community health workers: What do we know about them? The state of the evidence on programmes, activities, costs and impact on health outcomes of using community health workers. World Health Organisation 2007; p. 42.

[12] Zurn P, Codjia L, Sall FL, Braichet JM. How to recruit and retain health workers in underserved areas: the Senegalese experience. Bull World Health Organ 2010; 88(5): 386-9. [http://dx.doi.org/10.2471/BLT.09.070730] [PMID: 20461134]

[13] Perry HB, Zulliger R, Rogers MM. Community health workers in low-, middle-, and high-income countries: an overview of their history, recent evolution, and current effectiveness. Annu Rev Public Health 2014; 35(1): 399-421. [http://dx.doi.org/10.1146/annurev-publhealth-032013-182354] [PMID: 24387091]

[14] World Health Organisation. WHO guideline on health policy and system support to optimise community health worker programmes. Geneva: World Health Organisation 2018.

[15] Campbell J, Buchan J, Cometto G, *et al.* Human resources for health and universal health coverage: fostering equity and effective coverage. Bull World Health Organ 2013; 91(11): 853-63. [http://dx.doi.org/10.2471/BLT.13.118729] [PMID: 24347710]

[16] Global Health Workforce Alliance. Scaling up, saving lives. Geneva: World Health Organisation 2008.

[17] Saleh J-EA. Resilient Communities: Navigating Public Health Challenges in Developing Nations. Bentham Science Publishers 2025. [http://dx.doi.org/10.2174/97898153056091250101]

[18] World Health Organisation. Working for health: A global approach to health workforce planning. Geneva 2018.

[19] Federal Ministry of Health, Nigeria. (2023). National Health Workforce Accounts (NHWA), Nigeria profile. Abuja.

[20] Bauchi State Ministry of Health. (2023). Health Workforce Profile 2023. Available from: https://phcworkforcehub.org.ng/wp-content/uploads/2024/04/Bauchi-State-Health-Workforce-Profile_March-2023.pdf?utm

CHAPTER 7

Immunisation and Disease Prevention: Overcoming Coverage Gaps

Abstract: Immunisation remains one of the most effective public health interventions, yet in Nigeria, significant gaps in coverage persist, leaving millions vulnerable to preventable diseases. This chapter examines the current state of immunisation in Nigeria, highlighting the challenges that hinder widespread coverage, including cultural, economic, and geographical barriers. It explores strategies for reaching zero-dose children, emphasising the importance of integrating immunisation efforts with other health services. Additionally, the chapter discusses the role of disease surveillance and early detection systems in preventing outbreaks. By analysing success stories and best practices, this chapter offers insights into overcoming the barriers to achieving high immunisation coverage in Nigeria and other developing nations.

Keywords: Cultural barriers, Disease surveillance, Disease prevention, Geographical barriers, Health integration, Immunisation coverage, Nigeria, Public health, Vaccination strategies, Zero-dose children.

INTRODUCTION

Immunisation is one of the most cost-effective public health interventions, significantly reducing morbidity and mortality from preventable diseases. In Nigeria, however, immunisation coverage remains suboptimal, with wide disparities across regions and socio-economic groups. Despite global and national efforts, the country continues to struggle with low vaccination rates, particularly among "zero-dose" children who have not received any vaccines. This chapter explores the current state of immunisation in Nigeria, identifies the barriers to achieving comprehensive coverage, and discusses strategies to overcome these challenges. It also highlights the importance of integrating immunisation with other health services and examines successful case studies that have led to improved immunisation rates in similar contexts.

In Nigeria, routine immunisation coverage remains sub-optimal, incomplete, and often uneven across the states. The most recent national statistics on RI show an estimated coverage for key infant vaccines as BCG 74%, DTP3 56%, MCV1

Jalal-Eddeen Abubakar Saleh

60%, and PCV3 52% (latest WUENIC/WHO country profile). However, aggregating the data reveals wide subnational inequities and a substantial percentage of children who have not received even a single dose of a DTP-containing vaccine, tagged as zero-dose. The huge percentage of the zero-dose children, with estimates ranging from ~1.2 million (administrative) up to >2.2 million (WUENIC/UNICEF modelling), ranked Nigeria as one of the largest zero-dose populations in the world, most of whom are in the underserved population of the northern region [1].

THE STATE OF IMMUNISATION COVERAGE IN NIGERIA

Immunisation is one of the most cost-effective public health interventions, playing a crucial role in reducing mortality and morbidity from vaccine-preventable diseases. In Nigeria, however, achieving comprehensive immunisation coverage remains a significant challenge. Despite efforts to strengthen immunisation programs, the country continues to face substantial gaps in coverage, particularly among rural and marginalised populations. This section explores the current state of immunisation coverage in Nigeria, highlighting the progress made, the challenges that persist, and the implications for public health [2 - 4].

Progress in Immunisation Coverage

Over the past few decades, Nigeria has made considerable strides in expanding access to immunisation services. Despite these achievements, Nigeria's immunisation coverage remains uneven, with significant disparities between regions, states, and socio-economic groups. Key achievements include [2 - 4]:

1. **Introduction of New Vaccines:** Nigeria has introduced several new vaccines into its national immunisation program, including the pentavalent vaccine, which protects against five major diseases (diphtheria, tetanus, pertussis, hepatitis B, and Haemophilus influenzae type b), and the rotavirus vaccine, which prevents severe diarrhoea in children.
2. **Expanded Program on Immunisation (EPI):** The Expanded Program on Immunisation (EPI) in Nigeria has been instrumental in increasing vaccine coverage rates. The program has focused on reaching children under five years of age with essential vaccines, including those for measles, polio, and tuberculosis.
3. **Polio Eradication Efforts:** Nigeria's efforts to eradicate polio have been particularly noteworthy. The country was declared free of wild poliovirus in 2020, a significant public health milestone achieved through intense vaccination campaigns and surveillance.

4. **Strengthened Routine Immunisation:** Routine immunisation services have been strengthened through initiatives such as the National Immunisation Plus Days (NIPDs) and the introduction of the Reaching Every Ward (REW) strategy, which aims to improve vaccine delivery at the local level.

Current Coverage Levels

Nigeria's immunisation coverage levels vary widely, with national averages masking substantial regional differences. According to the 2023/24 NDHS data [2 - 4], there is a wide variation between the six geopolitical regions as highlighted below:

1. **National Coverage Rates:** The 2023 National Demographic and Health Survey (NDHS) report shows that, overall, 39% of children aged 12–23 months are fully vaccinated with basic antigens. Nationally, coverage rates for key vaccines such as DPT-HepB-Hib and measles remain below the recommended 90% threshold. The 2023/24 NDHS reported that sixty-seven per cent of children aged 12–23 months received the BCG vaccine, 53% received the third dose of DPT-HepB-Hib, 46% received the third dose of OPV, and 51% received a dose of measles vaccine.
2. **Regional Disparities:** Immunisation coverage is significantly higher in the southern regions of Nigeria compared to the northern regions. For example, while the south-south region has achieved a coverage rate above 60%, the north-central region reported a coverage as low as 30%.
3. **Urban-Rural Divide:** There is a pronounced urban-rural divide in immunisation coverage, with children in urban areas more likely to be fully immunised than those in rural areas. This disparity is driven by factors such as better access to health services in urban centres and higher levels of education and awareness among urban populations.
4. **Socio-Economic Factors:** Immunisation coverage is also influenced by socio-economic factors. Children from wealthier households are more likely to be fully vaccinated than those from poorer households. Additionally, maternal education plays a critical role, with children of mothers who have secondary or higher education being more likely to receive complete vaccinations.

Challenges to Achieving Full Coverage

Several challenges continue to hinder the achievement of full immunisation coverage in Nigeria. Some of these include [2 - 4]:

1. **Inadequate Health Infrastructure:** Many parts of Nigeria, particularly in the northern and rural areas, suffer from inadequate health infrastructure. Health

facilities are often poorly equipped, understaffed, and difficult to access, limiting the reach of immunisation services.

2. **Vaccine Hesitancy and Misinformation:** Vaccine hesitancy remains a significant barrier to achieving high immunisation coverage. Misinformation, cultural beliefs, and religious opposition have led to resistance in some communities, particularly in the North. This has been exacerbated by historical events, such as the polio vaccine boycott in 2003.
3. **Logistical and Supply Chain Issues:** The distribution of vaccines across Nigeria is hampered by logistical challenges, including inadequate cold chain systems, transportation difficulties, and supply chain disruptions. These issues often result in vaccine stockouts or delays, affecting coverage rates.
4. **Security Concerns:** Insecurity in certain regions, particularly in the North East, has severely impacted immunisation efforts. The presence of insurgent groups, communal conflicts, and banditry has made it difficult for health workers to reach children in these areas, leading to low coverage.
5. **Funding Gaps:** Insufficient funding for immunisation programs is another critical challenge. While Nigeria has received substantial support from international partners, domestic financing for immunisation remains inadequate. This has led to gaps in program implementation and sustainability.

Implications for Public Health

The gaps in immunisation coverage in Nigeria have significant public health implications, including the following [2 - 4]:

1. **Outbreaks of Vaccine-Preventable Diseases:** Low coverage rates have contributed to outbreaks of vaccine-preventable diseases, such as measles and yellow fever, particularly in regions with poor immunisation uptake. These outbreaks place additional strain on an already overstretched health system and result in preventable deaths, especially among children.
2. **Increased Child Mortality:** Inadequate immunisation coverage is a major contributor to high child mortality rates in Nigeria. Vaccine-preventable diseases remain a leading cause of death among children under five, undermining efforts to achieve the Sustainable Development Goals (SDGs) related to child health.
3. **Economic and Social Impact:** The economic and social impact of low immunisation coverage is profound. Outbreaks of preventable diseases lead to increased healthcare costs, loss of productivity, and a cycle of poverty for affected families. Additionally, the failure to fully immunize the population undermines Nigeria's human capital development, with long-term consequences for the country's economic growth and stability.

CONCLUSION

While Nigeria has made progress in expanding immunisation coverage, significant challenges remain. The current state of immunisation coverage in the country is characterised by wide regional, socio-economic, and urban-rural disparities, with coverage rates falling short of global targets. Addressing these challenges requires a concerted effort from the government, development partners, and communities to strengthen the immunisation system, tackle vaccine hesitancy, and ensure that all children, regardless of where they live, have access to life-saving vaccines. The health and future of Nigeria's children depend on it.

BARRIERS TO IMMUNISATION: CULTURAL, ECONOMIC, AND GEOGRAPHICAL

Despite the proven effectiveness of immunisation in preventing life-threatening diseases, a significant portion of Nigeria's population remains under-immunised. This section delves into the key barriers that impede immunisation efforts in Nigeria, focusing on cultural, economic, and geographical challenges. Understanding these barriers is crucial for developing targeted strategies to improve vaccine uptake and ensure that all children have access to life-saving immunisations [5 - 7].

Cultural Barriers

Cultural beliefs and practices play a significant role in shaping attitudes toward immunisation in Nigeria. These barriers are often deeply rooted in traditions, religious beliefs, and misinformation, leading to vaccine hesitancy or outright refusal [5, 6].

1. **Religious Beliefs:** In certain regions, particularly in northern Nigeria, religious beliefs can influence attitudes towards immunisation. Some religious leaders and communities view vaccines with suspicion, associating them with foreign intervention or harmful intentions. This has been evident in past resistance to polio vaccination campaigns, where misinformation fueled fears that vaccines were designed to harm or sterilise children.
2. **Misinformation and Myths:** Misinformation about vaccines is pervasive in many parts of Nigeria. Myths such as vaccines causing infertility, spreading diseases, or being unnecessary for healthy children contribute to vaccine hesitancy. Social media and word-of-mouth often perpetuate these myths, making it difficult for health authorities to counteract them.
3. **Traditional Practices:** Some communities prioritise traditional healing methods over modern medical interventions, including immunisation. In such

cases, reliance on herbal remedies and spiritual healers can lead to delays in seeking vaccinations or complete avoidance. Additionally, there is a belief in some areas that diseases preventable by vaccines are a natural part of childhood, and therefore, do not require intervention.

4. **Gender Norms and Roles:** Gender norms also influence immunisation coverage. In many rural areas, women may need permission from their husbands or male relatives to take their children to health facilities. If the male decision-makers are sceptical about vaccines, this can result in children missing out on immunisations. Furthermore, women's limited autonomy and restricted mobility can make it difficult for them to access health services, including immunisation clinics.

Economic Barriers

Economic factors significantly impact immunisation coverage in Nigeria, particularly in underserved and low-income communities. These barriers often intersect with other challenges, exacerbating the difficulties in achieving high vaccination rates [5, 6].

1. **Poverty and Financial Constraints:** Poverty remains a major barrier to accessing immunisation services. While vaccines are generally provided free of charge through national programs, indirect costs such as transportation, loss of income from taking time off work, and associated healthcare costs can deter families from seeking immunisation services. These costs can be prohibitive for families living in extreme poverty, leading to lower vaccination rates among children from poorer households.
    1. **Health System Financing:** Nigeria's health system is underfunded, which affects the availability and quality of immunisation services. Insufficient resources lead to vaccine stockouts, logistical challenges affecting vaccine deliveries, inadequate cold chain infrastructure, and understaffed health facilities. These failures often result in missed opportunities, even discouraging caregivers from bringing their children for vaccination, disproportionately affecting rural and underserved areas, where health services are already limited.
    2. **Economic Inequality:** Economic disparities within Nigeria also contribute to uneven immunisation coverage. Children from wealthier families are more likely to receive all necessary vaccinations compared to those from poorer backgrounds. This inequality is compounded by better access to healthcare, education, and information among higher-income groups, while the poor remain marginalised.
    3. **Workforce Challenges:** Economic challenges also affect the health workforce, which is critical for delivering immunisation services. Low

wages, poor working conditions, and inadequate training can lead to a demotivated and understaffed workforce, particularly in remote areas. This results in reduced outreach and lower vaccine coverage, especially in hard-to-reach communities.

Geographical Barriers

Nigeria's vast and diverse geography presents significant challenges to achieving uniform immunisation coverage. Remote, rural, and conflict-affected areas are particularly difficult to reach, resulting in geographical disparities in vaccine access. Similarly, access to functioning PHCs is hindered because of poor road networks and seasonal flooding that cut off catchment populations [5 - 7].

1. **Remote and Rural Areas:** Many parts of Nigeria, particularly in the North East and North West regions, are characterised by difficult terrain and limited infrastructure. In these remote areas, health facilities are often sparse, and the distance to the nearest clinic can be a major deterrent for families. Poor road networks, especially during the rainy season, can make it nearly impossible to transport vaccines or reach these communities consistently.
2. **Conflict and Insecurity:** Ongoing conflict and insecurity, particularly in the North East, pose significant barriers to immunisation. Insecurity prevents health workers from safely accessing conflict zones, while the displacement of populations disrupts routine immunisation schedules. The presence of insurgent groups, such as Boko Haram, has also led to the targeting of health workers and vaccination campaigns, further hindering efforts to achieve high coverage in these areas.
3. **Urban Slums:** Although urban areas generally have better access to health services, the rapid growth of urban slums presents a unique challenge. These densely populated areas often lack adequate health infrastructure, sanitation, and clean water, leading to higher disease transmission rates. Moreover, the transient nature of slum populations and the lack of formal healthcare facilities make it difficult to maintain accurate records and ensure consistent immunisation coverage.
4. **Nomadic Populations:** Nigeria is home to a significant number of nomadic communities, particularly in the northern regions. These populations are highly mobile, often moving in search of pasture or seasonal work, making it challenging to provide regular immunisation services. The lack of fixed health infrastructure and the difficulties in tracking these populations further complicate efforts to ensure that all children are vaccinated.

Implications and the Way Forward

The cultural, economic, and geographical barriers to immunisation in Nigeria have profound implications for public health. Addressing these barriers is essential for improving immunisation coverage and preventing outbreaks of vaccine-preventable diseases. A multi-faceted approach is needed, involving [5 - 7]:

1. **Community Engagement and Education:** Engaging with local communities to address cultural beliefs and misinformation is crucial. This involves working with religious and traditional leaders, leveraging social media, and implementing targeted education campaigns that build trust in vaccines and counteract myths.
2. **Strengthening Health Systems:** Improving health system financing and infrastructure, particularly in rural and underserved areas, is essential. This includes ensuring a reliable supply of vaccines, expanding cold chain capacity, and investing in the health workforce to improve service delivery.
3. **Innovative Service Delivery Models:** Reaching remote and mobile populations requires innovative service delivery models. This could include mobile clinics, outreach programs, and the use of technology to track immunization coverage and schedule follow-up visits.
4. **Addressing Economic Barriers:** Reducing the financial burden on families is key to improving vaccine uptake. This could involve providing transportation subsidies, integrating immunisation services with other health interventions, and ensuring that health services are accessible and affordable for all.
5. **Conflict-Sensitive Approaches:** In conflict-affected areas, adopting conflict-sensitive approaches to immunisation is critical. This includes negotiating access with all parties to the conflict, ensuring the safety of health workers, and adapting immunisation strategies to the realities of conflict zones.

CONCLUSION

By addressing these barriers through targeted interventions and sustained efforts, Nigeria can make significant progress toward achieving universal immunisation coverage and protecting the health of its population.

STRATEGIES FOR REACHING ZERO-DOSE CHILDREN

In Nigeria, the challenge of reaching zero-dose children, those who have not received any routine vaccines, remains a critical issue. These children are often the most vulnerable, living in hard-to-reach areas, underserved communities, or conflict zones, where health services are limited or nonexistent. Addressing the needs of zero-dose children is essential for closing immunisation gaps and preventing outbreaks of vaccine-preventable diseases. This section explores strategies that can be employed to identify, reach, and immunise these children effectively [8 - 10].

In Fig. (**1**), I have presented a snapshot of Routine immunisation coverage in Nigeria, which remains incomplete and highly uneven, using the data from the WHO/UNICEF (WUENIC) country estimates report modest coverage for key infant vaccines (most recent country profile).

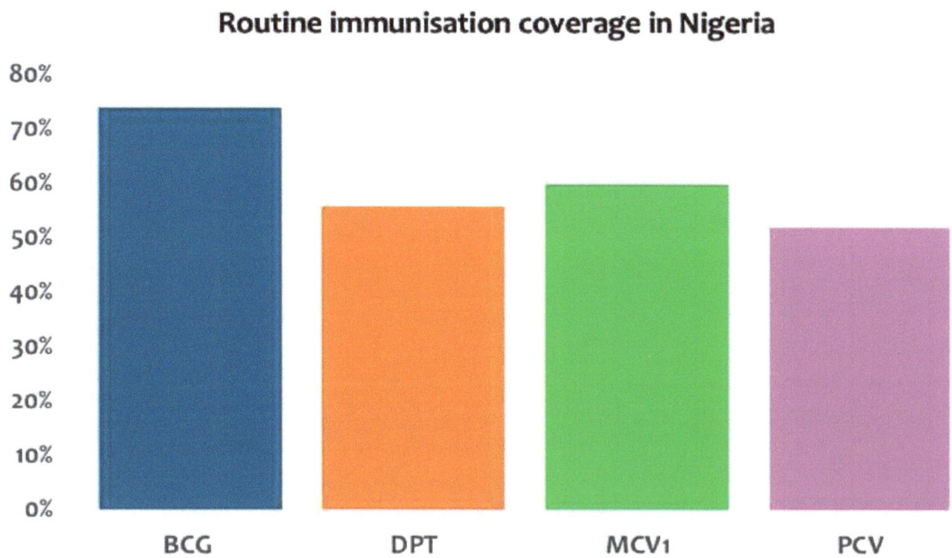

Fig. (1). Shows selected routine immunisation coverage in Nigeria (WUENIC/WHO estimates).

The national average, presented in Fig. (**1**), masks very wide subnational inequities and a substantial population of "zero-dose" children. It is on record that Nigeria has one of the largest zero-dose populations in the world, with estimates ranging from ~1.2 million (administrative) up to >2.2 million (WUENIC/UNICEF modelling), concentrated in a small number of high-burden states and urban poor settlements [11].

Identifying Zero-Dose Children

Accurate identification of zero-dose children is the first step in addressing immunisation gaps. This requires robust data collection, monitoring, and reporting systems that can track immunisation status at the community level [7, 8].

1. **Strengthening Health Information Systems:** A strong health information system is crucial for tracking the immunisation status of children. This involves integrating immunisation data into national health information systems, using digital tools for real-time data collection, and ensuring that data is disaggregated by geographic location, gender, and socioeconomic status to identify zero-dose children accurately.
2. **Community-Based Surveys and Outreach:** Conducting regular community-based surveys and outreach activities can help identify zero-dose children, particularly in remote and underserved areas. These surveys should be designed to capture information on immunisation status, barriers to access, and reasons for non-vaccination, enabling targeted interventions.
3. **Leveraging Community Health Workers (CHWs):** Community health workers (CHWs) play a critical role in identifying zero-dose children. They have the advantage of being embedded within communities, allowing them to track immunisation status, follow up with families, and refer children to health facilities. Training and empowering CHWs to use digital tools for tracking and reporting can enhance their effectiveness in reaching zero-dose children.

Enhancing Service Delivery in Hard-to-Reach Areas

Reaching zero-dose children often requires innovative approaches to service delivery, particularly in remote, rural, and conflict-affected areas where traditional health services are inaccessible [8, 9].

1. **Mobile Clinics and Outreach Services:** Deploying mobile clinics and outreach services is an effective strategy for reaching children in remote and underserved areas. These clinics can bring immunisation services directly to communities, reducing the distance and time families need to travel to access vaccines. Mobile teams can also provide other essential health services, making immunisation more attractive to families.
2. **Task-Shifting and Task-Sharing:** Task-shifting and task-sharing involve delegating immunisation-related tasks to less specialised health workers or CHWs, enabling a broader reach of services. This approach is particularly useful in areas with a shortage of skilled health workers. Training CHWs and other local health workers to administer vaccines can help bridge gaps in service delivery.
3. **Use of Technology and Innovation:** Technology can play a transformative role in reaching zero-dose children. The use of digital health tools, such as electronic immunisation registries, GPS mapping for service delivery planning, and mobile applications for appointment reminders, can improve the efficiency and effectiveness of immunisation campaigns. In areas with limited connec-

tivity, low-tech solutions like solar-powered cold chain equipment can ensure vaccine viability in remote locations.

4. **Partnerships with Local Organisations:** Partnering with local non-governmental organisations (NGOs), community-based organisations (CBOs), and religious institutions can enhance immunisation efforts. These organisations often have deep community ties and can mobilise resources and volunteers to support vaccination campaigns, ensuring that zero-dose children are reached even in the most challenging environments.

Addressing Social and Cultural Barriers

Social and cultural barriers often prevent families from seeking immunisation services for their children. Overcoming these barriers requires culturally sensitive and community-driven approaches [8 - 10].

1. **Community Engagement and Education:** Engaging communities through education and dialogue is key to overcoming vaccine hesitancy and resistance. This involves working with local leaders, religious figures, and influencers to promote the benefits of immunisation and dispel myths and misinformation. Community-based education campaigns, tailored to the specific cultural and religious context, can build trust and encourage vaccine acceptance.
2. **Incentives and Conditional Cash Transfers:** Providing incentives or conditional cash transfers to families who complete the full immunisation schedule can be an effective strategy to increase vaccine uptake. These incentives can offset the indirect costs associated with immunisation, such as transportation or lost income, making it easier for families to prioritise their children's health.
3. **Gender-Sensitive Approaches:** Addressing gender-related barriers is crucial for reaching zero-dose children. This includes empowering women with the knowledge and autonomy to make decisions about their children's health, as well as involving men in immunisation campaigns to ensure family-wide support for vaccination. Gender-sensitive approaches should also consider the unique challenges faced by adolescent mothers, who may require additional support to access immunisation services for their children.

Ensuring Sustainability and Long-Term Impact

Achieving and sustaining high immunisation coverage requires a long-term commitment to strengthening health systems and ensuring that zero-dose children are consistently reached [8 - 10].

1. **Integrating Immunisation with Other Health Services:** Integrating immunisation with other health services, such as maternal and child health programs, nutrition services, and antenatal care, can improve coverage and reduce missed opportunities. This integrated approach ensures that immunisation is part of a comprehensive package of care, making it more accessible and acceptable to families.
2. **Building Resilient Health Systems:** Strengthening the overall resilience of health systems is critical for sustaining immunisation efforts. This includes improving the availability of vaccines, ensuring a reliable cold chain, and building the capacity of health workers. Resilient health systems are better equipped to adapt to challenges such as pandemics, natural disasters, and conflicts, ensuring that immunisation services are maintained even in times of crisis.
3. **Monitoring and Evaluation:** Continuous monitoring and evaluation are essential for assessing the effectiveness of strategies to reach zero-dose children. This involves regularly reviewing data on immunisation coverage, identifying gaps, and adapting strategies as needed. Monitoring should also include community feedback mechanisms to ensure that immunisation services are responsive to local needs and challenges.
4. **Sustaining Political Commitment and Funding:** High-level political commitment and sustained funding are crucial for the success of immunisation programs. Governments, donors, and international organisations must prioritise immunisation as a key component of public health and allocate adequate resources to support ongoing efforts. Advocacy and public awareness campaigns can help maintain political commitment and ensure that immunisation remains a priority on the national health agenda.

CONCLUSION

By implementing these strategies, Nigeria can make significant progress in reaching zero-dose children, closing immunisation gaps, and moving closer to achieving universal immunisation coverage. This will not only protect children from vaccine-preventable diseases but also contribute to broader health and development goals, ensuring a healthier future for all.

DISEASE SURVEILLANCE AND EARLY DETECTION SYSTEMS

In the fight against vaccine-preventable diseases, robust disease surveillance and early detection systems are critical components of a comprehensive public health strategy. These systems not only help in identifying and responding to outbreaks promptly but also play a vital role in maintaining and improving immunisation coverage by providing the necessary data to guide targeted interventions. This section explores the key elements of effective disease surveillance and early detection systems and their importance in ensuring public health security in Nigeria and other developing nations [12 - 14].

Strengthening Disease Surveillance Systems

An effective disease surveillance system is the backbone of public health efforts to control and eliminate vaccine-preventable diseases. It involves the systematic collection, analysis, and interpretation of health data essential for planning, implementation, and evaluation of public health practices [12].

The Nigerian Centre for Disease Control (NCDC) coordinates event-based and indicator-based surveillance for vaccine-preventable outbreaks (measles, polio, Yellow Fever) and supports laboratory networks. Linkage between case surveillance and immunisation coverage data has enabled rapid outbreak response immunisation in recent years. Integrating surveillance, laboratory confirmation, and immunisation data (DHIS2 + NCDC workflows) strengthens both prevention and response [15].

Similarly, Nigeria's national routine health information platform for facility reporting is the DHIS2. It hosts routine immunisation modules and is used for near-real-time monitoring of doses administered. The real-time dashboards and automated reports help programme managers detect low-coverage districts and stockouts [16, 17].

1. **Integrated Disease Surveillance and Response (IDSR):** The IDSR framework is a crucial tool for strengthening surveillance systems. By integrating multiple surveillance functions into a single system, IDSR enhances the efficiency and effectiveness of disease monitoring. This approach involves collecting data from various levels of the health system, ranging from local health facilities to national health authorities, enabling the rapid detection and response to outbreaks.
2. **Community-Based Surveillance:** Engaging communities in surveillance activities is essential, especially in areas where access to formal health facilities is limited. Community-based surveillance involves training community health workers and volunteers to identify and report cases of vaccine-preventable diseases. This approach not only increases the reach of surveillance systems but also fosters trust and cooperation between communities and health authorities.
3. **Laboratory Networks and Diagnostic Capacity:** Strengthening laboratory networks and enhancing diagnostic capacity are critical for confirming cases of vaccine-preventable diseases and monitoring the effectiveness of immunisation programs. Ensuring that laboratories are equipped with the necessary tools and

trained personnel to conduct accurate and timely tests is vital for early detection and response to outbreaks.

Early Detection and Response Mechanisms

Timely detection and rapid response are key to preventing the spread of vaccine-preventable diseases. Effective early detection systems rely on the prompt identification of cases, swift reporting, and immediate action to contain outbreaks [12 - 14].

1. **Real-Time Data Reporting:** Implementing real-time data reporting systems is essential for early detection of outbreaks. Digital tools, such as mobile applications and electronic reporting systems, can facilitate the rapid transmission of health data from the field to central authorities. This allows for quicker analysis and response, reducing the time between detection and intervention.
2. **Rapid Response Teams:** Establishing and training rapid response teams is crucial for effective outbreak management. These teams, composed of epidemiologists, healthcare workers, and logistics experts, should be equipped to investigate and respond to disease outbreaks immediately. Their role includes case management, contact tracing, and coordination with local health authorities to ensure that containment measures are implemented promptly.
3. **Use of Geospatial Technology:** Geospatial technology, such as Geographic Information Systems (GIS), can be used to map disease outbreaks and identify patterns of spread. This technology enables public health officials to visualise hotspots, track the movement of diseases, and allocate resources more effectively. GIS can also be integrated with other data sources to provide a comprehensive view of the epidemiological situation.

Enhancing Data Quality and Use

High-quality data is the foundation of effective surveillance and early detection systems. Ensuring the accuracy, completeness, and timeliness of data collection and reporting is essential for informed decision-making [12 - 14].

1. **Data Quality Audits:** Conducting regular data quality audits helps to identify and address gaps in surveillance data. These audits involve reviewing the processes of data collection, reporting, and analysis to ensure that the information used for public health decision-making is reliable. Improving data quality not only enhances surveillance but also builds confidence in the health system among stakeholders.

2. **Capacity Building for Health Workers:** Training health workers on data management and the importance of accurate reporting is critical for improving surveillance systems. Capacity-building initiatives should focus on enhancing skills in data collection, analysis, and use, ensuring that health workers at all levels are equipped to contribute effectively to disease surveillance efforts.
3. **Data-Driven Decision-Making:** Promoting a culture of data-driven decision-making within health systems is essential for the effective use of surveillance data. Health authorities should utilise the data collected through surveillance systems to inform public health policies, allocate resources effectively, and design targeted interventions. This approach ensures that immunisation programs are responsive to the specific needs and challenges identified through surveillance activities.

Collaborations and Partnerships

Collaborations and partnerships are vital for strengthening disease surveillance and early detection systems. Engaging with various stakeholders, including international organisations, governments, and local communities, enhances the capacity to detect and respond to outbreaks [12 - 14].

1. **International Collaboration:** Collaboration with international health organisations, such as the World Health Organisation (WHO) and the Centers for Disease Control and Prevention (CDC), provides access to technical expertise, funding, and resources necessary for strengthening surveillance systems. These partnerships also facilitate the sharing of data and best practices across borders, contributing to global health security.
2. **Public-Private Partnerships:** Public-private partnerships can play a significant role in enhancing disease surveillance and early detection systems. The private sector can provide technological innovations, logistical support, and financial resources to complement government efforts. Collaborating with technology companies, for example, can lead to the development of advanced data collection and analysis tools.
3. **Community Engagement:** Engaging communities in surveillance efforts not only improves data collection at the grassroots level but also fosters a sense of ownership and responsibility among community members. This can lead to increased vigilance and timely reporting of potential outbreaks, enabling quicker responses and reducing the spread of diseases.

Sustaining and Scaling Surveillance Efforts

For disease surveillance and early detection systems to be effective in the long term, they must be sustainable and scalable. This requires continuous investment in infrastructure, human resources, and technology [12 - 14].

1. **Long-Term Funding and Resource Allocation:** Securing long-term funding and resources is essential for maintaining and expanding surveillance systems. Governments and donors must prioritise investment in surveillance infrastructure, including laboratories, data systems, and training programs. Ensuring consistent funding helps to avoid disruptions in surveillance activities and maintains the system's readiness to respond to outbreaks.
2. **Scalability of Surveillance Systems:** Designing surveillance systems with scalability in mind allows them to be adapted to different contexts and challenges. Whether dealing with a localised outbreak or a widespread epidemic, scalable systems can be adjusted to meet the demands of the situation. This flexibility is crucial for maintaining effective disease control in both routine and emergencies.
3. **Innovation and Adaptation:** Encouraging innovation and the adaptation of new technologies and methods is key to keeping surveillance systems effective and relevant. As new challenges and opportunities arise, surveillance systems must evolve to incorporate the latest advancements in data collection, analysis, and reporting. Continuous innovation ensures that these systems remain robust and capable of addressing emerging public health threats.

CONCLUSION

By strengthening disease surveillance and early detection systems, Nigeria can enhance its ability to prevent and control vaccine-preventable diseases. This will not only protect the health of its population but also contribute to global efforts to eradicate these diseases, ensuring a safer and healthier future for all.

INTEGRATING IMMUNISATION WITH OTHER HEALTH SERVICES

Integrating immunisation with other health services is a strategic approach that enhances the efficiency and effectiveness of public health interventions. This integration not only improves vaccine coverage but also strengthens the overall health system by ensuring that a broader range of health needs are addressed during a single healthcare visit. For countries like Nigeria, where healthcare resources are often limited and access to services can be challenging, integrating immunisation with other health services presents an opportunity to maximise the impact of health interventions, reduce costs, and improve health outcomes. This section explores the various dimensions of integrating immunisation with other health services and its implications for public health in developing nations [18 - 22].

The Rationale for Integration

The rationale behind integrating immunisation with other health services is grounded in the principles of efficiency, accessibility, and holistic care. By delivering multiple health interventions simultaneously, health systems can reduce the logistical and financial burdens on both providers and recipients of care. For example, during routine immunisation visits, healthcare workers can also provide nutrition screenings, distribute vitamin A supplements, administer deworming medications, and offer antenatal care services. This approach not only saves time and resources but also increases the likelihood that individuals, especially children and pregnant women, will receive the comprehensive care they need [18 - 22].

1. **Enhancing Efficiency of Service Delivery:** Integrating immunisation with other health services enables more efficient use of both human and material resources within the healthcare system. Instead of organising separate outreach sessions for immunisation, nutrition, antenatal care, and deworming, a single, coordinated visit allows health workers to deliver multiple interventions simultaneously. This approach reduces duplication of logistics, minimises transportation and staffing costs, and conserves cold chain and storage infrastructure. In resource-limited settings, such efficiency can be pivotal in expanding the reach of services without significantly increasing operational costs.
2. **Improving Accessibility and Reducing Missed Opportunities:** By bundling services together, integration reduces the number of visits required by individuals, particularly mothers and caregivers, to access essential healthcare for themselves and their children. In rural or hard-to-reach communities, where accessing a health facility may involve long travel distances or high opportunity costs, integrated service delivery minimises barriers to care. This, in turn, reduces missed opportunities for immunisation and other preventive interventions, ensuring that more children and vulnerable groups receive the full spectrum of recommended health services during each contact with the health system.
3. **Promoting Comprehensive and Person-Centred Care:** Health conditions do not occur in silos, and integrated services recognise the need for holistic care. For example, immunisation appointments can serve as an opportunity to provide growth monitoring, nutrition assessments, vitamin A supplementation, family planning counselling, or malaria prevention education. Such

comprehensive care meets individuals' broader health needs and fosters a person-centred approach that treats patients as whole beings rather than recipients of isolated interventions. This model builds trust and satisfaction among service users, ultimately encouraging ongoing engagement with health services.

4. **Strengthening Health System Resilience and Coordination:** Integration fosters collaboration across different health programs, reducing fragmentation and building a more coordinated health system. Rather than operating as parallel vertical programs with separate funding, staffing, and data systems, integrated models promote joint planning, pooled resources, and shared indicators of success. This enhances system-wide resilience, particularly during emergencies or disease outbreaks, by enabling health systems to maintain essential services while responding to emerging needs. Moreover, integration encourages capacity-building across health cadres and improves workforce adaptability.
5. **Accelerating Progress Toward UHC and the SDGs:** The integrated delivery of health services directly contributes to broader national and global health goals. It aligns with the vision of Universal Health Coverage (UHC) by ensuring that essential services are available, accessible, and affordable to all, particularly the most vulnerable. Integration also supports the achievement of Sustainable Development Goal 3 (Good Health and Well-being) by addressing multiple determinants of health through a unified platform. In doing so, it strengthens the impact and sustainability of health interventions, making them more cost-effective and equitable.

Models of Integrated Service Delivery

Several models of integrated service delivery have been successfully implemented in various contexts. These models can be adapted to suit the specific needs and circumstances of different regions, ensuring that immunisation and other health services are delivered in a coordinated and efficient manner [18 - 22].

1. **One-Stop-Shop Model:** The one-stop-shop model involves providing multiple health services during a single visit to a health facility. This model is particularly effective in settings where access to healthcare is limited, as it reduces the need for multiple visits. In this model, immunisation services are integrated with maternal and child health services, such as antenatal care, postnatal care, and growth monitoring. By offering a range of services in one location, this model enhances the convenience for patients and encourages higher utilisation of health services.
2. **Outreach and Mobile Clinics:** In remote or underserved areas, outreach and mobile clinics can deliver integrated health services to communities that might

otherwise have limited access to healthcare. These clinics can be equipped to provide immunisations, along with other essential health services like family planning, HIV testing and counselling, and basic curative care. By bringing services directly to the community, this model increases coverage and ensures that hard-to-reach populations receive the care they need.

3. **Integrated Health Campaigns:** Integrated health campaigns combine immunisation drives with other public health interventions, such as mass drug administration for neglected tropical diseases, health education campaigns, and distribution of insecticide-treated nets. These campaigns are often organised on a large scale and can reach a significant portion of the population in a short period. The advantage of this model is its ability to leverage the logistical and operational resources of immunisation programs to deliver multiple interventions simultaneously.

Benefits of Integration

Integrating immunisation with other health services offers several benefits that can enhance the effectiveness of public health programs in developing nations. Some of these benefits include [18 - 22]:

1. **Improved Coverage and Access:** By offering multiple services in one visit, integration can improve access to healthcare and increase the coverage of both immunisation and other health services. This is particularly important in areas where healthcare facilities are scarce or where transportation and financial barriers prevent frequent visits to health centres.
2. **Cost-Effectiveness:** Integration can lead to significant cost savings by reducing the duplication of efforts, optimising the use of resources, and lowering operational costs. For example, the shared use of cold chain infrastructure for vaccines and other temperature-sensitive health products can reduce costs while maintaining service quality.
3. **Enhanced Health Outcomes:** Providing a range of health services together can lead to better health outcomes, as it addresses multiple health needs simultaneously. For instance, integrating immunisation with nutrition services ensures that children receive both vaccines and nutritional support, which are critical for their overall development and protection against disease.
4. **Strengthened Health Systems:** Integration can contribute to the strengthening of health systems by promoting collaboration between different health programs, improving data collection and management, and enhancing the skills of healthcare workers. This holistic approach ensures that health systems are more resilient and capable of responding to a variety of health challenges.

Challenges and Considerations

While integration offers numerous benefits, some challenges must be addressed to ensure its success. Some of the ways to address the challenges include [18 - 22]:

1. **Coordination and Management:** Effective integration requires strong coordination and management across different health programs and services. This includes aligning objectives, timelines, and resources, as well as ensuring clear communication and collaboration among stakeholders. Without proper coordination, integration efforts can lead to inefficiencies and fragmented service delivery.
2. **Training and Capacity Building:** Healthcare workers need to be adequately trained to deliver integrated services. This includes not only technical skills related to immunisation and other health services but also the ability to manage multiple tasks during a single visit. Continuous capacity building is essential to ensure that healthcare workers can effectively implement integrated service delivery models.
3. **Resource Allocation:** Integration requires careful planning and allocation of resources to ensure that all services are delivered effectively. This includes ensuring that there are sufficient supplies, equipment, and personnel to support integrated service delivery. In resource-constrained settings, this can be a significant challenge, requiring innovative solutions and prioritisation.
4. **Monitoring and Evaluation:** Integrated services must be monitored and evaluated to assess their impact and effectiveness. This requires the development of indicators that can capture the performance of multiple services and the outcomes of integration efforts. Data collection and analysis must be robust to inform decision-making and continuous improvement.

Policy Implications and Recommendations

To successfully integrate immunisation with other health services, policymakers must create an enabling environment that supports integration efforts at all levels of the health system. The following could be considered [18 - 22]:

1. **Policy Frameworks:** Governments should develop and implement policy frameworks that promote the integration of health services. These frameworks should provide clear guidelines for the coordination of different health programs, resource allocation, and monitoring and evaluation of integrated services.
2. **Financing Mechanisms:** Sustainable financing mechanisms are essential to support the integration of health services. This includes securing funding for

both immunisation and other health services, as well as ensuring that resources are allocated in a way that supports integrated service delivery. Innovative financing models, such as performance-based funding, can incentivise integration and ensure that services are delivered efficiently.

3. **Stakeholder Engagement:** Engaging stakeholders, including communities, healthcare providers, and development partners, is crucial for the success of integration efforts. Stakeholder engagement ensures that integration strategies are responsive to the needs of the population and that there is broad support for integration initiatives.
4. **Continuous Learning and Adaptation:** Integration efforts should be guided by continuous learning and adaptation. This involves regularly reviewing and adjusting integration strategies based on the outcomes of monitoring and evaluation activities. By fostering a culture of learning and innovation, health systems can continuously improve the delivery of integrated services.

CONCLUSION

Integrating immunisation with other health services is a powerful strategy for enhancing the reach and impact of public health interventions in Nigeria and other developing nations. By addressing multiple health needs in a coordinated manner, integration can improve access to care, increase efficiency, and strengthen health systems. However, to achieve these benefits, integration efforts must be carefully planned, adequately resourced, and supported by strong policy frameworks and stakeholder engagement. As countries strive to improve health outcomes and achieve universal health coverage, integrating immunisation with other health services will play a crucial role in ensuring that no one is left behind.

SUCCESS STORIES: IMPROVING IMMUNISATION RATES

Success stories from around the world offer valuable lessons on how to improve immunisation rates, particularly in challenging contexts like Nigeria and other developing nations. These stories demonstrate that with the right strategies, community engagement, and political will, significant progress can be made in increasing vaccine coverage and protecting populations from vaccine-preventable diseases. This section highlights several success stories from different regions, illustrating how innovative approaches, partnerships, and persistence have led to remarkable improvements in immunisation rates [22 - 25].

Rwanda: A Model for Universal Immunisation

Rwanda's success in achieving high immunisation coverage rates is often cited as a model for other developing nations. Despite its history of conflict and limited resources, Rwanda has managed to achieve over 90% coverage for key vaccines, including the measles, mumps, and rubella (MMR) vaccine, and the pentavalent vaccine [22 - 25]. This success can be attributed to several key factors:

1. **Strong Political Commitment:** Rwanda's government has demonstrated an unwavering commitment to improving public health, with immunisation being a top priority. This political will has translated into sustained investment in health infrastructure, human resources, and vaccine procurement. The government's leadership has also fostered a culture of accountability and results-oriented programming, ensuring that immunisation targets are met.
2. **Community Health Worker Program:** Rwanda's robust Community Health Worker (CHW) program has been instrumental in reaching even the most remote communities. CHWs are trained to provide a range of health services, including immunisation, and are supported by a well-organised supply chain that ensures vaccines are available even in hard-to-reach areas. Their deep integration into communities has built trust and improved vaccine uptake.
3. **Use of Data and Technology:** Rwanda has effectively leveraged data and technology to improve immunisation coverage. The country's health information system allows for real-time tracking of immunisation rates, helping to identify gaps and respond quickly. Additionally, Rwanda has implemented mobile health (mHealth) initiatives, such as SMS reminders for parents, to ensure timely vaccinations.

India: Polio Eradication

India's successful eradication of polio is a landmark achievement in global health. Once considered the most challenging country in the world for polio eradication due to its large population and diverse geography, India was declared polio-free in 2014. The strategies employed in this campaign provide critical insights into improving immunisation rates [22 - 25]:

1. **Intensified Immunisation Campaigns:** India launched extensive immunisation campaigns, known as Pulse Polio Immunisation (PPI) drives, which mobilised millions of health workers, volunteers, and community members to vaccinate children under the age of five. These campaigns were conducted multiple times a year, ensuring that all children were reached.
2. **Addressing Social and Cultural Barriers:** India's polio eradication efforts involved intensive community engagement to overcome social and cultural barriers. Religious leaders, community influencers, and celebrities were enlisted to promote the benefits of vaccination, dispel myths, and encourage participation. This community-based approach was key to reaching hesitant or resistant populations.

3. **Surveillance and Rapid Response:** India's success was also due to its robust surveillance and rapid response mechanisms. The country established a comprehensive Acute Flaccid Paralysis (AFP) surveillance system to detect potential polio cases early. When cases were identified, rapid response teams were deployed to conduct mass immunisation in the affected areas, preventing further spread.

Nigeria: Overcoming Challenges in Polio Eradication

Nigeria's journey towards polio eradication is a story of overcoming immense challenges. As one of the last countries to eradicate polio, Nigeria's experience offers valuable lessons in persistence, innovation, and community engagement. Nigeria was declared polio-free in 2020, marking a significant milestone in global health [22 - 25].

1. **Tackling Insecurity and Access Issues:** Insecurity, particularly in the northern regions, posed significant challenges to Nigeria's polio eradication efforts. Despite these challenges, Nigeria implemented innovative strategies to reach children in conflict-affected areas. These included the use of "hit-and-run" immunisation campaigns, where teams would enter insecure areas briefly to vaccinate children and then withdraw. Additionally, negotiations with local leaders and armed groups were conducted to allow access to vaccination teams.
2. **Building Trust and Countering Misinformation:** Misinformation and distrust in vaccines were significant barriers in Nigeria's polio eradication campaign. To address this, Nigeria invested in extensive social mobilisation efforts. Religious and traditional leaders were engaged to advocate for vaccination, and community dialogues were held to address concerns and misinformation. These efforts helped build trust and increase vaccine acceptance.
3. **Integrating Polio Immunisation with Other Health Services:** To maximise the reach of polio immunisation, Nigeria integrated it with other health services, such as routine immunisation, nutrition programs, and maternal and child health services. This approach ensured that children received comprehensive care and that immunisation efforts were not limited to polio alone.

The Gambia: Leveraging Partnerships for Immunisation Success

The Gambia has achieved impressive immunisation coverage rates, thanks in large part to strong partnerships and international support. The country's success highlights the importance of collaboration in improving immunisation rates [22 - 25].

1. **Partnership with GAVI:** The Gambia has been a beneficiary of Gavi, the Vaccine Alliance, which has provided financial and technical support to strengthen the country's immunisation program. This partnership has enabled The Gambia to introduce new vaccines, improve cold chain infrastructure, and train healthcare workers.
2. **Community Involvement and Ownership:** The Gambia has successfully engaged communities in its immunisation efforts, ensuring that local populations take ownership of health interventions. This community-driven approach has led to high levels of vaccine acceptance and coverage, even in remote areas.
3. **Comprehensive Health Campaigns:** The Gambia has implemented comprehensive health campaigns that integrate immunisation with other public health interventions, such as vitamin A supplementation and deworming. These campaigns have been effective in reaching large numbers of children and improving overall health outcomes.

Practical Recommendations

In bridging Nigeria's immunisation gaps, I have presented in Table **1** a few practical recommendations for integrating immunisation into the primary care system. Effective integration of immunisation into primary healthcare requires both structural and operational reforms. The table below presents some practical recommendations to strengthen routine immunisation delivery through PHCs in Nigeria.

Table 1. Recommendations for integrating immunisation into the primary care system.

Strategic Area	Recommendations	Expected Outcomes
1. Improve Financing and Accountability Mechanisms	1. Ring-fence routine immunisation funds (transport, outreach, cold chain) at state and LGA levels. 2. Publish quarterly coverage scorecards and enforce managerial accountability.	Predictable financing, transparent resource use, and stronger local ownership of immunisation outcomes.
2. Integrate Service Delivery Platforms	Combine immunisation sessions with other services such as nutrition screening, vitamin A supplementation, deworming, and antenatal care.	Increased service uptake, reduced missed opportunities, and enhanced efficiency of PHC delivery.
3. Strengthen PHC Infrastructure and Reliability	1. PHCs to serve as a reliable immunisation point through monthly outreach sessions, cold-chain functionality, and prepositioned buffer stocks. 2. Link PHC performance metrics to immunisation KPIs.	Increased immunisation coverage and reduced stockouts; improved accountability at the facility level.

(Table 1) cont.....

Strategic Area	Recommendations	Expected Outcomes
4. Institutionalise Community Engagement	1. Recognise the volunteer community mobiliser as part of PHC staffing and provide basic training, stipends, and supervision. 2. Link mobilisation with RMNCH services.	Sustained community ownership and improved demand generation for immunisation.
5. Target Zero-Dose and Underserved Populations	1. Use DHIS2 and geospatial mapping to identify and prioritise zero-dose hotspots. 2. Deploy mobile teams and community mobilisers to reach those wards.	Reduction in zero-dose children and improved equity in immunisation access.
6. Strengthen Data Systems and Use	1. Strengthen DHIS2 and improve denominator estimation. 2. Conduct quarterly LQAS and household surveys to validate administrative data. 3. Link NCDC surveillance alerts to catch-up immunisation.	Reliable data for decision-making and prompt outbreak response; reduced discrepancies between administrative and survey data.

CONCLUSION

These success stories demonstrate that improving immunisation rates is possible, even in the most challenging environments. Whether through strong political commitment, innovative service delivery models, or effective community engagement, these examples provide valuable lessons for other countries striving to improve vaccine coverage. By learning from these experiences and adapting successful strategies to local contexts, Nigeria and other developing nations can make significant strides in protecting their populations from vaccine-preventable diseases and achieving universal immunisation coverage.

REFERENCES

[1] WHO and UNICEF. Estimates of National Immunisation Coverage (WUENIC) – Nigeria Country Summary. Geneva, New York: WHO/UNICEF 2024.

[2] Federal Ministry of Health and Social Welfare of Nigeria. (FMoHSW), National Population Commission (NPC) [Nigeria], and ICF. 2024. Nigeria Demographic and Health Survey 2023–24: Key Indicators Report. Abuja, Nigeria and Rockville, Maryland, USA: NPC and ICF.

[3] World Health Organisation. (2023). Closing immunisation gaps in Nigeria through a primary healthcare approach. Available from: https://www.who.int/about/accountability/results/who-result--report-2020-mtr/country-story/2023/strong-collaboration-for-better-health--closing-i-munization-gaps-in-nigeria-through-a-primary-health-care-approach

[4] UNICEF. State of the World's Children 2023: Immunisation. New York: UNICEF 2023.

[5] Jegede AS. What led to the Nigerian boycott of the polio vaccination campaign? PLoS Med 2007; 4(3): e73.
[http://dx.doi.org/10.1371/journal.pmed.0040073] [PMID: 17388657]

[6] Mohammed Y, Reynolds HW, Waziri H, *et al.* Exploring the landscape of routine immunization in Nigeria: A scoping review of barriers and facilitators. Vaccine X 2024; 20: 100563.

[http://dx.doi.org/10.1016/j.jvacx.2024.100563] [PMID: 39430738]

[7] Okwaraji YB, Cousens S, Berhane Y, Mulholland K, Edmond K. Effect of geographical access to health facilities on child mortality in rural Ethiopia: a community based cross sectional study. PLoS One 2012; 7(3): e33564.
[http://dx.doi.org/10.1371/journal.pone.0033564] [PMID: 22428070]

[8] Lydon P, Beyai PL, Chaudhri I, Cakmak N, Satoulou A, Dumolard L. Government financing for health and specific national budget lines: The case of vaccines and immunization. Vaccine 2008; 26(51): 6727-34.
[http://dx.doi.org/10.1016/j.vaccine.2008.06.090] [PMID: 18625279]

[9] GAVI, The Vaccine Alliance. Zero-dose children and missed communities. Retrieved from the GAVI website, 2021.

[10] Ingle EA, Shrestha P, Seth A, Lalika MS, Azie JI, Patel RC. Interventions to vaccinate zero-dose children: A narrative review and synthesis. Viruses 2023; 15(10): 2092.
[http://dx.doi.org/10.3390/v15102092] [PMID: 37896868]

[11] WHO and UNICEF. (2023). Nigeria Estimates of Immunisation Coverage. Available from: https://cdn.who.int/media/docs/default-source/country-profiles/immunization/2024-coun-ry-profiles/immunization-2024-nga.pdf?download=true&sfvrsn=dad4f722_3

[12] World Health Organisation. Early detection, assessment and response to acute public health events: Implementation of early warning and response with a focus on event-based surveillance. Geneva: WHO 2020.

[13] NCDC. National Action Plan for Health Security (NAPHS) 2018-2022. Abuja: NCDC 2018.

[14] Lee LM, Teutsch SM, Thacker SB, St. Louis ME. Principles and Practice of Public Health Surveillance. Oxford: Oxford University Press 2010.
[http://dx.doi.org/10.1093/acprof:oso/9780195372922.001.0001]

[15] NCDC. Integrated Disease Surveillance and Response (IDSR) Annual Bulletin. Abuja: NCDC 2023.

[16] World Health Organisation. (2023). Immunisation Agenda 2030: A Global Strategy to Leave No One Behind. Geneva.

[17] GAVI, the Vaccine Alliance. (2023). Zero-Dose Learning Hub: Nigeria Country Progress Brief. Geneva.

[18] World Health Organisation. Integrated health services. Geneva 2018.

[19] Ophori EA, Tula MY, Azih AV, Okojie R, Ikpo PE. Current trends of immunization in Nigeria: prospect and challenges. Trop Med Health 2014; 42(2): 67-75.
[http://dx.doi.org/10.2149/tmh.2013-13] [PMID: 25237283]

[20] Wallace A, Dietz V, Cairns KL. Integration of immunization services with other health interventions in the developing world: what works and why? Systematic literature review. Trop Med Int Health 2009; 14(1): 11-9.
[http://dx.doi.org/10.1111/j.1365-3156.2008.02196.x] [PMID: 19017307]

[21] PAHO. Maternal and Neonatal Immunisation Field Guide for Latin America and the Caribbean. Washington, D.C. 2017.

[22] John TJ, Samuel R. Herd immunity and herd effect: new insights and definitions. Eur J Epidemiol 2000; 16(7): 601-6.
[http://dx.doi.org/10.1023/A:1007626510002] [PMID: 11078115]

[23] Duclos P. A global perspective on vaccine safety. Vaccine 2004; 22(15-16): 2059-63.
[http://dx.doi.org/10.1016/j.vaccine.2004.01.010] [PMID: 15121323]

[24] Nasir UN, Bandyopadhyay AS, Montagnani F, *et al.* Polio elimination in Nigeria: A review. Hum Vaccin Immunother 2016; 12(3): 658-63.

[http://dx.doi.org/10.1080/21645515.2015.1088617] [PMID: 26383769]

[25] Saleh J-EA. Resilient Communities: Navigating Public Health Challenges in Developing Nations. Bentham Science Publishers 2025.
[http://dx.doi.org/10.2174/97898153056091250101]

CHAPTER 8

Tackling Corruption and Improving Accountability in Public Health

Abstract: Corruption within the public health sector is a significant barrier to achieving equitable and effective healthcare, particularly in developing nations like Nigeria. This chapter examines the pervasive impact of corruption on health outcomes, demonstrating how misallocation of resources, embezzlement, and lack of transparency compromise the delivery of essential health services. The chapter explores the importance of transparency in health budgets and expenditures as a critical measure to combat corruption, highlighting the need for robust monitoring and evaluation systems to ensure accountability. Additionally, the role of civil society and community participation in health governance is discussed as a means of strengthening public oversight and enhancing accountability mechanisms. The chapter also delves into the legal and institutional frameworks necessary to combat corruption in the health sector, offering case studies of successful anti-corruption initiatives that provide valuable lessons for other contexts. Ultimately, this chapter underscores the urgent need for comprehensive reforms to tackle corruption and build a more accountable and transparent public health system in Nigeria and other developing nations.

Keywords: Anti-corruption initiatives, Accountability, Civil society participation, Corruption, Health governance, Legal frameworks, Monitoring and evaluation, Nigeria, Public health, Transparency.

INTRODUCTION

Corruption is a pervasive challenge in many sectors, and public health is no exception. It undermines the efficiency of health systems, distorts health priorities, and ultimately compromises the delivery of essential services. In developing nations, where resources are already limited, corruption exacerbates inequalities, disproportionately affecting the most vulnerable populations. In the health sector, it undermines service delivery by diverting scarce resources and eroding public trust. The WHO estimates that, globally, up to US$500 billion of health spending is lost annually to inefficiencies and corrupt practices, equivalent to 6–7 per cent of total health expenditure [1, 2].

Jalal-Eddeen Abubakar Saleh

The term 'Corruption' could be referred to as the misuse of entrusted power for personal gain, and one of the ways to checkmate corruption in the health sector is by institutionalising 'Transparency' and 'Accountability.' The term 'Transparency' refers to the openness and accessibility of information, whereas 'Accountability' refers to the obligation of public officials to justify actions and accept responsibility [1 - 3]. The impact in Nigeria and other Low- and Middle-Income Countries (LMICs) is even severe, translating into preventable deaths, stockouts of drugs and other hospital consumables, and persistent under-performance of public health programmes. It is important to note that corruption in the health sector occurs at multiple levels. It is best understood through clear typologies, allowing targeted prevention and accountability mechanisms.

This chapter explores the multifaceted impact of corruption on health outcomes, highlighting the urgent need for transparency, accountability, and robust governance structures in the public health sector.

THE IMPACT OF CORRUPTION ON HEALTH OUTCOMES

Corruption is a pervasive issue that undermines the effectiveness of public health systems worldwide, particularly in developing nations like Nigeria. It diverts scarce resources, erodes trust in public institutions, and exacerbates health inequalities, ultimately leading to poorer health outcomes. Understanding the impact of corruption on health is crucial for devising strategies to combat it and improve public health [4 - 6].

Table **1** identifies major areas within the health system where corruption risks are most prevalent: procurement, human resources, service delivery, and financing. By mapping specific vulnerabilities, such as bribery during drug procurement or ghost workers on payrolls, the table helps illuminate how systemic inefficiencies are perpetuated by unethical practices. Each corruption point is linked to tangible impacts, like drug shortages or the collapse of patient trust. This clear mapping of corruption risks serves as a foundation for targeted reforms and policy responses. It advocates for greater transparency, robust oversight, and institutional checks across vulnerable functions. Furthermore, it positions anti-corruption as a health issue, not merely an administrative one, by illustrating how corrupt practices directly undermine service quality, financial integrity, and ultimately, population health outcomes.

Resource Diversion and Its Consequences

Corruption often leads to the misallocation and diversion of resources intended for healthcare, severely hampering the delivery of essential services. This diversion can occur at multiple levels, from the misappropriation of funds by high-level officials to the theft of medical supplies by lower-level staff. These dire consequences include [4]:

Table 1. Corruption risk points in the health system.

Health System Component	Corruption Risk	Potential Impact
Procurement	Bribery, overpricing	Shortage of drugs and supplies
Human Resources	Ghost workers, favoritism	Inefficiency, low morale
Service Delivery	Informal payments	Reduced access, inequity
Finance	Misallocation of funds	Program failure, underfunding

1. **Reduced Access to Care:** When funds allocated for health infrastructure, equipment, and medicines are siphoned off, the availability and quality of healthcare services diminish. This can result in the closure of health facilities, shortages of essential drugs, and the deterioration of healthcare infrastructure, leaving communities, particularly the most vulnerable, with limited or no access to care.
2. **Increased Out-of-Pocket Costs:** Corruption often forces patients to pay out-of-pocket for services and medications that should be free or subsidised. These illegal payments, often in the form of bribes, disproportionately affect the poor, who may be unable to afford care, leading to delayed treatment, worsening of conditions, or even death.
3. **Wastage and Inefficiency:** Corruption fosters inefficiency within the health system, as funds are diverted from their intended purposes. This inefficiency results in the wastage of resources, such as the procurement of substandard or unnecessary medical supplies, and contributes to a lack of accountability in the management of public health funds.

Erosion of Trust in Public Institutions

Corruption undermines public trust in health systems and institutions, a critical component of effective healthcare delivery. When people perceive the health system as corrupt, they are less likely to seek care, follow medical advice, or participate in public health initiatives, such as immunisation campaigns [4].

1. **Distrust in Healthcare Providers:** When corruption is rampant, patients may lose trust in healthcare providers, fearing that their care is compromised by the providers' pursuit of illicit gains. This distrust can lead to reluctance in seeking care, self-medication, or turning to unqualified practitioners, all of which can have detrimental effects on health outcomes.

2. **Undermining Public Health Programs:** Corruption can sabotage public health programs, such as vaccination campaigns or disease prevention initiatives, by fostering scepticism and resistance among the population. If people believe that these programs are driven by corrupt motives rather than public interest, they may refuse to participate, undermining efforts to control and eradicate diseases.
3. **Weakening Health Governance:** Corruption weakens the governance structures that are essential for an effective health system. It erodes the rule of law, making it difficult to enforce regulations, monitor health services, and hold individuals accountable for malpractice. This lack of accountability creates an environment where corruption can flourish, further deteriorating the health system.

Exacerbation of Health Inequalities

Corruption disproportionately affects marginalised and vulnerable populations, exacerbating existing health inequalities. These groups are often the most reliant on public health services and the least able to afford private alternatives, making them more vulnerable to the adverse effects of corruption [4, 5].

1. **Unequal Access to Services:** In corrupt systems, those with financial means or connections may gain preferential access to healthcare services, while the poor and marginalised are left with inadequate or no care. This creates a two-tiered health system, where the quality of care depends on one's ability to pay or influence, deepening social and health disparities.
2. **Geographic Disparities:** Corruption can lead to geographic disparities in health service delivery, with rural and remote areas often being the most neglected. Resources intended for these regions may be diverted to urban centres or embezzled, leaving rural populations without essential healthcare services and contributing to higher morbidity and mortality rates in these areas.
3. **Vulnerability of Specific Populations:** Specific populations, such as women, children, and people with disabilities, are particularly vulnerable to the impacts of corruption in health services. For example, corruption in maternal and child health programs can lead to higher maternal and infant mortality rates, while people with disabilities may face additional barriers in accessing the care they need.

Implications for Health Outcomes

The overall impact of corruption on health outcomes is profound and far-reaching. Corruption not only directly harms individuals by limiting access to necessary healthcare services but also weakens the entire health system, making it less resilient to crises and less capable of meeting the population's health needs [4 - 6].

1. **Higher Disease Burden:** Corruption contributes to a higher burden of disease, as it impedes efforts to prevent and control communicable and non-communicable diseases. For instance, corruption in vaccine procurement or distribution can lead to lower immunisation coverage, resulting in outbreaks of preventable diseases. Similarly, corruption in health campaigns can hinder the fight against diseases like HIV/AIDS, tuberculosis, and malaria.
2. **Poor Health Outcomes:** The inefficiencies and inequities caused by corruption directly translate into poorer health outcomes. These include higher mortality and morbidity rates, lower life expectancy, and an overall decline in the population's health. The impact is particularly severe in low- and middle-income countries, where health systems are already strained by limited resources.
3. **Economic Costs:** The economic costs of corruption in health are substantial. Corruption not only leads to waste of financial resources but also imposes high costs on individuals and families, who may face catastrophic health expenditures due to bribes or out-of-pocket payments. Additionally, poor health outcomes linked to corruption can reduce productivity and economic growth, creating a vicious cycle of poverty and poor health.

CONCLUSION

The impact of corruption on health outcomes is a critical issue that must be addressed to improve public health in Nigeria and other developing nations. By diverting resources, eroding trust, exacerbating inequalities, and weakening health systems, corruption poses a significant barrier to achieving universal health coverage and improving health outcomes. Tackling corruption in the health sector is not just a matter of governance; it is a matter of life and death for millions of people. The following sections will explore strategies to combat corruption and improve accountability in public health to build a more equitable and effective health system for all.

TRANSPARENCY IN HEALTH BUDGETS AND EXPENDITURES

Transparency in health budgets and expenditures is a fundamental pillar of good governance and a critical element in combating corruption within the public health sector. Ensuring that health budgets are transparent and expenditures are effectively monitored not only promotes accountability but also enhances the efficient use of resources, leading to better health outcomes. This section explores the importance of transparency in health financing, the challenges in achieving it, and strategies for fostering greater openness and accountability in the management of health funds [7 - 9].

The Importance of Transparency in Health Financing

Transparency in health financing is essential for several reasons, all of which contribute to the overall effectiveness and sustainability of health systems. Some of these include [7]:

1. **Accountability and Trust:** Transparent budgeting and expenditure processes help build public trust in health systems and government institutions. When citizens can see how health funds are allocated and spent, they are more likely to trust that resources are being used effectively and for their intended purposes. This trust is crucial for encouraging public participation in health programs and fostering a sense of ownership among the community.
2. **Efficient Resource Allocation:** Transparency ensures that resources are allocated based on need and effectiveness, rather than political influence or corruption. By making budgetary decisions open to scrutiny, health systems can prioritize spending on the most critical areas, such as primary healthcare, immunization programs, and disease prevention. This leads to more efficient use of limited resources and better health outcomes.
3. **Reducing Corruption:** Transparent budgeting and spending processes are powerful tools in the fight against corruption. When health budgets and expenditures are open to public scrutiny, it becomes more difficult for officials to engage in corrupt practices, such as embezzlement or the misallocation of funds. Transparency acts as a deterrent, reducing opportunities for corruption and ensuring that health resources reach their intended targets.
4. **Enhancing Donor Confidence:** In many developing countries, a significant portion of health funding comes from international donors. Transparency in how these funds are managed and spent is essential for maintaining donor confidence. Donors are more likely to continue supporting health programs if they can see that their contributions are being used effectively and transparently. This sustained funding is crucial for the long-term success of health initiatives.

Challenges to Achieving Transparency

While the benefits of transparency in health budgets and expenditures are clear, achieving it is often fraught with challenges, particularly in developing nations. The following challenges are worth noting [7]:

1. **Weak Institutional Frameworks:** Many developing countries lack the robust institutional frameworks necessary for enforcing transparency in health financing. Weak financial management systems, limited oversight mechanisms, and insufficient regulatory frameworks can all contribute to a lack of transparency. In such environments, it is difficult to track how health funds are allocated and spent, creating opportunities for corruption and mismanagement.
2. **Political Resistance:** Transparency often faces resistance from political elites who benefit from opaque financial systems. In some cases, powerful individuals or groups may have vested interests in maintaining the status quo, as it allows them to control the flow of resources and engage in corrupt practices. Overcoming this resistance requires strong political will and a commitment to reform.
3. **Limited Public Awareness and Engagement:** In many settings, the public is not adequately informed about how health budgets and expenditures are managed, and there may be limited opportunities for citizen engagement. Without public awareness and participation, there is little pressure on governments to be transparent, and corruption can continue unchecked. Educating the public about the importance of transparency and providing mechanisms for their involvement are essential steps in addressing this challenge.
4. **Inadequate Technology and Infrastructure:** The lack of technological infrastructure can also hinder transparency efforts. In many developing countries, financial records are still maintained manually, making it difficult to track and report expenditures accurately. The absence of modern financial management systems and digital tools can lead to inefficiencies, errors, and opportunities for corruption.

Strategies for Promoting Transparency

To overcome these challenges and promote transparency in health budgets and expenditures, several strategies can be implemented, each contributing to a more open and accountable health financing system. Some of these strategies include [7, 8]:

1. **Strengthening Financial Management Systems:** Developing and implementing robust financial management systems is a critical step towards achieving transparency. These systems should include clear procedures for budget preparation, approval, and execution, as well as mechanisms for monitoring and reporting expenditures. Investing in digital financial management tools can enhance accuracy, reduce errors, and provide real-time data on health spending.

2. **Enhancing Legislative Oversight:** Strengthening the role of legislative bodies in overseeing health budgets and expenditures is essential for promoting transparency. Parliaments and local councils should have the authority to review and approve health budgets, monitor expenditures, and hold the executive branch accountable for any discrepancies. This oversight can be further supported by independent audit institutions that conduct regular reviews of health finances.
3. **Increasing Public Participation and Engagement:** Engaging the public in the budgeting process is crucial for enhancing transparency and accountability. Governments can create platforms for citizen participation, such as public hearings, community consultations, and online forums, where people can provide input on budget priorities and monitor expenditures. Public access to information, including detailed reports on health budgets and spending, should be guaranteed by law.
4. **Implementing Open Budget Initiatives:** Open Budget Initiatives (OBIs) are programs designed to increase the transparency of government budgets by making budget information publicly available in an accessible format. These initiatives typically involve publishing detailed budget documents online, including planned and actual expenditures, and providing tools for citizens to track and analyse this data. OBIs have been successful in several countries, leading to greater accountability and reduced corruption in public spending.
5. **Fostering Collaboration with Civil Society Organisations (CSOs):** Civil society organisations play a vital role in promoting transparency and holding governments accountable for their spending. CSOs can conduct independent budget analyses, advocate for greater transparency, and educate the public on how to monitor health expenditures. Governments should collaborate with CSOs by providing them with access to budget information and involving them in the budgetary process.
6. **Leveraging Technology for Transparency:** Modern technology offers numerous tools that can enhance transparency in health budgets and expenditures. For example, e-procurement systems can be used to ensure that the procurement of health supplies is conducted transparently and competitively. Mobile applications and online platforms can be developed to allow citizens to report corruption and monitor health spending in real-time. The use of blockchain technology is also being explored as a way to create tamper-proof records of financial transactions, further reducing opportunities for corruption.

The Role of International Organisations

International organisations can play a crucial role in promoting transparency in health budgets and expenditures in developing countries. These organisations can provide technical assistance, funding, and expertise to help governments build capacity for transparent financial management. They can also promote best practices, set global standards for transparency, and hold governments accountable for their commitments [7 - 9].

1. **Technical Assistance and Capacity Building:** Organisations such as the World Health Organisation (WHO), the World Bank, and the International Monetary Fund (IMF) can provide technical assistance to help countries strengthen their financial management systems and implement transparency measures. This support can include training for government officials, the development of digital tools, and the establishment of monitoring and evaluation frameworks.
2. **Promoting Global Standards:** International organisations can set global standards for transparency in health financing, encouraging countries to adopt best practices and align with international norms. For example, the Open Government Partnership (OGP) promotes transparency, accountability, and citizen participation in governance, including in the management of public finances. By adhering to these standards, countries can improve their transparency and attract more investment and support from the international community.
3. **Monitoring and Accountability:** International organisations can also play a role in monitoring how countries manage their health budgets and expenditures, holding governments accountable for any lapses in transparency. Through mechanisms such as peer reviews, country assessments, and public reporting, these organisations can help ensure that governments remain committed to transparent financial practices.

CONCLUSION

Transparency in health budgets and expenditures is essential for building accountable and effective health systems. It not only reduces corruption and enhances trust in public institutions but also ensures that resources are used efficiently to improve health outcomes. While achieving transparency poses significant challenges, particularly in developing countries, these challenges can be overcome through a combination of strong institutional frameworks, public engagement, and the strategic use of technology. By fostering transparency, Nigeria and other developing nations can create more equitable and resilient health systems, ultimately contributing to better health and well-being for all citizens.

MONITORING AND EVALUATION IN HEALTH PROGRAMS

Monitoring and evaluation (M&E) are critical components of effective health programs, ensuring that initiatives achieve their intended outcomes and that resources are used efficiently. M&E provides the data needed to assess progress, identify challenges, and make informed decisions to improve program effectiveness [10].

It is worth noting that corruption in the health sector is not anecdotal but measurable and systemic. A few examples to buttress this fact are looking at some audit findings to help the reader understand the gravity. In Nigeria's Auditor-General report of 2023, there are irregular expenditures uncovered totalling ₦ 6.8 billion across federal health institutions between 2020–2022, including unretired advances and non-compliant procurements [11 - 13].

Similarly, the analyses of the Public Procurement Bureau (2022) revealed that in the absence of competitive bidding, there was an average inflation cost of 25–35% in selected hospital equipment procurements. In another example, the Health Facility Monitoring & Accreditation Agency (HEFAMAA) spot checks in Lagos State (2021) found that 12% of sampled facilities were dispensing expired medicines, a pointer to poor regulatory oversight [11 - 15].

This section explores the importance of M&E in health programs, the challenges involved, and strategies for strengthening M&E systems in Nigeria and other developing nations [10, 16, 17].

The Importance of Monitoring and Evaluation

Monitoring and evaluation serve several essential functions in health programs, contributing to better health outcomes and more efficient use of resources. The importance of M&E includes [10]:

1. **Accountability and Transparency:** M&E systems promote accountability by providing a transparent record of how resources are used and what results are achieved. By regularly tracking progress and outcomes, M&E ensures that health programs are held accountable to stakeholders, including government agencies, donors, and the public. This transparency builds trust and confidence in the health system.
2. **Data-Driven Decision-Making:** Effective M&E systems generate reliable data that can be used to guide decision-making at all levels of the health system. By analysing data on program performance, health officials can identify what works, what doesn't, and why. This evidence-based approach allows for the

timely adjustment of strategies, policies, and interventions to improve program outcomes.

3. **Enhancing Program Effectiveness:** M&E helps to identify strengths and weaknesses in health programs, allowing for continuous improvement. By regularly assessing program implementation and outcomes, M&E provides the feedback needed to refine interventions, optimise resource allocation, and maximise impact. This process of continuous learning is essential for adapting to changing circumstances and ensuring that health programs remain effective over time.
4. **Measuring Impact and Sustainability:** Evaluating the impact of health programs is crucial for understanding their long-term effects on health outcomes. M&E systems provide the tools to assess whether programs are achieving their intended goals and contributing to sustainable improvements in public health. This information is vital for scaling successful interventions and ensuring that health programs have a lasting impact.

Challenges in Monitoring and Evaluation

Despite its importance, implementing effective M&E systems in health programs can be challenging, particularly in developing countries. Some of the challenges include [10]:

1. **Limited Resources and Capacity:** One of the primary challenges in M&E is the lack of resources and capacity. Many health programs in developing countries operate with limited funding, and M&E activities are often underfunded or overlooked. Additionally, there may be a shortage of trained personnel with the skills needed to design, implement, and analyse M&E systems, leading to gaps in data collection and reporting.
2. **Inadequate Data Collection Systems:** Reliable data is the foundation of effective M&E, but in many developing countries, data collection systems are inadequate. Health information systems may be fragmented, outdated, or lacking in coverage, resulting in incomplete or inaccurate data. This makes it difficult to monitor program progress or evaluate outcomes effectively. Furthermore, the lack of standardized data collection methods can lead to inconsistencies and reduce the comparability of data across different programs or regions.
3. **Political and Institutional Barriers:** Political and institutional barriers can also hinder effective M&E. In some cases, there may be resistance to M&E efforts due to fears that negative findings could lead to reduced funding or damage reputations. Additionally, weak institutional frameworks and poor governance can limit the effectiveness of M&E activities. Without strong

political support and institutional commitment, M&E systems may be underutilised or ignored.

4. **Lack of Stakeholder Engagement:** Effective M&E requires the active involvement of all stakeholders, including government agencies, health workers, donors, and the communities served by health programs. However, in many cases, there is limited engagement of these stakeholders in M&E activities. This can lead to a lack of ownership, reduced buy-in, and missed opportunities for learning and improvement. Ensuring that all relevant stakeholders are involved in the M&E process is essential for its success.

Strategies for Strengthening Monitoring and Evaluation

To overcome these challenges and enhance the effectiveness of M&E systems in health programs, several strategies can be implemented. Some of these strategies include [10, 16]:

1. **Building Capacity for M&E:** Investing in capacity building for M&E is crucial for improving the quality and effectiveness of these systems. This includes training health workers, program managers, and data analysts in M&E methods, data collection, and analysis. Strengthening the capacity of institutions responsible for M&E, such as health ministries and research organizations, is also essential. Capacity-building efforts should focus on developing the skills and knowledge needed to design, implement, and use M&E systems effectively.
2. **Enhancing Health Information Systems:** Improving health information systems is vital for collecting reliable data needed for M&E. This includes modernizing data collection methods, integrating different data sources, and ensuring that data systems are interoperable and scalable. Investing in digital health technologies, such as electronic health records and mobile data collection tools, can enhance data accuracy, timeliness, and accessibility. Strengthening the infrastructure for data management, storage, and analysis is also critical for supporting M&E activities.
3. **Promoting a Culture of Learning and Improvement:** Encouraging a culture of learning and improvement within health programs is essential for the success of M&E. This involves fostering an environment where data is valued and used to inform decision-making, rather than being seen as a burden or threat. Health officials and program managers should be encouraged to view M&E as a tool for learning and continuous improvement, rather than as a punitive measure. This mindset shift can help to overcome resistance to M&E and promote the use of data for program enhancement.
4. **Engaging Stakeholders in M&E:** Engaging stakeholders in the M&E process is essential for ensuring its relevance and effectiveness. This includes involving

communities, health workers, and program beneficiaries in the design and implementation of M&E activities. Stakeholder engagement can be facilitated through participatory approaches, such as community-based monitoring and feedback mechanisms. By involving stakeholders in M&E, programs can ensure that the data collected is meaningful, the findings are actionable, and the process fosters a sense of ownership and accountability.

5. **Ensuring Political and Institutional Support:** Strong political and institutional support is critical for the success of M&E systems. Governments and health ministries must prioritize M&E in their health policies and allocate sufficient resources for its implementation. This includes establishing clear guidelines, standards, and frameworks for M&E and ensuring that these are enforced. Additionally, fostering partnerships with international organisations, donors, and academic institutions can provide the technical and financial support needed to strengthen M&E systems.
6. **Leveraging Technology for M&E:** The use of technology can significantly enhance M&E systems by improving data collection, analysis, and reporting. Digital tools, such as mobile health applications, online dashboards, and Geographic Information Systems (GIS), can facilitate real-time data collection and provide visualisations that make it easier to track program progress. Technology can also be used to automate routine M&E tasks, reduce human error, and improve data accuracy. By embracing technological innovations, health programs can make M&E more efficient, effective, and accessible.

The Role of International Partners in Strengthening M&E

International partners, including donors, non-governmental organisations (NGOs), and multilateral agencies, play a crucial role in supporting M&E efforts in developing countries. Some of these roles include [16, 17]:

1. **Providing Technical Assistance:** International partners can offer technical assistance to help countries build and strengthen their M&E systems. This includes providing expertise in M&E design, data collection methods, and analysis techniques. Technical assistance can also involve training programs, workshops, and mentorship opportunities to build local capacity for M&E.
2. **Supporting Funding and Resource Mobilisation:** Financial support from international partners is often critical for the establishment and maintenance of robust M&E systems. Donors can provide funding for M&E activities, including the development of health information systems, training programs, and data collection tools. Additionally, international partners can help mobilize resources by advocating for the inclusion of M&E in health program budgets and policies.

3. **Facilitating Knowledge Sharing and Collaboration:** International partners can facilitate knowledge sharing and collaboration between countries, helping to spread best practices and lessons learned in M&E. This can be achieved through regional networks, online platforms, and international conferences that bring together M&E practitioners, policymakers, and researchers. By promoting cross-country learning and collaboration, international partners can help countries overcome common challenges and improve the effectiveness of their M&E systems.
4. **Promoting Global Standards and Best Practices:** International organizations, such as the World Health Organization (WHO) and the Global Fund, can play a key role in setting global standards and promoting best practices in M&E. These organizations can guide M&E frameworks, indicators, and methodologies, helping countries align their M&E systems with international standards. By adhering to these standards, countries can improve the comparability and reliability of their M&E data, facilitating global efforts to monitor and evaluate health programs.

CONCLUSION

Monitoring and evaluation are essential components of effective health programs, providing the data and insights needed to improve program outcomes and ensure accountability. Despite the challenges involved, strengthening M&E systems is crucial for achieving better health outcomes in Nigeria and other developing nations. By building capacity, enhancing data collection systems, promoting stakeholder engagement, and leveraging technology, health programs can develop robust M&E systems that support data-driven decision-making and continuous improvement. International partners also have a vital role to play in providing technical assistance, funding, and support for knowledge sharing. By prioritizing M&E, countries can ensure that their health programs are effective, accountable, and capable of delivering sustainable improvements in public health.

CIVIL SOCIETY AND COMMUNITY PARTICIPATION IN HEALTH GOVERNANCE

Civil society and community participation are essential components of effective health governance. Involving communities and civil society organisations (CSOs) in the design, implementation, and monitoring of health programs ensures that these initiatives are more responsive to the needs of the population, promote transparency, and foster accountability.

This section explores the critical role that civil society and communities play in health governance, the challenges they face, and strategies to enhance their participation in Nigeria and other developing nations [18 - 20].

The Role of Civil Society in Health Governance

Civil society organisations, including non-governmental organisations (NGOs), faith-based organisations (FBOs), professional associations, and advocacy groups, play a vital role in health governance. Their involvement is crucial for several reasons [18]:

1. **Advocacy and Policy Influence:** CSOs are instrumental in advocating for policies that prioritise public health and address the needs of marginalised populations. They serve as a bridge between communities and policymakers, amplifying the voices of those who may otherwise be unheard. By engaging in policy dialogue, CSOs can influence the development of health policies that are equitable, inclusive, and aligned with the needs of the population.
2. **Accountability and Oversight:** CSOs often act as watchdogs, holding governments and health institutions accountable for their actions. By monitoring the implementation of health programs and expenditures, CSOs help ensure that resources are used effectively and that services reach those who need them most. This oversight role is crucial for preventing corruption, improving service delivery, and fostering transparency in health governance.
3. **Service Delivery and Capacity Building:** In many developing countries, CSOs are directly involved in delivering health services, particularly in underserved areas where government presence may be limited. They often provide essential services such as immunization, maternal and child health care, and HIV/AIDS prevention and treatment. Additionally, CSOs play a significant role in capacity building, training health workers, and empowering communities to take charge of their health.
4. **Promoting Community Engagement:** CSOs are key players in promoting community engagement in health governance. By organising and mobilising communities, CSOs encourage participation in decision-making processes, ensuring that health programs are more attuned to the specific needs and preferences of the people they serve. This grassroots involvement is essential for creating health systems that are responsive and inclusive.

Community Participation in Health Governance

Community participation is fundamental to achieving effective and sustainable health governance. When communities are actively involved in the planning, implementation, and monitoring of health programs, the outcomes are more likely to be positive and long-lasting [18, 19].

1. **Empowering Communities:** Empowering communities to take an active role in health governance involves building their capacity to participate in decision-making processes. This includes providing education and training on health issues, rights, and governance structures. Empowered communities are better equipped to advocate for their needs, demand accountability, and contribute to the design and implementation of health programs.
2. **Participatory Planning and Decision-Making:** Involving communities in the planning and decision-making stages of health programs ensures that these initiatives are more relevant and effective. Participatory approaches, such as community health committees or participatory rural appraisal (PRA) techniques, allow communities to express their needs, set priorities, and contribute to the design of interventions. This collaborative approach leads to programs that are better suited to local contexts and more likely to be accepted and supported by the community.
3. **Monitoring and Feedback Mechanisms:** Community participation in monitoring and evaluation is critical for ensuring that health programs are responsive and accountable. Establishing feedback mechanisms, such as community scorecards or citizen report cards, allows communities to assess the quality of health services, provide input on their experiences, and hold service providers accountable. This feedback is invaluable for identifying areas for improvement and ensuring that health programs meet the needs of the population.
4. **Strengthening Social Accountability:** Social accountability mechanisms, such as public hearings, community audits, and social audits, are effective tools for involving communities in health governance. These mechanisms enable communities to scrutinise health programs, budgets, and expenditures, ensuring that resources are used efficiently and transparently. Strengthening social accountability fosters a sense of ownership among community members and encourages them to actively participate in the governance of health services.

Challenges to Civil Society and Community Participation

Despite the critical role of civil society and community participation in health governance, several challenges hinder their effective involvement. Some of these include [18 - 20]:

1. **Limited Resources and Capacity:** Many CSOs and community groups operate with limited resources and capacity, which can constrain their ability to participate meaningfully in health governance. This includes financial limitations, a lack of technical expertise, and insufficient access to information. Without adequate support, these organisations may struggle to engage in advocacy, service delivery, or monitoring activities effectively.

2. **Political and Institutional Barriers:** Political and institutional barriers can also impede civil society and community participation. In some contexts, governments may be reluctant to involve CSOs and communities in health governance, fearing criticism or loss of control. Additionally, weak institutional frameworks and bureaucratic hurdles can limit opportunities for participation and reduce the effectiveness of CSOs and community involvement.
3. **Social and Cultural Constraints:** Social and cultural factors can also pose challenges to community participation in health governance. In some societies, hierarchical structures, gender norms, and power dynamics may limit the ability of certain groups, such as women or marginalised communities, to participate in decision-making processes. Overcoming these barriers requires targeted efforts to promote inclusivity and ensure that all voices are heard.
4. **Lack of Coordination and Collaboration:** The lack of coordination and collaboration between CSOs, communities, and government agencies can weaken the impact of participation efforts. When actors work in silos, opportunities for synergy and collective action are missed, reducing the effectiveness of health programs. Strengthening partnerships and fostering collaboration is essential for maximising the contributions of civil society and communities to health governance.

Strategies for Enhancing Civil Society and Community Participation

To overcome these challenges and enhance the role of civil society and community participation in health governance, several strategies can be implemented, including [18 - 20]:

1. **Strengthening Capacity and Resources:** Investing in the capacity and resources of CSOs and community groups is crucial for enabling effective participation in health governance. This includes providing financial support, technical training, and access to information and technology. Capacity-building efforts should focus on enhancing skills in advocacy, service delivery, monitoring, and evaluation, ensuring that these organisations can contribute meaningfully to health governance.
2. **Promoting Enabling Environments:** Creating an enabling environment for civil society and community participation involves addressing political and institutional barriers to involvement. Governments should establish legal and policy frameworks that support the participation of CSOs and communities in health governance, including mechanisms for consultation, representation, and feedback. Additionally, efforts should be made to reduce bureaucratic hurdles and promote a culture of openness and collaboration.
3. **Ensuring Inclusivity and Equity:** Ensuring that participation is inclusive and equitable requires targeted efforts to engage marginalized groups, such as

women, youth, and ethnic minorities, in health governance. This can be achieved through targeted outreach, capacity-building programs, and the establishment of inclusive decision-making bodies. Promoting gender equity and social inclusion is essential for ensuring that all members of the community have a voice in health governance.

4. **Fostering Partnerships and Collaboration:** Strengthening partnerships and collaboration between CSOs, communities, and government agencies is essential for enhancing the effectiveness of participation efforts. Multi-stakeholder platforms, such as health forums or coalitions, can facilitate dialogue, coordination, and joint action. By working together, actors can pool resources, share knowledge, and leverage their respective strengths to achieve better health outcomes.
5. **Leveraging Technology for Participation:** The use of technology can enhance civil society and community participation in health governance by improving access to information, facilitating communication, and enabling virtual participation. Digital platforms, such as social media, online forums, and mobile applications, can provide new avenues for engagement, particularly in remote or underserved areas. Technology can also be used to collect and disseminate data, allowing communities to monitor health programs and hold service providers accountable.
6. **Supporting Advocacy and Social Mobilisation:** Supporting advocacy and social mobilisation efforts is crucial for empowering civil society and communities to influence health governance. This includes funding advocacy campaigns, supporting grassroots movements, and providing platforms for dialogue and debate. Advocacy efforts should focus on raising awareness of health issues, promoting policy change, and ensuring that the voices of communities are heard at all levels of decision-making.

The Role of International Partners in Supporting Participation

International partners, including donors, NGOs, and multilateral agencies, play a vital role in supporting civil society and community participation in health governance. Some of these roles include [19, 20]:

1. **Providing Financial and Technical Support:** International partners can provide financial and technical support to strengthen the capacity of CSOs and community groups. This includes funding for capacity-building initiatives, technical assistance in advocacy and service delivery, and support for the development of participatory mechanisms. By investing in local organisations, international partners can help to build a strong and vibrant civil society that can effectively engage in health governance.

2. **Promoting Global Standards and Best Practices:** International organisations can promote global standards and best practices in civil society and community participation. This includes guiding participatory approaches, tools for community engagement, and frameworks for monitoring and evaluation. By aligning local participation efforts with international standards, countries can improve the quality and effectiveness of their health governance.
3. **Facilitating Knowledge Sharing and Collaboration:** International partners can facilitate knowledge sharing and collaboration between CSOs, communities, and governments. This includes supporting regional networks, online platforms, and international conferences that bring together stakeholders from different countries to share experiences, lessons learned, and best practices. By promoting cross-country learning and collaboration, international partners can help to strengthen civil society and community participation in health.

CONCLUSION

There is a wide range of mechanisms, piloted in Nigeria, as a way of addressing the issue of anti-corruption in the health sector. Some of these measures include 'Public Expenditure Tracking Surveys' (PETS) as one of the anti-corruption mechanisms to track public expenditure. This mechanism tracks budget allocations through the system to identify leakages. In Nigeria, PETS piloted by the World Bank and the Budget Office in 2019 found leakage rates of 22% in primary-care capital releases before reaching facilities [9 - 15].

Similarly, there is another anti-corruption mechanism, referred to as 'Open Contracting and E-Procurement.' In Nigeria, there is the **Nigeria Open Contracting Portal (NOCOPO)**, which mandates online publication of federal procurement data, including health tenders. However, this system at the sub-national level remains weak. Equally important to mention is the Performance-Based Financing (PBF), which has changed the narrative. It links facility funding to verified outputs and improves transparency through electronic disbursements and independent verification agents. The Digital Electronic Tools, especially the integration of the DHIS2 and GIFMIS (Government Integrated Financial Management Information System), allow cross-checking of expenditure with service outputs, enabling anomaly detection [9 - 15].

LEGAL AND INSTITUTIONAL FRAMEWORKS FOR COMBATING CORRUPTION

Effective legal and institutional frameworks are critical for combating corruption in public health. These frameworks establish the rules, regulations, and structures necessary to prevent, detect, and punish corrupt practices. By ensuring transparency, accountability, and integrity within the health system, they play a vital role in safeguarding public health resources and improving health outcomes. This section examines the key elements of legal and institutional frameworks for combating corruption in Nigeria and other developing nations, the challenges in implementing these frameworks, and strategies to strengthen them [21, 22].

Legal Frameworks for Anti-Corruption in Public Health

A robust legal framework is the foundation of any effort to combat corruption. It provides the legal basis for prosecuting corrupt practices, enforcing transparency, and ensuring accountability in the health sector [21, 22]. It is critical to note that sustained accountability in the health sector requires citizen voice. There are civil-society coalitions such as BudgIT, FollowTheMoney, and the Health Reform Foundation of Nigeria (HERFON) that conduct budget-tracking, data visualisation, and community audits. There are relevant laws and frameworks that the reader could refer to, and these include [23 - 27]:

- Public Procurement Act (2007)
- Fiscal Responsibility Act (2007)
- Freedom of Information Act (2011)
- Corrupt Practices and Other Related Offences Act (2000)
- Nigeria's Open Government Partnership National Action Plan (2023–2025).

1. **Anti-Corruption Laws and Regulations:** The existence of comprehensive anti-corruption laws and regulations is crucial for creating a legal environment that deters corruption. These laws should cover a wide range of corrupt practices, including bribery, embezzlement, fraud, and abuse of power. In Nigeria, laws such as the Corrupt Practices and Other Related Offences Act, the Public Procurement Act, and the Economic and Financial Crimes Commission (EFCC) Act provide the legal framework for addressing corruption in public health.
2. **Transparency and Accountability Laws:** Legal provisions that mandate transparency and accountability in government operations are essential for preventing corruption in the health sector. These laws often include requirements for public disclosure of health budgets, expenditures, and procurement processes. In Nigeria, the Freedom of Information (FOI) Act is a key legal tool that empowers citizens and civil society organizations to access information and hold public officials accountable.
3. **Whistleblower Protection Laws:** Protecting whistleblowers who expose corruption is critical for encouraging the reporting of corrupt practices. Whistleblower protection laws provide legal safeguards for individuals who

report corruption, ensuring that they are not subject to retaliation, harassment, or other negative consequences. Implementing strong whistleblower protection is essential for fostering a culture of transparency and accountability within the health system.

4. **Enforcement Mechanisms:** Legal frameworks must also include strong enforcement mechanisms to ensure that anti-corruption laws are effectively implemented. This includes the establishment of specialised anti-corruption agencies, the allocation of resources for investigations, and the empowerment of law enforcement agencies to prosecute corruption cases. In Nigeria, the EFCC and the Independent Corrupt Practices and Other Related Offences Commission (ICPC) are responsible for enforcing anti-corruption laws and investigating cases of corruption in the public sector.

Institutional Frameworks for Anti-Corruption in Public Health

In addition to legal frameworks, robust institutional frameworks are necessary to combat corruption effectively. These frameworks provide the organisational structures, policies, and processes that support anti-corruption efforts in the health sector [28, 29].

1. **Anti-Corruption Agencies and Bodies:** Specialised anti-corruption agencies and bodies play a central role in coordinating and implementing anti-corruption initiatives. These agencies are responsible for investigating corruption cases, enforcing anti-corruption laws, and promoting transparency and accountability within government institutions. In Nigeria, agencies such as the EFCC, ICPC, and the Code of Conduct Bureau (CCB) are tasked with addressing corruption in public institutions, including the health sector.
2. **Health Sector Regulatory Bodies:** Regulatory bodies within the health sector also have a critical role in preventing corruption. These institutions are responsible for overseeing the conduct of health professionals, regulating pharmaceutical companies, and ensuring compliance with health policies and standards. Strengthening the capacity and independence of regulatory bodies is essential for curbing corrupt practices, such as the misappropriation of health funds or the distribution of counterfeit medicines.
3. **Internal Audit and Compliance Units:** Internal audit and compliance units within health ministries and agencies are crucial for detecting and preventing corruption. These units conduct regular audits of health programs, budgets, and expenditures to ensure that resources are used appropriately and that financial irregularities are promptly addressed. Establishing robust internal audit mechanisms and ensuring their independence is vital for maintaining the integrity of health systems.

4. **Judicial and Law Enforcement Institutions:** An effective judiciary and law enforcement system are essential for prosecuting corruption cases and enforcing anti-corruption laws. These institutions must be independent, transparent, and free from political interference to function effectively. Strengthening the capacity of the judiciary to handle corruption cases, providing training for judges and prosecutors, and ensuring that law enforcement agencies have the necessary resources to investigate corruption are key components of an effective institutional framework.

Challenges in Implementing Anti-Corruption Frameworks

While legal and institutional frameworks are essential for combating corruption, their effectiveness is often undermined by various challenges [28, 29].

1. **Political Interference:** Political interference is a significant challenge in implementing anti-corruption frameworks. In many cases, political elites may seek to protect their interests by influencing anti-corruption agencies or the judiciary, undermining their independence and effectiveness. This interference can lead to selective enforcement of anti-corruption laws and hinder efforts to hold powerful individuals accountable.
2. **Limited Resources and Capacity:** Many anti-corruption institutions face constraints in terms of resources and capacity. Insufficient funding, inadequate staffing, and a lack of technical expertise can weaken the ability of these institutions to carry out their mandates effectively. This challenge is particularly pronounced in developing countries, where budgetary constraints and competing priorities may limit the resources available for anti-corruption efforts.
3. **Weak Enforcement of Laws:** The weak enforcement of anti-corruption laws is another significant challenge. Even when comprehensive legal frameworks are in place, the failure to enforce these laws consistently can create a culture of impunity. Factors contributing to weak enforcement include corruption within law enforcement agencies, bureaucratic inefficiencies, and a lack of political will to prosecute high-profile individuals.
4. **Public Perception and Trust:** Public perception and trust play a critical role in the effectiveness of anti-corruption efforts in public health. In many developing nations, historical experiences of corruption, mismanagement, and lack of transparency have eroded public confidence in health institutions. When citizens perceive that corruption is deeply entrenched and that anti-corruption initiatives are mere formalities, they may become disillusioned and disengaged. This distrust can manifest in reduced public participation in health programs, reluctance to comply with health policies, and scepticism toward government-led interventions.

Moreover, trust deficits can make whistleblower protections and reporting mechanisms less effective, as individuals may fear retaliation or believe that their complaints will not lead to meaningful action. Restoring public trust requires consistent enforcement of anti-corruption measures, visible accountability for offenders, and open communication with communities about efforts to enhance transparency. Without addressing these perception issues, even well-designed anti-corruption frameworks risk being undermined by public apathy or resistance.

Strategies for Strengthening Legal and Institutional Frameworks

To overcome the challenges outlined above and enhance the effectiveness of legal and institutional frameworks for combating corruption, several strategies can be implemented [28, 29].

1. **Ensuring Independence of Anti-Corruption Institutions:** Strengthening the independence of anti-corruption institutions is essential for reducing political interference and ensuring that these bodies can carry out their mandates effectively. This can be achieved by establishing clear legal protections for the autonomy of anti-corruption agencies, ensuring secure tenure for their leadership, and providing adequate resources to prevent dependence on political or external influences.
2. **Enhancing Capacity and Resources:** Increasing the capacity and resources of anti-corruption institutions is crucial for improving their effectiveness. This includes providing sufficient funding, training, and technical support to enable these institutions to conduct thorough investigations, enforce laws, and prosecute cases effectively. Investment in capacity-building programs for law enforcement, regulatory bodies, and the judiciary is also essential for strengthening the overall anti-corruption framework.
3. **Strengthening Legal Provisions for Enforcement:** Revising and strengthening legal provisions for the enforcement of anti-corruption laws can help address the issue of weak enforcement. This may involve introducing stricter penalties for corruption offenses, streamlining legal procedures to expedite the prosecution of corruption cases, and enhancing the powers of anti-corruption agencies to conduct investigations and enforce compliance.
4. **Promoting Public Awareness and Participation:** Public awareness and participation are critical for the success of anti-corruption efforts. Governments should engage in public education campaigns to raise awareness about anti-corruption laws, the importance of transparency, and the mechanisms available for reporting corruption. Encouraging citizen participation in monitoring public health expenditures and programs can also contribute to greater accountability and reduce opportunities for corruption.

5. **Strengthening International Cooperation:** International cooperation is essential for combating corruption, particularly in cases involving cross-border corruption or the illicit flow of funds. Collaborating with international organisations, such as the United Nations, the World Bank, and Interpol, can provide technical assistance, promote the sharing of best practices, and facilitate the recovery of stolen assets. Strengthening international legal frameworks, such as anti-money laundering laws, can also help to prevent and combat corruption.
6. **Leveraging Technology for Anti-Corruption Efforts:** Technology can be a powerful tool for enhancing transparency, accountability, and the effectiveness of anti-corruption efforts. Implementing digital platforms for public procurement, e-governance, and financial management can reduce opportunities for corruption by increasing transparency and reducing human discretion. Additionally, the use of data analytics and artificial intelligence can improve the detection of corrupt practices and enhance the efficiency of investigations.

The Role of Civil Society and Media in Supporting Anti-Corruption Frameworks

Civil society and the media play a crucial role in supporting and strengthening legal and institutional frameworks for combating corruption [29].

1. **Advocacy and Monitoring:** Civil society organisations are key players in advocating for stronger anti-corruption frameworks and monitoring their implementation. By engaging in advocacy, CSOs can influence the development and reform of anti-corruption laws and policies. Additionally, CSOs can act as watchdogs, monitoring government actions, conducting independent audits, and reporting on corruption cases.
2. **Investigative Journalism:** The media, particularly investigative journalists, play a vital role in exposing corruption and holding public officials accountable. Investigative journalism can uncover corruption scandals, raise public awareness, and put pressure on governments to take action. Protecting the freedom of the press and ensuring the safety of journalists are essential for enabling the media to fulfil this role.
3. **Public Engagement and Mobilisation:** Public engagement and mobilisation are essential components in the fight against corruption in public health. Civil society organisations (CSOs) and the media play a crucial role in raising awareness, educating citizens on their rights, and fostering a culture of accountability. When the public is informed about corruption risks and their impact on healthcare delivery, they are more likely to demand transparency and hold institutions accountable.

CASE STUDIES: ANTI-CORRUPTION INITIATIVES IN THE HEALTH SECTOR

Examining successful anti-corruption initiatives in the health sector provides valuable insights into effective strategies and practices for combating corruption. This section highlights case studies from various countries that have implemented innovative and impactful anti-corruption measures in their health systems. By analysing these examples, we can identify best practices, lessons learned, and strategies that can be adapted to other contexts, including Nigeria and other developing nations [28 - 30].

Case Study 1: Brazil's Health System Transparency and Accountability

Background: Brazil has faced significant challenges with corruption in its public health system, particularly in the procurement and distribution of medical supplies. To address these issues, Brazil implemented several anti-corruption initiatives aimed at increasing transparency and accountability.

Key Initiatives:

1. **e-SUS Strategy:** Brazil launched the e-SUS strategy, a digital platform designed to improve transparency and efficiency in the management of health resources. The platform integrates various health management systems, including procurement, inventory, and financial management. By centralising data and automating processes, e-SUS reduces opportunities for corruption and enhances oversight.
2. **Public Procurement Reforms:** The Brazilian government introduced reforms to public procurement processes, including mandatory electronic bidding and online publication of contract details. These measures increase transparency and reduce opportunities for fraud and favouritism in the procurement of medical supplies and services.
3. **Corruption Reporting Mechanisms:** Brazil established dedicated channels for reporting corruption, including hotlines and online platforms. These mechanisms allow citizens and health workers to report irregularities and corrupt practices anonymously, contributing to greater accountability and transparency.

Impact: The implementation of these initiatives has led to increased transparency in health procurement processes, reduced opportunities for corruption, and improved public trust in the health system. The e-SUS platform has enhanced data management and oversight, while public procurement reforms have made the bidding process more competitive and transparent.

Case Study 2: Kenya's Health Sector Integrity Program

Background: Kenya has faced challenges with corruption in its health sector, including the mismanagement of funds and procurement irregularities. In response, the Kenyan government, in collaboration with international partners, implemented the Health Sector Integrity Program to address these issues.

Key Initiatives:

1. **Integrated Financial Management System (IFMS):** Kenya introduced the Integrated Financial Management System (IFMS) to improve financial management and accountability in the health sector. The IFMS integrates budgeting, accounting, and reporting functions, providing real-time data on financial transactions and reducing opportunities for financial mismanagement and corruption.
2. **Enhanced Auditing and Oversight:** The Kenyan government strengthened auditing and oversight mechanisms by establishing an independent audit unit within the Ministry of Health. This unit conducts regular audits of health programs and expenditures, identifying irregularities and recommending corrective actions.
3. **Anti-Corruption Training and Capacity Building:** The Health Sector Integrity Program includes training and capacity-building initiatives for health workers and administrators. These programs focus on ethics, anti-corruption measures, and financial management, equipping personnel with the knowledge and skills to detect and prevent corruption.

Impact: The Health Sector Integrity Program has improved financial management and accountability in Kenya's health sector. The IFMS has enhanced transparency in financial transactions, while the independent audit unit has increased oversight and identified areas for improvement. Training and capacity-building efforts have strengthened the integrity and ethical standards of health personnel.

Case Study 3: India's National Health Mission and Accountability Measures

Background: India's National Health Mission (NHM) aims to improve health outcomes and strengthen the healthcare system across the country. To address corruption and enhance accountability, the NHM has implemented several initiatives focused on transparency and community involvement.

Key Initiatives:

1. **Online Public Disclosure:** The NHM introduced an online public disclosure system that provides information on health program budgets, expenditures, and performance. This system allows citizens to access information on health services and resources, promoting transparency and enabling public scrutiny.
2. **Community Monitoring:** The NHM established community monitoring mechanisms, including Village Health and Sanitation Committees (VHSCs) and Health Management Committees (HMCs). These committees involve community members in monitoring health services, identifying issues, and providing feedback. Community participation helps ensure that health programs are responsive to local needs and reduces opportunities for corruption.
3. **Performance-Based Funding:** The NHM implemented performance-based funding mechanisms that link funding to the achievement of specific health outcomes and targets. This approach incentivises effective program implementation and reduces the potential for misuse of funds.

Impact: The NHM's initiatives have led to greater transparency and accountability in health program management. The online public disclosure system has increased access to information, while community monitoring has enhanced local oversight and involvement. Performance-based funding has improved program efficiency and effectiveness, reducing opportunities for corruption.

Case Study 4: Nigeria's Public Procurement and Financial Management Reforms

Background: In response to challenges with corruption in the health sector, Nigeria has implemented several reforms aimed at improving public procurement and financial management. These initiatives focus on increasing transparency, reducing fraud, and enhancing oversight.

Key Initiatives:

1. **Public Procurement Act:** Nigeria's Public Procurement Act mandates transparent bidding processes and the use of electronic procurement systems. The Act requires public procurement processes to be competitive and open, reducing opportunities for corruption and favoritism in the procurement of health supplies and services.
2. **Treasury Single Account (TSA):** The implementation of the Treasury Single Account (TSA) aims to consolidate government revenues and expenditures into

a single account. This system improves financial management, reduces leakages, and enhances transparency in the handling of public funds, including those allocated to health programs.
3. **Independent Monitoring and Evaluation:** Nigeria has established independent monitoring and evaluation mechanisms to assess the performance of health programs and expenditures. These mechanisms involve external auditors and evaluators who provide unbiased assessments and recommendations for improving program implementation and financial management.

Impact: The Public Procurement Act and TSA reforms have increased transparency and reduced opportunities for financial mismanagement in Nigeria's health sector. Independent monitoring and evaluation mechanisms have improved oversight and accountability, contributing to more effective and efficient use of health resources.

Lessons Learned and Best Practices

The case studies presented highlight several key lessons and best practices for combating corruption in the health sector [28 - 30]:

1. **Promoting Transparency:** Implementing digital platforms and online disclosure systems enhances transparency and reduces opportunities for corruption by making information accessible to the public.
2. **Strengthening Oversight:** Independent auditing and oversight mechanisms are critical for detecting and addressing corruption. Establishing dedicated audit units and monitoring bodies can improve accountability and ensure the effective use of resources.
3. **Engaging Communities:** Community involvement in monitoring and evaluating health services helps ensure that programs are responsive to local needs and reduces opportunities for corruption. Engaging citizens in oversight processes fosters greater accountability and transparency.
4. **Implementing Reforms:** Comprehensive reforms in procurement, financial management, and performance-based funding can enhance the efficiency and effectiveness of health programs. Reforms should be designed to address specific vulnerabilities and promote integrity.
5. **Building Capacity:** Training and capacity-building initiatives for health workers, administrators, and auditors are essential for equipping personnel with the skills and knowledge needed to prevent and detect corruption.
6. **Leveraging Technology:** Technology can play a significant role in improving transparency, efficiency, and accountability. Digital tools for financial manage-

ment, procurement, and public disclosure can reduce opportunities for corruption and enhance oversight.

CONCLUSION

By applying these lessons and best practices, countries can strengthen their efforts to combat corruption in the health sector and improve the effectiveness and integrity of health systems.

REFERENCES

[1] World Health Organisation. Why corruption matters in health and how to tackle it. Geneva: WHO 2020.

[2] Transparency International. Global Corruption Barometer. Africa (Lond) 2023; •••: 2023.

[3] FMoH. (2022). Basic Health Care Provision Fund: Operational Guidelines and Accountability Framework. Abuja: FMoH.

[4] Glynn EH. Corruption in the health sector: A problem in need of a systems-thinking approach. Front Public Health 2022; 10: 910073. [http://dx.doi.org/10.3389/fpubh.2022.910073] [PMID: 36091569]

[5] Vian T. Review of corruption in the health sector: theory, methods and interventions. Health Policy Plan 2007; 23(2): 83-94. [http://dx.doi.org/10.1093/heapol/czm048] [PMID: 18281310]

[6] National Academies of Sciences, Engineering, and Medicine; Health and Medicine Division; Board on Health Care Services; Board on Global Health; Committee on Improving the Quality of Health Care Globally. (2018). Crossing the Global Quality Chasm: Improving Health Care Worldwide. Washington (DC): National Academies Press (US). The Critical Health Impacts of Corruption. Available from: https://www.ncbi.nlm.nih.gov/books/NBK535646/

[7] Lewis, M. (2006). Governance and corruption in public health care systems. Centre for Global Development Working Paper, (78). [http://dx.doi.org/10.2139/ssrn.984046]

[8] United Nations. 2012.The future we want: RIO+20. United Nations Conference on Sustainable Development.

[9] World Bank. World Development Report 2004: Making Services Work for Poor People. Washington, DC: World Bank 2004.

[10] Bamberger M, Rugh J, Mabry L. RealWorld Evaluation: Working under budget, time, data, and political constraints. SAGE Publications 2006.

[11] Federal Government of Nigeria, Office of the Auditor-General. (2023). Annual Audit Report on Federal Health Institutions, 2020–2022. Abuja: OAuGF.

[12] Budget Office of the Federation. (2019). Public Expenditure Tracking Survey in the Health Sector. Abuja: FGoN.

[13] Bureau of Public Procurement. Procurement Performance Report, Health Sector. Abuja: BPP 2022.

[14] Federal Ministry of Finance, Budget and National Planning. (2023). Government Integrated Financial Management Information System (GIFMIS) Implementation Report. Abuja: FMoFBNP.

[15] BudgIT Foundation. (2022). Health Budget Transparency Scorecard: Nigeria States 2022. Lagos: BudgIT.

[16] World Health Organisation. (2016). Framework on integrated, people-centred health services. World

Health Organisation.

[17] Brinkerhoff DW, Bossert TJ. Health governance: principal-agent linkages and health system strengthening. Health Policy Plan 2014; 29(6): 685-93. [http://dx.doi.org/10.1093/heapol/czs132] [PMID: 23411121]

[18] Gaventa J, Barrett G. Mapping the Outcomes of Citizen Engagement. World Dev 2012; 40(12): 2399-410. [http://dx.doi.org/10.1016/j.worlddev.2012.05.014]

[19] Cornwall A, Shankland A. Engaging citizens: Lessons from building Brazil's national health system. Soc Sci Med 2008; 66(10): 2173-84. [http://dx.doi.org/10.1016/j.socscimed.2008.01.038] [PMID: 18336976]

[20] WHO. World Health Report 2006—Working Together for Health, 2006. Available from: http://www.who.int/whr/2006/en/index.html

[21] Rose-Ackerman S, Palifka BJ. Corruption and Government: Causes, Consequences, and Reform. 2nd ed., Cambridge University Press 2016. [http://dx.doi.org/10.1017/CBO9781139962933]

[22] Adejumobi S. State, economy, and society in post-military Nigeria. Palgrave Macmillan 2011. [http://dx.doi.org/10.1057/9780230117594]

[23] Health Reform Foundation of Nigeria. Community Accountability for Health: Lessons from State-Level Implementation. Abuja: HERFON 2021.

[24] Improving Governance in the Health Sector of Sub-Saharan Africa. Washington, DC: World Bank 2020.

[25] United Nations Office on Drugs and Crime. Nigeria: Corruption Risk Assessment in the Health Sector. Vienna: UNODC 2021.

[26] Federal Republic of Nigeria. Public Procurement Act. Abuja: Federal Government Printer 2007.

[27] Open Government Partnership. Nigeria National Action Plan II (2023–2025). Abuja: OGP Secretariat 2023.

[28] Gaitonde R, Oxman AD, Okebukola PO, Rada G. Interventions to reduce corruption in the health sector. Cochrane Libr 2016; 2016(8): CD008856. [http://dx.doi.org/10.1002/14651858.CD008856.pub2] [PMID: 27528494]

[29] Olken BA. Monitoring corruption: Evidence from a field experiment in Indonesia. J Polit Econ 2007; 115(2): 200-49. [http://dx.doi.org/10.1086/517935]

[30] DFID. DFID's Anti-corruption strategies for Nigeria. Department for International Development 2013.

CHAPTER 9

Innovations in Public Health

Abstract: This chapter explores the transformative role of innovation in public health, focusing on case studies from Nigeria and other developing nations. It highlights how technological advancements, public-private partnerships, community-driven initiatives, and mobile health services have reshaped healthcare delivery, making it more accessible, efficient, and effective. The chapter also examines innovative financing mechanisms that have enabled the scaling of health interventions and presents key lessons from successful public health innovations. These insights offer valuable guidance for policymakers, practitioners, and stakeholders aiming to improve health outcomes in resource-constrained settings.

Keywords: Community-driven health initiatives, Case studies, Developing countries, Healthcare delivery, Innovative financing, Mobile health, Nigeria, Public health innovation, Public-private partnerships, Technological advancements.

INTRODUCTION

In public health, innovation extends beyond technology; it encompasses new approaches, partnerships, and financing models that solve persistent health challenges in more effective and sustainable ways. In Nigeria and other developing nations, innovations are bridging long-standing gaps in access, data visibility, financing, and workforce distribution. Innovation is the lifeblood of progress, and nowhere is this more evident than in the field of public health. In Nigeria and other developing nations, the need for creative solutions to overcome entrenched health challenges has never been more urgent. From technological advancements to novel financing mechanisms, innovative approaches are reshaping the landscape of healthcare delivery, making it more accessible, efficient, and effective. This chapter explores a range of innovations that have been instrumental in addressing public health challenges in Nigeria and beyond. It delves into the role of technology, public-private partnerships, community-driven initiatives, and mobile health services in revolutionising healthcare. It highlights both technological and community-driven innovations, showing how they contribute to health-system transformation when embedded within supportive

Jalal-Eddeen Abubakar Saleh

governance and accountability frameworks. The chapter also examines innovative financing mechanisms that have enabled the scaling of health interventions and draws lessons from successful public health innovations that can be applied in other contexts [1, 2].

TECHNOLOGICAL INNOVATIONS IN HEALTHCARE DELIVERY

Technological innovations have the potential to revolutionise healthcare delivery, making it more efficient, accessible, and responsive to populations' needs. This section explores key technological innovations in healthcare delivery, focusing on successful case studies from Nigeria and other regions. Highlighting these innovations aims to illustrate how technology can address critical public health challenges and improve health outcomes [1, 2]. Undoubtedly, digital transformation has reshaped how health services are delivered, monitored, and financed. Recent advances in Nigeria illustrate the growing impact of telemedicine, mobile health (mHealth), and drone technology on access and efficiency [3 - 5].

Table **1** showcases some innovative public health interventions successfully piloted or implemented in Nigeria. Each innovation, ranging from mobile health apps to drone deliveries of medical supplies, is described alongside its sponsor and observed outcomes. This structured presentation underscores the diversity of approaches being deployed to bridge healthcare access gaps and improve service efficiency. By capturing both government-led and private-sector-driven initiatives, the table illustrates how innovation thrives at the intersection of need, technology, and collaboration. The examples reinforce that scalable success is often rooted in context-appropriate solutions, like task-shifting to community pharmacies or leveraging mobile technology in remote regions. The table ultimately invites policymakers to institutionalise and scale these innovations while fostering a supportive environment for experimentation and adaptive learning.

Table 1. Selected Public Health Innovations.

Innovation	Description	Examples	Impact/Outcome
mHealth Apps (by NGOs, MOH)	Use of mobile apps for health messaging	The *mTRAC* and *CommCare* platforms enable community health workers to report data in real time.	Increased awareness
Telemedicine (by the private sector)	Remote diagnosis and treatment	*Dokita247* and *CribMD* provide remote consultations and e-prescriptions through mobile platforms.	Improved rural access

(Table 1) cont.....

Innovation	Description	Examples	Impact/Outcome
Artificial Intelligence (AI) and Data Analytics	**Real-time disease surveillance** across national and subnational levels.	NCDC's use of predictive models for outbreak detection through the *Surveillance Outbreak Response Management and Analysis System (*SORMAS) and DHIS2 integration.	Enables faster response to infectious disease alerts and resource optimisation.
Community Pharmacies (by Govt., NAFDAC)	Task-shifting to licensed pharmacies	*Community Pharmacy Scheme* to improve access to essential health services in urban and peri-urban communities.	Improved drug access
Drone Delivery (by private firms)	Medical supply delivery to remote areas	*Zipline* (in Ghana and Kaduna State, Nigeria) delivers vaccines and blood products to hard-to-reach areas.	Faster response

Telemedicine and Digital Health Platforms

Telemedicine and digital health platforms have emerged as transformative tools in healthcare delivery, particularly in underserved and remote areas. These technologies facilitate remote consultations, diagnostics, and treatment, bridging the gap between patients and healthcare providers [1 - 5].

Case Study: Telemedicine Initiative in Nigeria

Background: The telemedicine initiative in Nigeria, spearheaded by various organisations, including the government and private sector partners, aims to improve healthcare access in remote and underserved regions.

Key Features:

1. **Remote Consultations:** Telemedicine platforms enable patients to consult with healthcare providers remotely via video calls, reducing the need for travel and minimising the strain on local healthcare facilities.
2. **Integrated Health Records:** Digital health platforms often include electronic health records (EHR) systems that store patient information securely and allow seamless data sharing between healthcare providers.
3. **Specialised Services:** Telemedicine services in the country include specialised consultations in areas such as cardiology, dermatology, and mental health, addressing gaps in local expertise.

Impact: The telemedicine initiative has improved healthcare access for individuals in remote areas, reducing travel times and associated costs. It has also enhanced the capacity of local health workers by providing them with access to specialist consultations and continuing education.

Mobile Health (mHealth) Applications

Mobile health (mHealth) applications utilise mobile technology to deliver health services, information, and support directly to users' smartphones. These apps can promote health education, facilitate disease monitoring, and support self-management of chronic conditions [1 - 5].

Case Study: mHealth in Nigeria's Maternal Health Program

Background: Nigeria has implemented several mHealth programs aimed at improving maternal health outcomes. One notable example is the "mHealth for Maternal and Child Health" program, which leverages mobile technology to provide vital health information and support.

Key Features:

1. **Health Information:** The mHealth program provides pregnant women with access to educational content on prenatal care, childbirth, and postnatal care through SMS and mobile apps.
2. **Appointment Reminders:** Mobile applications send reminders for antenatal visits, vaccinations, and follow-up appointments, helping to ensure that mothers and infants receive timely care.
3. **Data Collection and Monitoring:** mHealth tools collect data on maternal and child health, enabling health authorities to monitor trends and identify areas for intervention.

Impact: The mHealth program has improved maternal health by increasing awareness and knowledge among pregnant women. It has also enhanced the management of maternal care and contributed to better health outcomes through timely interventions and support.

Health Information Systems (HIS)

Health Information Systems (HIS) integrate various aspects of health data management, including patient records, inventory management, and health service delivery. These systems improve the efficiency and effectiveness of healthcare operations [1 - 5].

Case Study: HIS Implementation in Kenya

Background: Kenya's health sector has adopted Health Information Systems to streamline healthcare delivery and improve data management. The Kenyan government, along with international partners, has implemented HIS across various health facilities.

Key Features:

1. **Electronic Health Records (EHR):** HIS in Kenya includes EHR systems that enable the digital recording of patient data, facilitating better coordination of care and reducing paperwork.
2. **Supply Chain Management:** The HIS also manages the inventory of medical supplies and pharmaceuticals, ensuring timely procurement and distribution to prevent stockouts.
3. **Data Analytics:** Advanced data analytics capabilities allow for the analysis of health trends, identification of disease outbreaks, and informed decision-making.

Impact: The implementation of HIS has enhanced the efficiency of health service delivery in Kenya. By digitising patient records and improving supply chain management, the system has reduced errors, improved resource allocation, and supported better health outcomes.

Innovative Diagnostic Technologies

Innovative diagnostic technologies offer new ways to detect and diagnose diseases, often at earlier stages and with greater accuracy. These technologies can significantly improve disease management and patient outcomes [1 - 6].

Case Study: Portable Diagnostic Devices in India

Background: India has seen the adoption of portable diagnostic devices that enable rapid and accurate testing for various diseases, including diabetes, tuberculosis, and infectious diseases.

Key Features:

1. **Point-of-Care Testing:** Portable diagnostic devices allow for point-of-care testing, providing immediate results and facilitating timely diagnosis and treatment.
2. **Remote Monitoring:** Some devices are equipped with remote monitoring capabilities, allowing healthcare providers to track patients' health metrics and make data-driven decisions.

3. **Affordability and Accessibility:** Many portable diagnostic devices are designed to be affordable and easy to use, making them accessible to healthcare providers in low-resource settings.

Impact: The use of portable diagnostic devices has improved the accuracy and speed of disease diagnosis in India. These technologies have enabled earlier detection of conditions, improved patient management, and increased access to diagnostic services in remote areas.

Electronic Health Records and Data Management

Electronic Health Records (EHR) systems are central to modern healthcare delivery, enabling the digital management of patient information and facilitating the exchange of health data across healthcare providers [1 - 6].

Case Study: EHR Implementation in South Africa

Background: South Africa has made significant strides in implementing Electronic Health Records (EHR) systems to enhance healthcare delivery and data management across the country.

Key Features:

1. **Centralised Data Repository:** EHR systems in South Africa centralise patient data, making it accessible to healthcare providers across different facilities and improving continuity of care.
2. **Patient Portals:** Patient portals allow individuals to access their health records, schedule appointments, and communicate with healthcare providers, empowering patients to take an active role in their health.
3. **Data Security and Privacy:** The EHR system includes robust security measures to protect patient information and ensure compliance with privacy regulations.

Impact: The EHR system in South Africa has enhanced the quality of care by providing healthcare providers with comprehensive and up-to-date patient information. It has also improved patient engagement and contributed to better health outcomes through coordinated and informed care.

CONCLUSION

Technological innovations have the potential to significantly improve healthcare delivery by enhancing access, efficiency, and quality of care. The case studies presented highlight the diverse ways in which technology can address public health challenges and contribute to better health outcomes. As technology continues to evolve, healthcare systems in Nigeria and other developing nations must embrace these innovations and adapt them to local contexts. By leveraging technology effectively, we can advance public health and work towards achieving equitable and sustainable healthcare for all.

PUBLIC-PRIVATE PARTNERSHIPS IN HEALTH

Public-Private Partnerships (PPPs) have become increasingly important in addressing complex public health challenges by combining resources, expertise, and innovation from both the public and private sectors. These collaborations can enhance the efficiency, effectiveness, and sustainability of health initiatives. This section explores the role of PPPs in health, highlighting successful examples from Nigeria and other regions to illustrate how these partnerships can drive improvements in healthcare delivery and outcomes [7 - 9].

Overview of Public-Private Partnerships in Health

Public-Private Partnerships (PPPs) in health care are collaborative arrangements between government entities and private sector organisations aimed at improving health services and outcomes. These partnerships leverage the strengths of each sector to address gaps in healthcare delivery, enhance service quality, and expand access to health services.

Key Objectives of PPPs:

1. **Resource Mobilisation:** Mobilising additional financial and technical resources from the private sector to complement public health funding.
2. **Innovation and Efficiency:** Introducing innovative solutions and improving operational efficiency through private sector expertise and technologies.
3. **Service Expansion:** Expanding access to health services, particularly in underserved and remote areas, through joint initiatives and infrastructure development.
4. **Quality Improvement:** Enhancing the quality of health services by incorporating private sector standards and practices.

Successful Case Studies of PPPs in Health

Case Study 1: Nigeria's Health Insurance Authority and Private Sector Involvement

Background: Nigeria has implemented the National Health Insurance Authority (NHIA) to improve access to healthcare services and reduce out-of-pocket expenses for citizens. The NHIA includes collaboration with private sector insurance companies to expand coverage and improve service delivery.

Key Features:

1. **Insurance Partnerships:** Private insurance companies partner with the government to provide health insurance coverage, offering a range of health services to insured individuals. These partnerships help increase enrollment and expand coverage options.
2. **Health Management Organisations (HMOs):** HMOs play a crucial role in managing health insurance plans, coordinating care, and ensuring service quality. They work with both public and private healthcare providers to deliver services to insured patients.
3. **Performance Monitoring:** The NHIA includes mechanisms for monitoring the performance of insurance providers and healthcare facilities to ensure that quality standards are met and services are delivered efficiently.

Impact: The collaboration between the government and private insurance companies has expanded health insurance coverage in Nigeria, improved access to healthcare services, and increased the efficiency of service delivery. The involvement of private sector players has also introduced innovative approaches to health insurance management.

Case Study 2: The Global Fund and Private Sector Collaboration

Background: The Global Fund to Fight AIDS, Tuberculosis, and Malaria (Global Fund) has partnered with private sector organisations to enhance the fight against these diseases. The collaboration aims to leverage private sector expertise, funding, and resources to support health initiatives in developing countries.

Key Features:

1. **Resource Mobilization:** Private sector contributions, including financial donations and in-kind support, complement the Global Fund's resources, enabling larger-scale interventions and expanded reach.
2. **Innovation and Technology:** Private sector partners contribute technological innovations and expertise, such as advanced diagnostic tools and treatment options, to improve disease prevention and management.
3. **Capacity Building:** The collaboration includes capacity-building initiatives to strengthen health systems, improve service delivery, and enhance the effectiveness of disease control programs.

Impact: The partnership between the Global Fund and private sector organizations has led to significant advancements in the fight against AIDS, tuberculosis, and malaria. The collaboration has resulted in increased funding, improved access to essential services, and the introduction of innovative technologies and practices.

Case Study 3: India's PPPs in Healthcare Infrastructure Development

Background: India has leveraged public-private partnerships to develop and upgrade healthcare infrastructure, including the construction of new hospitals and the enhancement of existing facilities. These partnerships aim to improve the quality and accessibility of healthcare services.

Key Features:

1. **Hospital Development:** Private sector entities invest in the construction and management of hospitals, providing high-quality facilities and services in collaboration with government health authorities.
2. **Service Delivery Models:** PPPs involve innovative service delivery models, such as public-private hospital chains and integrated healthcare systems, to enhance efficiency and patient care.
3. **Training and Capacity Building:** Private partners contribute to training healthcare professionals and building capacity within the public health system, improving the overall quality of care.

Impact: The PPPs in healthcare infrastructure development in India have resulted in the establishment of modern healthcare facilities, increased access to services, and improved patient care. The collaboration has also enhanced the capacity of the public health system through training and capacity-building efforts.

Challenges and Considerations in PPPs

Challenges:

1. **Alignment of Goals:** Ensuring that the objectives of both public and private partners are aligned can be challenging. Differences in priorities and expectations may affect the success of the partnership.
2. **Regulatory and Legal Framework:** Establishing clear regulations and legal agreements is essential for the smooth operation of PPPs. Ambiguities or inconsistencies in the legal framework can lead to disputes and inefficiencies.
3. **Transparency and Accountability:** Maintaining transparency and accountability in PPPs is crucial to preventing corruption and ensuring that

resources are used effectively. Robust oversight mechanisms are needed to monitor performance and outcomes.

4. **Sustainability:** Ensuring the long-term sustainability of PPPs requires ongoing commitment from both sectors. Long-term planning and resource allocation are necessary to maintain the benefits of the partnership.

Considerations:

1. **Stakeholder Engagement:** Engaging all relevant stakeholders, including government agencies, private sector partners, and community representatives, is important for the success of PPPs. Effective communication and collaboration can enhance the effectiveness of the partnership.
2. **Clear Objectives and Metrics:** Establishing clear objectives and performance metrics is essential for measuring the success of PPPs. Well-defined goals and evaluation criteria help ensure that the partnership delivers the desired outcomes.
3. **Capacity Building:** Building the capacity of both public and private sector partners is important for effective collaboration. Training and support can enhance the ability of partners to contribute effectively to the partnership.

CONCLUSION

Public-Private Partnerships (PPPs) play a crucial role in advancing healthcare delivery by combining the strengths of both sectors. Successful case studies from Nigeria and other regions demonstrate the potential of PPPs to improve access to healthcare, enhance service quality, and drive innovation. While challenges exist, careful planning, clear objectives, and effective stakeholder engagement can help ensure the success of PPPs. As countries continue to address public health challenges, leveraging PPPs can contribute to more effective and sustainable healthcare solutions.

COMMUNITY-DRIVEN HEALTH INITIATIVES

Community-driven health initiatives empower local populations to take an active role in improving their health outcomes. By engaging communities in the design, implementation, and evaluation of health programs, these initiatives leverage local knowledge, resources, and enthusiasm to address health challenges effectively. This section explores the concept of community-driven health initiatives, highlights successful case studies, and discusses the key elements that contribute to their success [7 - 10].

Concept and Importance of Community-Driven Health Initiatives

Community-driven health initiatives are grassroots approaches in which local populations play a central role in designing, implementing, and sustaining health interventions. These initiatives harness local knowledge, cultural relevance, and social capital to deliver more responsive and equitable healthcare services. Their importance lies in enhancing trust, fostering ownership, and promoting sustainability by ensuring that solutions are aligned with community priorities and values [7 - 10].

Concept: Community-driven health initiatives are programs and interventions designed and implemented by local communities with the support of health organisations and government bodies. These initiatives focus on addressing health issues that are specific to the community, using locally appropriate solutions and strategies.

Importance:

1. **Local Relevance:** Community-driven initiatives are tailored to address the specific health needs and priorities of the local population, ensuring that interventions are relevant and effective.
2. **Empowerment:** By involving community members in health initiatives, these programs empower individuals to take control of their health and contribute to the well-being of their community.
3. **Sustainability:** Initiatives driven by community involvement are often more sustainable, as they build on local resources and capacities, fostering a sense of ownership and commitment among participants.
4. **Enhanced Outreach:** Community-driven programs can reach underserved populations more effectively, as local networks and relationships facilitate trust and engagement.

Successful Case Studies of Community-Driven Health Initiatives

Across Africa and beyond, numerous community-driven health projects have yielded impressive results. In Ethiopia, the Health Extension Program empowered female health workers at the village level to improve maternal and child health outcomes. In Nigeria, community-based surveillance for polio eradication has significantly contributed to early case detection and rapid response. These examples demonstrate the transformative impact of local engagement in improving access and outcomes [10 - 12].

Case Study 1: Nigeria's Community Health Influencers, Promoters, and Services (CHIPS) Program

Background: The CHIPS program in Nigeria aims to improve access to primary health care services through community health workers who are trained to provide essential health services and information.

Key Features:

1. **Training and Deployment:** Local community members are trained as CHIPs agents to deliver health services, including immunisation, antenatal care, and health education, within their communities.
2. **Integrated Services:** CHIPs agents provide a range of services, from basic health care to disease prevention and health promotion, integrating with existing health systems to enhance coverage.
3. **Community Engagement:** The program emphasises community involvement in identifying health needs and developing strategies to address them, ensuring that interventions are aligned with local priorities.

Impact: The CHIPs program has significantly improved access to health services in remote and underserved areas. By utilising local community members as health workers, the program has enhanced service delivery, increased immunisation rates, and promoted better health practices.

Case Study 2: Bangladesh's Oral Rehydration Therapy (ORT) Program

Background: Bangladesh's ORT program was developed to address the high rates of diarrheal diseases, particularly among children, through community-based education and the promotion of oral rehydration solutions.

Key Features:

1. **Community Education:** Community health workers educate families on the preparation and use of oral rehydration solutions to treat and prevent dehydration caused by diarrhoea.
2. **Local Production:** ORT solutions are produced locally, making them more accessible and affordable for communities.
3. **Village-Based Distribution:** ORT is distributed through local health posts and community centres, ensuring that the solutions reach the households in need.

Impact: The ORT program has been highly successful in reducing mortality and morbidity from diarrheal diseases in Bangladesh. The community-driven approach has enabled widespread adoption of ORT and empowered local communities to take action against preventable diseases.

Case Study 3: India's ASHA (Accredited Social Health Activist) Program

Background: India's ASHA program aims to improve maternal and child health by training community health workers to provide a range of health services and support within their communities.

Key Features:

1. **Training and Support:** ASHA workers receive training to provide health education, conduct home visits, and facilitate access to health services, including immunization and antenatal care.
2. **Community-Based Approach:** ASHA workers are selected from within the communities they serve, ensuring that they understand local health issues and cultural practices.
3. **Incentive-Based System:** The program includes a performance-based incentive system to motivate ASHA workers and ensure the delivery of high-quality services.

Impact: The ASHA program has significantly improved maternal and child health outcomes in India. By leveraging local knowledge and networks, the program has increased access to essential health services, improved health education, and enhanced community engagement.

Key Elements of Successful Community-Driven Health Initiatives

The success of community-driven health efforts depends on several core elements: meaningful community participation, strong leadership, adequate training and resources, and alignment with broader health system goals. Additionally, regular feedback loops, transparent decision-making, and respect for local customs enhance effectiveness and sustainability. Institutional support and policy frameworks are also vital for scaling such models [10 - 12].

1. **Community Involvement:** Active involvement of community members in all stages of the health initiative, from planning to implementation and evaluation, is crucial. This ensures that the initiative addresses local needs and gains the support and trust of the community.
2. **Capacity Building:** Providing training and resources to community members enhances their ability to contribute effectively to health initiatives. Capacity

building also helps to ensure that community-driven programs are sustainable and adaptable.

3. **Local Leadership:** Engaging local leaders and influencers can facilitate community buy-in and support. Local leaders play a key role in mobilising resources, advocating for health initiatives, and addressing potential challenges.
4. **Culturally Appropriate Interventions:** Health interventions should be designed to respect and align with local cultural practices and beliefs. This increases the likelihood of acceptance and successful implementation.
5. **Monitoring and Evaluation:** Regular monitoring and evaluation of community-driven initiatives are essential for assessing their effectiveness and making necessary adjustments. Involving the community in evaluation processes helps to ensure that feedback is used to improve the program.
6. **Collaboration with Health Authorities:** Collaboration with local and national health authorities ensures that community-driven initiatives are integrated into the broader health system and that resources and support are available.

CONCLUSION

Community-driven health initiatives play a vital role in improving health outcomes by leveraging local knowledge, resources, and commitment. The case studies from Nigeria, Bangladesh, and India demonstrate the effectiveness of these initiatives in addressing health challenges and enhancing service delivery. By engaging communities in the design and implementation of health programs, these initiatives not only address local needs but also foster a sense of ownership and empowerment. As public health systems continue to evolve, community-driven approaches will remain essential for achieving equitable and sustainable health improvements.

LEVERAGING MOBILE TECHNOLOGY FOR HEALTH SERVICES

Mobile technology has revolutionised the delivery of healthcare services, providing innovative solutions to reach underserved populations, enhance service delivery, and improve health outcomes. Mobile health (mHealth) applications and platforms utilise mobile phones and other portable devices to provide health information, deliver services, and collect data. This section explores the impact of mobile technology on health services, highlights successful case studies, and discusses key considerations for effectively leveraging mobile technology in healthcare [13 - 15].

Overview of Mobile Technology in Health

Mobile technology is revolutionising health service delivery, especially in resource-constrained settings. Through mobile phones and digital platforms, health information, appointment reminders, telemedicine, and disease surveillance can now reach remote communities. mHealth solutions bridge geographical and infrastructure gaps, offering real-time communication and improving efficiency across health systems [13].

Concept: Mobile technology in health, or mHealth, encompasses the use of mobile devices and applications to support health and healthcare delivery. It includes a wide range of activities, such as remote consultations, health information dissemination, data collection, and disease monitoring.

Key Benefits:

1. **Enhanced Access:** Mobile technology extends the reach of health services to remote and underserved areas, overcoming geographical and logistical barriers to healthcare access.
2. **Real-Time Communication:** Mobile platforms facilitate real-time communication between healthcare providers and patients, enabling timely medical advice, follow-up, and support.
3. **Data Collection and Management:** Mobile tools enable efficient data collection, management, and analysis, supporting public health surveillance, program evaluation, and decision-making.
4. **Health Education:** Mobile applications provide health information and educational resources, promoting health literacy and encouraging preventive practices.

Successful Case Studies of Mobile Technology in Health

There are several examples of mobile health successes. In Uganda, the mTrac system has improved health data reporting from rural facilities via SMS. In Nigeria, mobile apps like SmartHealth have enabled frontline health workers to track immunisation coverage and maternal health indicators more effectively. These case studies illustrate how mobile technology enhances data accuracy, service delivery, and responsiveness [13 - 15].

Case Study 1: Kenya's M-Pesa and Health Services

Background: M-Pesa, a mobile money transfer service, has been adapted to support health services in Kenya by enabling cashless transactions and facilitating financial services related to health.

Key Features:

1. **Mobile Payments for Health Services:** M-Pesa allows patients to pay for health services and purchase medications using mobile money, reducing the need for cash transactions and improving financial accessibility.
2. **Health Insurance Payments:** The platform supports the payment of health insurance premiums, making it easier for individuals to access coverage and healthcare services.
3. **Emergency Fund Transfers:** M-Pesa enables quick transfers of funds for emergency health needs, ensuring that individuals can access necessary care without delay.

Impact: M-Pesa has improved financial access to health services in Kenya by providing a convenient and secure method for payments and transactions. This has increased the affordability and accessibility of healthcare for many individuals.

Case Study 2: India's mHealth Initiative for Maternal and Child Health

Background: India's mHealth initiative focuses on improving maternal and child health outcomes through mobile technology, providing vital information and support to pregnant women and new mothers.

Key Features:

1. **Health Information Services:** Mobile applications deliver information on prenatal care, nutrition, and postnatal care to expectant and new mothers, enhancing their knowledge and self-care practices.
2. **Appointment Reminders:** The initiative includes automated reminders for medical appointments and vaccination schedules, helping to ensure timely care and adherence to health recommendations.
3. **Teleconsultations:** Mobile platforms facilitate teleconsultations with healthcare providers, allowing women in remote areas to access medical advice and support.

Impact: The mHealth initiative has improved maternal and child health by providing accessible and relevant health information, reducing missed appointments, and increasing access to medical consultations.

Case Study 3: Tanzania's mHealth Program for Disease Surveillance

Background: Tanzania has implemented a mHealth program for disease surveillance, utilizing mobile technology to monitor and respond to outbreaks of communicable diseases.

Key Features:

1. **Real-Time Reporting:** Health workers use mobile devices to report cases of communicable diseases in real-time, allowing for prompt detection and response to outbreaks.
2. **Data Collection and Analysis:** Mobile applications facilitate the collection and analysis of health data, providing valuable insights into disease patterns and trends.
3. **Response Coordination:** The program includes tools for coordinating response efforts, including resource allocation and communication with field teams.

Impact: The mHealth program has enhanced disease surveillance and response capabilities in Tanzania, leading to more effective management of outbreaks and improved public health outcomes.

Key Considerations for Leveraging Mobile Technology in Health

Effectively leveraging mobile technology requires infrastructure readiness, digital literacy, data privacy safeguards, and inclusive design that considers gender and accessibility. Interoperability with existing health systems, cost-effectiveness, and local language support are also crucial. Stakeholder engagement, from policymakers to users, is key to successful adoption and scale-up [13 - 15].

1. **Accessibility and Inclusivity:** Ensuring that mobile health solutions are accessible to all individuals, including those in remote and low-resource settings, is crucial. Considerations include language options, device compatibility, and user-friendly interfaces.
2. **Data Security and Privacy:** Protecting the privacy and security of health data is essential. Mobile health platforms must comply with data protection regulations and employ robust security measures to safeguard sensitive information.
3. **Integration with Existing Systems:** Mobile health solutions should be integrated with existing health systems and infrastructure to ensure seamless operation and data sharing. Integration enhances the efficiency and effectiveness of health interventions.

4. **User Training and Support:** Providing training and support for users, including healthcare providers and patients, is important for the successful adoption and utilisation of mobile health tools. Training should cover the use of technology, data entry, and interpretation of health information.
5. **Evaluation and Adaptation:** Regular evaluation of mobile health programs is necessary to assess their impact, identify challenges, and make improvements. Adaptation based on feedback and evaluation results ensures that the technology remains effective and relevant.
6. **Partnership and Collaboration:** Collaborating with technology providers, health organisations, and government bodies is essential for the successful implementation and scaling of mobile health initiatives. Partnerships can provide technical expertise, funding, and support for program development. Table **2** below shows some distinctions in health innovation between community-driven and technology-driven models. However, integrating these two approaches would be useful in addressing public health challenges, as seen in polio surveillance and COVID-19 risk communication in Northeast Nigeria [16, 17].

Table 2. shows community-driven versus technology-driven innovations.

Dimension	Community-Driven Innovations	Technology-Driven Innovations
Definition	Locally developed solutions grounded in social capital, community participation, and indigenous knowledge.	Innovations leveraging digital tools, hardware, or software to enhance health outcomes.
Examples	Community-led WASH interventions in Borno; women's cooperatives promoting maternal nutrition in Kebbi; participatory malaria surveillance in Ghana.	Use of telemedicine platforms, mobile data apps, and drones for logistics or diagnosis.
Strengths	High local ownership, sustainability, and context relevance.	Scalability, efficiency, and precision.
Limitations	Limited funding, slower diffusion.	Requires infrastructure, literacy, and maintenance support.

Table **3** shows the distinction between community-driven and technology-driven models. The key distinction in health innovation lies between these two models. It is important to underscore that integrating both approaches, community leadership supported by digital tools, has proven most effective, as seen in polio surveillance and COVID-19 risk communication in Northeast Nigeria.

Table 3. shows the distinction between community-driven and technology-driven models.

Dimension	Community-Driven Innovations	Technology-Driven Innovations
Definition	Locally developed solutions grounded in social capital, community participation, and indigenous knowledge.	Innovations leveraging digital tools, hardware, or software to enhance health outcomes.
Examples	Community-led WASH interventions in Borno; women's cooperatives promoting maternal nutrition in Kebbi; participatory malaria surveillance in Ghana.	Use of telemedicine platforms, mobile data apps, and drones for logistics or diagnosis.
Strengths	High local ownership, sustainability, and context relevance.	Scalability, efficiency, and precision.
Limitations	Limited funding, slower diffusion.	Requires infrastructure, literacy, and maintenance support.

CONCLUSION

Leveraging mobile technology for health services offers significant opportunities to improve healthcare delivery, enhance access to services, and support public health initiatives. Successful case studies from Kenya, India, and Tanzania demonstrate the transformative impact of mobile health tools in addressing various health challenges. By addressing key considerations such as accessibility, data security, and integration, mobile technology can be effectively utilised to advance health outcomes and support sustainable healthcare solutions. As mobile technology continues to evolve, its role in enhancing health services will become increasingly important, offering new avenues for improving health and well-being globally.

INNOVATIVE FINANCING MECHANISMS FOR HEALTH

Innovative financing mechanisms are critical for addressing the complex challenges faced by health systems, particularly in resource-constrained settings. These mechanisms aim to diversify funding sources, improve financial efficiency, and ensure the sustainability of health programs. This section explores various innovative financing approaches, highlights successful case studies, and discusses key considerations for implementing these mechanisms effectively [18 - 20].

Innovative financing is reshaping how public health programs are funded and sustained, addressing the traditional challenge of dependence on donor funding. These approaches align financial incentives with measurable health outcomes, an essential step toward sustainability [18 - 20].

1. **Results-Based Financing (RBF):** Used in the World Bank–supported Nigeria State Health Investment Project (NSHIP) in Adamawa and Nasarawa, where facilities receive funds based on verified service outputs. Independent verification has led to a **30% increase in antenatal visits** and improved staff motivation.
2. **Health Bonds and Social Impact Investing:** Emerging tools such as *Development Impact Bonds (DIBs)* for maternal and child health, piloted in Rwanda and India, offer performance-linked returns to investors while ensuring measurable outcomes.
3. **Blended Finance and Crowdsourced Funding:** Platforms like *Sterling One Foundation* and *HelpMum* have leveraged corporate social responsibility funds to expand vaccine access and maternal care innovations.
4. **Basic Health Care Provision Fund (BHCPF) Disbursement Digitisation:** The shift toward electronic payments to facilities and verification agents is improving transparency and performance tracking.

Overview of Innovative Financing Mechanisms

Innovative financing mechanisms refer to non-traditional approaches that mobilise new resources for health, improve efficiency, or incentivise better outcomes. These include mechanisms like health bonds, results-based financing, community health insurance, and public-private partnerships. Such approaches are increasingly essential for bridging funding gaps in health, especially in developing countries [18].

Concept: Innovative financing mechanisms involve new and creative approaches to raising, managing, and utilising financial resources for health. These mechanisms aim to supplement traditional funding sources, improve financial sustainability, and enhance the effectiveness of health interventions.

Key Approaches:

1. **Performance-Based Financing (PBF):** PBF links financial incentives to the achievement of specific health outcomes or performance targets. This approach motivates healthcare providers to improve service quality and coverage by tying payments to measurable results.
2. **Health Impact Bonds:** Health impact bonds are financial instruments where investors provide upfront capital for health interventions and receive returns based on the achievement of predetermined health outcomes. This approach attracts private investment and aligns financial interests with health goals.

3. **Crowdfunding:** Crowdfunding involves raising small amounts of money from a large number of people, typically via online platforms. This method can mobilize public support and resources for specific health projects or programs.
4. **Social Impact Investing:** Social impact investing focuses on generating positive social outcomes alongside financial returns. Investors provide capital to health initiatives with the expectation of achieving measurable social impact and receiving financial returns.
5. **Blended Finance:** Blended finance combines public and private funding sources to support health initiatives. By leveraging public funds to attract private investment, blended finance can increase the overall financial resources available for health.

Successful Case Studies of Innovative Financing Mechanisms

Rwanda's community-based health insurance scheme has significantly expanded access to care and reduced out-of-pocket spending. In Nigeria, the Basic Health Care Provision Fund is an example of pooled funding that supports primary healthcare delivery. Elsewhere, the Global Financing Facility has leveraged donor and domestic funds to improve maternal and child health outcomes. These cases reflect how innovation in financing can drive equity and efficiency [18, 19].

Case Study 1: Rwanda's Performance-Based Financing Program

Background: Rwanda's Performance-Based Financing (PBF) program aims to improve healthcare service delivery by linking payments to the achievement of health targets at the facility level.

Key Features:

1. **Target-Based Payments:** Health facilities receive financial incentives based on their performance in delivering essential health services, such as immunisation and maternal care.
2. **Quality and Coverage Metrics:** Performance metrics include service quality, patient satisfaction, and coverage rates. Facilities are evaluated and rewarded based on their performance against these indicators.
3. **Community Involvement:** Community-based health committees are involved in monitoring and evaluating facility performance, ensuring that incentives align with local needs and priorities.

Impact: The PBF program has improved healthcare service delivery in Rwanda by motivating facilities to enhance their performance and achieve better health outcomes. The approach has led to increased service coverage and improved quality of care.

Case Study 2: The Global Fund's Health Impact Bonds

Background: The Global Fund has utilised health impact bonds to raise capital for health programs focused on combating diseases such as malaria and tuberculosis.

Key Features:

1. **Investor Engagement:** Investors provide upfront capital for health interventions, with returns tied to the achievement of specific health outcomes, such as reduced disease incidence or increased treatment adherence.
2. **Outcome-Based Returns:** Returns are based on the measurable impact of the interventions, ensuring that financial interests are aligned with health goals.
3. **Partnerships:** The initiative involves partnerships between investors, governments, and health organizations to ensure effective implementation and monitoring of the programs.

Impact: Health impact bonds have mobilized significant private investment for disease control programs, leading to improved health outcomes and increased funding for critical health interventions.

Case Study 3: India's Crowdfunding for Healthcare Projects

Background: Crowdfunding platforms in India have been used to raise funds for various healthcare projects, including the construction of health facilities and the purchase of medical equipment.

Key Features:

1. **Online Fundraising:** Crowdfunding platforms allow individuals and organisations to contribute small amounts of money to support specific health projects.
2. **Public Engagement:** Campaigns are often promoted through social media and other online channels, engaging the public and raising awareness about health issues.
3. **Transparency:** Platforms provide transparency in how funds are used, ensuring that contributors are informed about the impact of their donations.

Impact: Crowdfunding has successfully mobilised resources for healthcare projects in India, enabling the development of infrastructure and the provision of medical services. The approach has increased public involvement in health financing and supported community-driven initiatives.

Key Considerations for Implementing Innovative Financing Mechanisms

Implementing innovative financing mechanisms requires strong governance, transparency, and accountability to build trust among stakeholders. Clear outcome indicators, risk-sharing frameworks, and mechanisms for community involvement are vital. Additionally, ensuring alignment with national health priorities and legal frameworks helps institutionalise and sustain these mechanisms over time [18 - 20].

1. **Alignment with Health Priorities:** Innovative financing mechanisms should align with national and local health priorities to ensure that funds are used effectively to address pressing health needs.
2. **Capacity Building:** Building the capacity of health systems and stakeholders to manage and implement innovative financing mechanisms is essential. Training and support are needed to ensure the effective use of resources and the achievement of desired outcomes.
3. **Risk Management:** Assessing and managing risks associated with innovative financing mechanisms is crucial. This includes financial risks, operational challenges, and potential impacts on health programs.
4. **Monitoring and Evaluation:** Implementing robust monitoring and evaluation systems is necessary to track the performance of innovative financing mechanisms. This includes measuring the impact on health outcomes, financial efficiency, and overall program effectiveness.
5. **Stakeholder Engagement:** Engaging stakeholders, including government agencies, healthcare providers, and community organisations, is important for the successful implementation of innovative financing mechanisms. Collaboration and communication help to ensure alignment and address potential challenges.
6. **Sustainability:** Ensuring the sustainability of innovative financing mechanisms requires long-term planning and resource management. Mechanisms should be designed to provide ongoing support for health programs and adapt to changing needs and contexts.

CONCLUSION

Innovative financing mechanisms offer significant opportunities to enhance the funding and sustainability of health programs, particularly in resource-limited settings. Successful case studies from Rwanda, the Global Fund, and India demonstrate the potential of performance-based financing, health impact bonds, and crowdfunding to mobilise resources and improve health outcomes. By considering key factors such as alignment with health priorities, capacity building, and risk management, innovative financing approaches can effectively support and sustain health initiatives, contributing to the advancement of global health goals. As the landscape of health financing continues to evolve, these mechanisms will play an increasingly important role in addressing health challenges and promoting sustainable development.

LESSONS FROM SUCCESSFUL PUBLIC HEALTH INNOVATIONS

Public health innovations often lead to transformative changes in healthcare delivery, improving access, quality, and outcomes. Learning from successful public health innovations provides valuable insights for scaling up and replicating effective strategies. This section highlights key lessons derived from successful public health innovations, focusing on their implementation, impact, and sustainability. The aim is to guide the leveraging of these lessons to enhance public health efforts globally [21 - 24].

Emphasise Evidence-Based Approaches

Successful innovations are rooted in rigorous data and research. Evidence-based approaches ensure that interventions are relevant, effective, and scalable. Policymakers and implementers must prioritise data collection, pilot testing, and impact evaluation to guide decision-making and resource allocation [21].

Lesson: Successful public health innovations are grounded in robust evidence and research. Evidence-based approaches ensure that interventions are effective, efficient, and tailored to the needs of the target population.

Implementation:

1. **Research and Data Collection:** Conduct thorough research and data collection to identify health needs, determine the effectiveness of interventions, and guide decision-making.
2. **Pilot Testing:** Pilot test innovations in selected settings to evaluate their impact, refine strategies, and gather feedback before broader implementation.
3. **Continuous Evaluation:** Implement ongoing monitoring and evaluation to assess the effectiveness of innovations, adapt to changing circumstances, and ensure continuous improvement.

Impact: Evidence-based approaches enhance the likelihood of achieving desired health outcomes, ensuring that resources are used effectively and interventions are responsive to the needs of the population.

Foster Community Engagement and Ownership

Public health innovations thrive when communities are not passive recipients but active partners. Engaging communities in co-creation fosters local buy-in, adapts solutions to cultural contexts, and enhances accountability. Ownership also facilitates sustainability long after external support ends [21, 22].

Lesson: Engaging communities in the design, implementation, and evaluation of public health innovations leads to greater acceptance, ownership, and sustainability of interventions.

Implementation:

1. **Participatory Approaches:** Involve community members in decision-making processes, ensuring that their perspectives and needs are considered in the development of health interventions.
2. **Local Partnerships:** Establish partnerships with local organisations, leaders, and stakeholders to facilitate community engagement and support for public health initiatives.
3. **Capacity Building:** Provide training and support to community members and local organisations to build their capacity to implement and sustain health innovations.

Impact: Community engagement fosters trust, increases the relevance of interventions, and enhances the likelihood of successful implementation and long-term sustainability.

Leverage Technology and Innovation

Technology, whether digital health tools, diagnostics, or logistics systems, can accelerate impact and efficiency. Successful innovations often integrate simple, scalable technologies that address real-world challenges. Ensuring user-friendliness and adaptability is crucial to wide adoption [21 - 24].

Lesson: Technology and innovation play a critical role in enhancing public health interventions, improving access to services, and increasing efficiency.

Implementation:

1. **Adopt New Technologies:** Integrate technological advancements, such as mobile health apps, telemedicine, and electronic health records, into public health programs to improve service delivery and data management.

2. **Promote Innovation:** Encourage innovative solutions and approaches to address health challenges, leveraging creativity and technological advancements to enhance health outcomes.
3. **Ensure Accessibility:** Design technology-based interventions with accessibility in mind, making sure they are usable by diverse populations, including those in low-resource settings.

Impact: Leveraging technology and innovation improves the efficiency and effectiveness of health interventions, expands access to services, and supports better health outcomes.

Prioritise Sustainability and Scalability

Pilot projects must be designed with sustainability in mind. This includes securing long-term funding, embedding innovations in national systems, and planning for scale from the outset. Flexible models that can adapt to varying contexts also support broader replication [22 - 24].

Lesson: Sustainability and scalability are essential for the long-term success of public health innovations. Ensuring that interventions can be maintained and expanded helps to maximise their impact.

Implementation:

1. **Develop Sustainable Models:** Design innovations with sustainability in mind, including strategies for securing long-term funding, building local capacity, and integrating interventions into existing health systems.
2. **Plan for Scaling Up:** Develop strategies for scaling up successful innovations to reach larger populations or different regions, ensuring that they can be adapted to various contexts.
3. **Monitor and Adapt:** Continuously monitor the performance of innovations, identify challenges, and make necessary adjustments to ensure their sustainability and scalability.

Impact: Prioritising sustainability and scalability ensures that public health innovations can have a lasting impact, reaching broader populations and contributing to long-term health improvements.

Foster Multisectoral Collaboration

Health outcomes are influenced by sectors beyond healthcare, education, water and sanitation, agriculture, and more. Effective innovations often merge from cross-sector collaboration that leverages diverse expertise, shares resources, and addresses root determinants of health [21 - 24].

Lesson: Multisectoral collaboration is crucial for addressing complex health challenges and implementing effective innovations. Collaboration between various sectors enhances the effectiveness and reach of public health interventions.

Implementation:

1. **Engage Diverse Stakeholders:** Involve stakeholders from different sectors, including government, private sector, civil society, and academia, in the development and implementation of health innovations.
2. **Build Partnerships:** Establish partnerships and networks to leverage resources, expertise, and support for public health initiatives.
3. **Coordinate Efforts:** Ensure coordination and alignment of efforts across sectors to avoid duplication, maximise impact, and address health challenges comprehensively.

Impact: Multisectoral collaboration enhances the effectiveness and reach of public health innovations, ensuring a comprehensive approach to addressing health challenges and achieving positive outcomes.

Adapt to Local Contexts

No innovation succeeds without sensitivity to the social, cultural, and political environment. Contextual adaptation ensures relevance and acceptability. Successful programs are those that listen to communities, respect local norms, and tailor interventions accordingly [21 - 25].

Lesson: Public health innovations should be tailored to local contexts to ensure their relevance and effectiveness. Adapting interventions to the specific needs, cultures, and conditions of target populations enhances their success.

Implementation:

1. **Conduct Contextual Assessments:** Assess local conditions, including cultural, social, and economic factors, to understand the context in which innovations will be implemented.
2. **Adapt Interventions:** Modify innovations to fit local needs and preferences, ensuring that they are culturally appropriate and aligned with community values, language, and practices. This includes engaging local stakeholders in

the design and delivery of interventions to build trust, ownership, and sustainability.

CONCLUSION

There are several cross-cutting lessons and scalability factors that emerge from Nigeria's evolving innovation landscape and global experience. Some of these are:

1. **Institutionalisation:** Innovations must be embedded within national systems (FMoH, NPHCDA, or NCDC frameworks) to ensure continuity after pilot phases.
2. **Data Interoperability:** Linking innovations with DHIS2, LMIS, and HRH databases enhances scalability and monitoring.
3. **Public–Private Trust:** Strong governance frameworks and transparent contracts are vital to sustain PPPs.
4. **Community Engagement:** Local ownership ensures acceptance, adaptation, and equitable impact.
5. **Capacity Building:** Human capital development remains the backbone of technology adoption and scale.
6. **Adaptive Financing:** Diversifying funding sources and aligning incentives to results sustains innovation momentum.

It is important to underscore that the most successful innovations are context-specific, evidence-driven, and equity-oriented, ensuring that technological progress translates into tangible health gains for all.

REFERENCES

[1] World Health Organisation. (2021). Global Strategy on Digital Health 2020-2025. WHO. Available from: https://www.who.int/publications/i/item/9789240020924

[2] Kolawole JA, Edward OO. Issues on E-health Adoption in Nigeria. International Journal of Modern Education and Computer Science 2014; 6(9): 36-46. [http://dx.doi.org/10.5815/ijmecs.2014.09.06]

[3] Pharmacists Council of Nigeria. Community Pharmacy Initiative: Strengthening access to primary health care services through community pharmacies in Nigeria. Abuja: Federal Ministry of Health 2021.

[4] World Health Organisation. Nigeria Health System Review 2023. Geneva: WHO Regional Office for Africa 2023.

[5] Nigeria Centre for Disease Control and Prevention. Harnessing data science and artificial intelligence for public health surveillance in Nigeria. Abuja: NCDC 2023.

[6] Babatunde, A. O., Abdulkareem, A. A., Akinwande, F. O., Adebayo, A. O., Omenogor, E. T., Adebisi, Y. A., & Ilesanmi, E. B. (2021). Leveraging mobile health technology towards Achieving Universal Health Coverage in Nigeria. Public health in practice (Oxford, England), 2, 100120. [http://dx.doi.org/10.1016/j.puhip.2021.100120]

[7] Mackintosh M, Channon A, Karan A, Selvaraj S, Cavagnero E, Zhao H. What is the private sector? Understanding private provision in the health systems of low-income and middle-income countries. Lancet 2016; 388(10044): 596-605.
[http://dx.doi.org/10.1016/S0140-6736(16)00342-1] [PMID: 27358253]

[8] Anyaehie USB, Nwakoby BAN, Chikwendu C, *et al.* Constraints, challenges and prospects of public-private partnership in health-care delivery in a developing economy. Ann Med Health Sci Res 2014; 4(1): 61-6.
[http://dx.doi.org/10.4103/2141-9248.126615] [PMID: 24669333]

[9] The National Policy on Public Private Partnerships. Abuja, Nigeria: The Infrastructure Concession Regulatory Commission 2009.

[10] Okafor C. Improving Outcomes in the Nigeria Healthcare Sector through Public- Private Partnership. African Research Review 2016; 10(4): 1-17.
[http://dx.doi.org/10.4314/afrrev.v10i4.1]

[11] Rifkin SB. Examining the links between community participation and health outcomes: a review of the literature. Health Policy Plan 2014; 29(Suppl 2) (Suppl. 2): ii98-ii106.
[http://dx.doi.org/10.1093/heapol/czu076] [PMID: 25274645]

[12] Adepoju LA, Onafuye BA, Megbuwon T, Ogunseye OO. The Role of Community Health Workers in Enhancing Rural Primary Healthcare and Health Outcomes in Nigeria: A Review. Journal of Medicine and Health Research 2025; 10(1): 9-19.
[http://dx.doi.org/10.56557/jomahr/2025/v10i19082]

[13] World Health Organization. (2016). Framework on Integrated People-Centred Health Services. WHO. Available from: https://www.who.int/servicedeliverysafety/areas/people-centred-care/framework/en/

[14] GSMA. (2020). State of Mobile Internet Connectivity 2020. GSMA Intelligence. Retrieved from: https://www.gsma.com/r/wp-content/uploads/2020/09/GSMA-State-of-Mobile-Internet-Connec-ivity-Report-2020.pdf

[15] Labrique AB, Vasudevan L, Kochi E, Fabricant R, Mehl G. mHealth innovations as health system strengthening tools: 12 common applications and a visual framework. Glob Health Sci Pract 2013; 1(2): 160-71.
[http://dx.doi.org/10.9745/GHSP-D-13-00031] [PMID: 25276529]

[16] United Nations Development Programme. Financing the Future of Health: Innovative Models in Africa. New York: UNDP 2022.

[17] World Health Organisation. 2022.Innovation for Health in Africa: Scaling Local Solutions.

[18] Nwafor EC, Ogomegbulam M. Leveraging Technology to Enhance Healthcare Delivery and Reduce Brain Drain in Nigeria. Nigerian Health Journal 2024; 24(4): 1647-55.
[http://dx.doi.org/10.60787/tnhj.v24i4.893]

[19] Guarnaschelli, S., Lampert, S., Marsh, E., & Johnson, L. (2014). Innovative Financing for Development: Scalable Business Models that Produce Economic, Social, and Environmental Outcomes. Aspen Network of Development Entrepreneurs, 2300 N St. NW, #700, Washington, DC 20037.

[20] Federal Ministry of Health. (2017). Nigeria Health Financing Policy and Strategy. Achieving Universal Health Coverage and Rebuilding Nigeria's Economy through Efficient Health Investment. https://p4h.world/app/uploads/2023/02/Nigeria-Health-Financing-Pol-cy-Strategy21032019.x23411.pdf

[21] Abdullah F, Naledi T, Nettleship E, *et al.*. First social impact bond for the SAMRC: A novel financing strategy to address the health and social challenges facing adolescent girls and young women in South Africa. S Afr Med J 2019; 109(11b): 57-62.
[http://dx.doi.org/10.7196/SAMJ.2019.v109i11b.14254]

[22] Kruk ME, Gage AD, Arsenault C, *et al.* High-quality health systems in the Sustainable Development Goals era: time for a revolution. Lancet Glob Health 2018; 6(11): e1196-252. [http://dx.doi.org/10.1016/S2214-109X(18)30386-3] [PMID: 30196093]

[23] World Innovation Summit for Health. (2015). Global Diffusion Healthcare Innovation: Accelerating the Journey.

[24] Jamison DT, Gelband H, Horton S, *et al.* Disease Control Priorities: Improving Health and Reducing Poverty. 3rd ed. Washington (DC): The International Bank for Reconstruction and Development / The World Bank; 2017 Nov 27. [http://dx.doi.org/10.1596/978-1-4648-0527-1] [PMID: 30212058]

[25] Saleh J-EA. Resilient Communities: Navigating Public Health Challenges in Developing Nations. Bentham Science Publishers 2025. [http://dx.doi.org/10.2174/97898153056091250101]

CHAPTER 10

The Road Ahead: Strategies for Sustainable Health Transformation

Abstract: This chapter provides a comprehensive roadmap for sustainable health transformation in Nigeria and other developing nations. It emphasises the need for evidence-based policy recommendations, robust international partnerships, and the strengthening of health systems to tackle current and future public health challenges. The chapter aligns health transformation efforts with the Sustainable Development Goals (SDGs), particularly SDG 3. It explores the future of public health in the context of technological advancements, demographic changes, and environmental challenges. Finally, it calls for collective action across all sectors to mobilise for health transformation, ensuring that health gains are sustained for future generations.

Keywords: Collective Action, Future of Public Health, Health systems strengthening, Health Equity, International partnerships, Public health policy, Sustainable health transformation, Sustainable Development Goals (SDGs).

INTRODUCTION

As Nigeria and other developing nations navigate the complexities of public health, the journey toward sustainable health transformation is both challenging and promising. The road ahead demands a holistic approach that integrates policy innovation, international collaboration, and community engagement. The chapter explores the strategies necessary for sustaining the gains made in public health, strengthening health systems, and preparing for future challenges. It emphasises the importance of aligning with global health agendas, such as the SDGs, and mobilising all sectors of society to ensure that health transformation is not only achieved but sustained.

This concluding chapter summarises the lessons from the previous chapters. It distils lessons from the preceding chapters and emphasises that achieving sustainable health transformation in Nigeria and similar developing countries relies on the following:

Jalal-Eddeen Abubakar Saleh

- **Strong Governance and political will** that align policy with accountability.
- **Poverty reduction measures** and inclusive social protection mechanisms.
- **Strong, resilient health systems** anchored on infrastructure, workforce, and financing reforms.
- **Security, equity, and transparency**, ensuring health for all, even in fragile contexts.
- **Innovation and partnerships** that accelerate impact through technology and collaboration.

These insights once again reaffirmed that health transformation is not a linear journey but a continuous cycle of learning, adapting, and reinforcing systemic resilience.

Fig. (**1**) is a flowchart of the Roadmap to Health Transformation. It outlines a systematic pathway from policy formulation to measurable health outcomes. It begins with Policy Design and Strategic Planning, which lays the foundational vision and priorities for the health system. This leads to Stakeholder Engagement and Partnerships, ensuring inclusive collaboration across government agencies, communities, civil society, and the private sector. Resource Mobilisation and Sustainable Funding follows, highlighting the importance of securing and efficiently utilising financial, human, and material resources. At the core of operationalisation are Governance Structures and Institutional Capacity, which enable transparent coordination and resilient leadership. These elements feed into Program Implementation and Service Delivery, where interventions are rolled out, followed by Monitoring, Evaluation, and Accountability to assess performance and guide improvement. The outcome is Health Outcomes and Impact, which reflects the effectiveness and equity of the health transformation agenda.

Interwoven throughout the roadmap are essential cross-cutting enablers that sustain and amplify progress at every stage. Governance and Leadership provide vision, legitimacy, and coordination. Funding and Financial Sustainability ensure continuity and responsiveness in health interventions. Partnerships and Collaboration leverage multisectoral inputs and shared ownership, while Transparency and Accountability reinforce trust, drive results, and reduce inefficiencies. Together, these enablers create a robust ecosystem for achieving transformational change in health systems, particularly in low- and middle-income contexts.

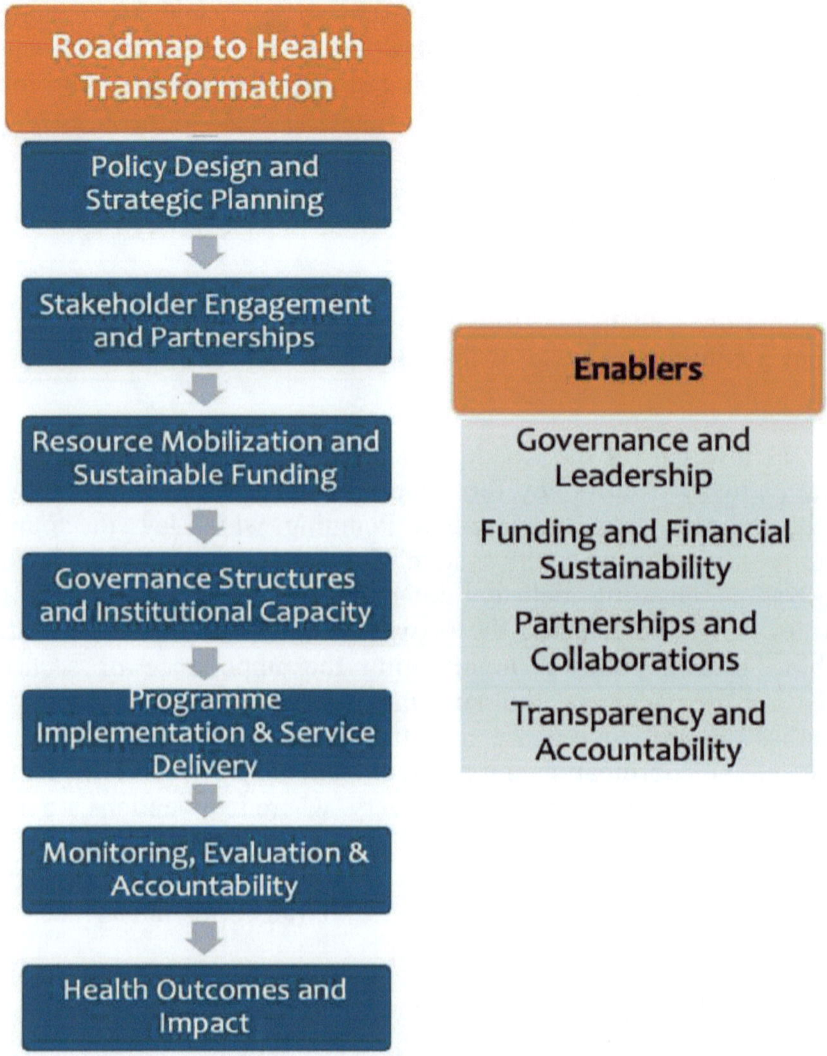

Fig. (1). Flowchart showing the roadmap to health transformation.

POLICY RECOMMENDATIONS FOR HEALTH TRANSFORMATION

The transformation of health systems in Nigeria and other developing nations requires comprehensive and well-coordinated policy interventions. Sustainable health transformation is not only about immediate improvements in health outcomes but also about creating a resilient system that can adapt to future challenges [1, 2].

This section outlines key policy recommendations and action steps that are essential for achieving sustainable health transformation, focusing on governance, financing, workforce development, infrastructure, and innovation. The Table **1** below presents some policy recommendations matching key actions with policy areas and a suggested timeline: short-term (1-2 years), medium-term (3-5 years), and long-term (> 5 years) [1, 2].

Table 1. shows the phased implementation of policy recommendations for health transformation in nigeria.

Policy Area	Action Steps	Timeline	Implementation Notes
10.1.1 Strengthening Governance and Accountability	• Develop and enforce anti-corruption policies. • Promote decentralization. • Enhance leadership capacity	**Short–Medium Term**	Governance reforms (anti-corruption and transparency) can begin immediately; decentralization and leadership development will mature over time.
10.1.2 Ensuring Sustainable Health Financing	• Increase public health investment. • Expand health insurance coverage. • Diversify funding sources	**Medium–Long Term**	Budgetary alignment can start short-term, but achieving UHC and diversified financing mechanisms requires gradual policy and structural reform.
10.1.3 Building a Resilient Health Workforce	• Invest in health education and training. • Improve working conditions and incentives. • Strengthen workforce planning and management.	**Medium–Long Term**	Workforce expansion and retention strategies need sustained funding and institutional reform; outcomes are visible over several years.
10.1.4 Enhancing Health Infrastructure	• Upgrade existing health facilities. • Expand infrastructure in underserved areas. • Leverage digital and telehealth technology	**Medium–Long Term**	Facility upgrades can start immediately, but full infrastructure expansion and digital integration require long-term investment and coordination.
10.1.5 Fostering Innovation and Research	• Support health research and development. • Encourage adoption of innovative technologies. • Facilitate knowledge sharing and collaboration	**Short–Medium Term**	Research funding and digital innovations can begin with modest resources; institutionalization and scale-up occur over time.
10.1.6 Promoting Equity and Inclusivity in Health	• Address social determinants of health. • Target marginalised groups. • Monitor and evaluate equity outcomes.	**Short–Long Term**	Targeted interventions can start quickly; addressing social determinants and equity tracking will require multi-sectoral, sustained engagement.

Strengthening Governance and Accountability

Governance and accountability are the cornerstones of a well-functioning health system. In Nigeria and other developing nations, weak governance has led to inefficiencies, corruption, and mismanagement of resources, ultimately hampering health outcomes. Strengthening governance involves instituting transparent decision-making processes, enforcing regulatory frameworks, and ensuring that all stakeholders, government agencies, health professionals, and the public are held accountable for service delivery. Strong leadership at all levels of government is crucial in driving reforms that improve efficiency, oversight, and patient-centeredcare [1].

Recommendation: In strengthening governance and accountability, a critical requirement is to implement robust governance frameworks that enhance transparency, accountability, and efficiency in the health sector. Effective governance is the cornerstone of a well-functioning health system, ensuring that resources are used efficiently and that health services are delivered equitably. The action steps are as outlined below [1]:

Action Steps:

1. **Develop and Enforce Anti-Corruption Policies:** Implement strict anti-corruption measures and establish independent bodies to monitor and enforce these policies within the health sector. This includes regular audits, transparent procurement processes, and clear reporting mechanisms.
2. **Promote Decentralisation:** Encourage the decentralisation of health governance, empowering local health authorities to make decisions that reflect the needs and priorities of their communities. This approach fosters accountability and responsiveness at the local level.
3. **Enhance Leadership Capacity:** Invest in leadership training programs for health sector managers and policymakers to strengthen their ability to implement and sustain health reforms. Strong leadership is critical for driving the transformation agenda and ensuring that policies are effectively translated into action.

Ensuring Sustainable Health Financing

Health financing remains a critical challenge for many developing nations, where underfunding leads to inadequate healthcare access, poor infrastructure, and workforce shortages. Relying heavily on out-of-pocket payments creates financial hardship for many households and limits service utilisation. Sustainable financing models, such as increasing domestic budgetary allocations, implementing Universal Health Coverage (UHC) schemes, and leveraging innovative financing mechanisms (e.g., public-private partnerships), are essential to ensuring that healthcare services remain accessible, affordable, and of high quality [1].

Recommendation: Establishing sustainable health financing mechanisms that ensure equitable access to quality healthcare for all citizens, regardless of their socio-economic status, is a critical requirement. Adequate and sustainable financing is essential for the long-term viability of health systems. The action steps are as outlined below [1, 2]:

Action Steps:

1. **Increase Public Health Investment:** Advocate for increased government spending on health, ensuring that health budgets are aligned with national health priorities and the needs of the population. This includes committing a significant portion of the national budget to health, as recommended by the Abuja Declaration.
2. **Expand Health Insurance Coverage:** Implement Universal Health Coverage (UHC) through expanded health insurance schemes that are accessible to all, particularly the poor and vulnerable populations. This can be achieved by scaling up community-based health insurance programs and integrating them into a national framework.
3. **Diversify Funding Sources:** Explore innovative financing mechanisms, such as health bonds, public-private partnerships, and international aid, to supplement domestic funding and reduce reliance on out-of-pocket payments. Diversified funding sources ensure that the health sector is financially resilient and capable of withstanding economic shocks.

Building a Resilient Health Workforce

The availability of skilled healthcare professionals is fundamental to health system performance, yet Nigeria faces persistent workforce shortages, brain drain, and uneven distribution of healthcare workers. A resilient workforce requires strategic investments in training, retention incentives, and equitable deployment, particularly in underserved areas. Policies must prioritise continuous professional development, improved working conditions, and stronger community health workforce integration to ensure that services reach even the most remote populations [1, 2].

Recommendation: Developing and implementing strategies to build a resilient and motivated health workforce capable of delivering quality healthcare services across all levels of the health system must be incorporated. A well-trained and adequately supported workforce is crucial for the success of health transformation efforts. The action steps are as outlined below [1, 2]:

Action Steps:

1. **Invest in Health Education and Training:** Expand and improve health education and training programs to produce a sufficient number of skilled healthcare professionals. This includes upgrading medical and nursing schools, offering continuous professional development, and addressing gaps in the training of specialised healthcare workers.
2. **Improve Working Conditions and Incentives:** Enhance the working conditions of healthcare workers by providing competitive salaries, safe working environments, and career development opportunities. Incentives such as rural service allowances and housing benefits can attract and retain healthcare professionals in underserved areas.
3. **Strengthen Workforce Planning and Management:** Implement effective workforce planning and management systems to ensure that healthcare workers are deployed where they are most needed. This includes leveraging data to forecast workforce needs and ensuring an equitable distribution of healthcare personnel across regions.

Enhancing Health Infrastructure

Deficient health infrastructure, including inadequate health facilities, outdated medical equipment, and poor transportation networks, poses a significant barrier to quality healthcare in many developing nations. Addressing these challenges requires a multi-sectoral approach that includes targeted infrastructure investments, improved supply chain management for essential medicines, and expansion of healthcare facilities, particularly in rural and peri-urban areas. Strengthening primary healthcare centers as the first point of contact for communities is essential for ensuring widespread health access [1, 2].

Recommendation: Investing in the development and maintenance of health infrastructure to support the delivery of quality healthcare services is sacrosanct. Adequate infrastructure, including health facilities, medical equipment, and technology, is fundamental to achieving sustainable health transformation. The action steps are as outlined below [1, 2]:

Action Steps:

1. **Upgrade Existing Health Facilities:** Renovate and equip existing health facilities to meet modern standards of care. This includes ensuring the availability of essential medical equipment, reliable electricity, clean water, and sanitation facilities.
2. **Expand Health Infrastructure in Underserved Areas:** Prioritize the construction of new health facilities in underserved and remote areas to improve access to healthcare. Mobile clinics and telemedicine initiatives can also be employed to reach populations in hard-to-access regions.
3. **Leverage Technology for Infrastructure Development:** Incorporate digital health technologies, such as electronic health records (EHRs) and telehealth platforms, into the health infrastructure to enhance service delivery and data management. Technology can also facilitate the integration of health services and improve overall system efficiency.

Fostering Innovation and Research

Innovation and research are pivotal for driving health transformation, yet many developing nations struggle with weak research capacity and limited investment in medical and public health innovation. Encouraging local research, supporting indigenous solutions, and fostering partnerships between academia, industry, and government can accelerate advancements in healthcare delivery. Digital health technologies, Artificial Intelligence (AI) in diagnostics, and telemedicine offer promising pathways to expanding healthcare access and improving service efficiency [1, 2].

Recommendation: Promoting innovation and research in the health sector to drive continuous improvement and adaptation to emerging challenges must be considered. Innovation is key to developing new solutions that can address persistent health issues and improve the effectiveness of healthcare delivery. The action steps are as outlined below [1, 2]:

Action Steps:

1. **Support Health Research and Development:** Allocate funding and resources for health Research and Development (R&D) to foster innovation in disease prevention, treatment, and health system management. Collaboration with academic institutions and research organisations can enhance the quality and relevance of research efforts.
2. **Encourage the Adoption of Innovative Technologies:** Create an enabling environment for the adoption of innovative health technologies, including

regulatory frameworks that support the safe and effective use of new tools and treatments. This includes fast-tracking the approval and integration of new medical devices, pharmaceuticals, and digital health solutions.

3. **Facilitate Knowledge Sharing and Collaboration:** Establish platforms for knowledge sharing and collaboration among healthcare providers, researchers, and policymakers. This can include conferences, workshops, and online forums that promote the exchange of ideas and best practices in health innovation.

Promoting Equity and Inclusivity in Health

Health disparities remain a significant concern, particularly for marginalised groups, including women, children, people with disabilities, and rural communities. A commitment to equity means ensuring that all populations, regardless of socioeconomic status, have access to high-quality healthcare. Policies must address social determinants of health, remove financial and cultural barriers to care, and strengthen community engagement in health decision-making to promote inclusive health systems [1, 2].

Recommendation: Ensuring that health policies and programs are designed and implemented with a focus on equity and inclusivity, addressing the needs of all population groups, especially the most vulnerable, is the global norm. Equity is central to achieving health transformation that benefits the entire population. The action steps are as outlined below [1, 2]:

Action Steps:

1. **Address Social Determinants of Health:** Develop policies that address the social determinants of health, such as poverty, education, and housing, which contribute to health disparities. Multi-sectoral approaches are necessary to tackle these underlying factors and promote health equity.
2. **Target Interventions for Marginalised Groups:** Design targeted health interventions that address the specific needs of marginalised and vulnerable populations, including women, children, people with disabilities, and rural communities. This includes ensuring access to essential health services and reducing barriers to care.
3. **Monitor and Evaluate Equity Outcomes:** Implement monitoring and evaluation systems that track health outcomes across different population groups, ensuring that progress is being made toward greater equity. Data disaggregation by factors such as gender, age, and socio-economic status is essential for identifying and addressing health inequities.

CONCLUSION

The transformation of health systems requires a comprehensive approach that addresses governance, financing, workforce development, infrastructure, innovation, and equity. By implementing these policy recommendations, Nigeria and other developing nations can build resilient health systems capable of delivering high-quality, equitable healthcare to all citizens. Sustainable health transformation is not an endpoint but an ongoing process that requires continuous commitment, adaptation, and collaboration across all sectors of society.

THE ROLE OF INTERNATIONAL PARTNERSHIPS AND COLLABORATIONS

International partnerships and collaborations are vital for achieving sustainable health transformation, especially in developing nations like Nigeria. In the public health space, international partnerships have been catalytic in health system strengthening and emergency response. Examples of some key partners working in the health space include:

- The World Health Organisation (WHO): The WHO jointly developed the Nigeria Country Cooperation Strategy 4, a medium-term strategic framework covering 2023–2027, which aims to support Nigeria in attaining the Universal Health Coverage and emergency preparedness.
- World Bank (WB): The WB collaborates with Nigeria through the Nigeria State Health Investment Project (NSHIP) and Accelerating Nutrition Results in Nigeria (ANRiN).
- Global Fund (GF): The GF partners with the Nigerian Government to contribute to reducing the burden of HIV, TB, and malaria, and enabling continuity of essential services.

These partnerships aim to achieve SDG 17, and in this context, with a focus on SDG 3 (Good Health and Well-being), leveraging resources, technical expertise, and innovative solutions that can significantly enhance national efforts to improve public health [3, 4]. This section explores the critical role that international collaborations play in strengthening health systems, facilitating knowledge exchange, and addressing global health challenges.

Strengthening Health Systems Through Global Support

International organisations, donor agencies, and global health initiatives have played a crucial role in supporting Nigeria's health system, particularly in disease control, maternal health, and emergency response. However, aid dependency can be counterproductive if not aligned with national priorities. Strengthening health systems through global support requires integrating external funding with national health strategies and ensuring that aid programs build long-term resilience rather than short-term fixes [3, 4].

Recommendation: Leverage international partnerships to strengthen national health systems by tapping into global expertise, financial resources, and technical assistance. These collaborations are essential for building the capacity needed to address complex health challenges and improve health outcomes. The action steps are as outlined below [3, 4]:

Action Steps:

1. **Engage with Multilateral Organisations:** Collaborate with multilateral organisations such as the World Health Organisation (WHO), the World Bank, and the Global Fund to Fight AIDS, Tuberculosis, and Malaria. These organisations provide crucial support in the form of funding, technical assistance, and policy guidance, helping countries strengthen their health systems and achieve their health goals.
2. **Participate in Global Health Initiatives:** Actively participate in global health initiatives and programs, such as Gavi, the Vaccine Alliance, and the Global Health Security Agenda (GHSA). These initiatives offer valuable resources and expertise to improve immunisation coverage, disease surveillance, and health security, contributing to national health system resilience.
3. **Access to Innovative Technologies and Practices:** Through international partnerships, countries can gain access to cutting-edge technologies and innovative practices that may not be readily available domestically. For example, partnerships with countries and organisations leading in digital health can help introduce and scale up electronic health records (EHRs), telemedicine, and mobile health solutions in low-resource settings.

Facilitating Knowledge Exchange and Capacity Building

One of the most significant benefits of global partnerships is the opportunity for knowledge exchange and workforce capacity building. Collaborations with academic institutions, professional networks, and multilateral organisations can help bridge skill gaps, improve clinical training, and strengthen research capabilities. Investing in South-South and triangular cooperation models allows for experience-sharing between countries facing similar challenges [3, 4].

Recommendation: Promote knowledge exchange and capacity building through international collaborations to enhance the skills and competencies of health professionals and policymakers. Knowledge sharing is a powerful tool for fostering innovation and improving health system performance. The action steps are as outlined below [3, 4]:

Action Steps:

1. **South-South and Triangular Cooperation:** Engage in South-South and triangular cooperation, where countries with similar development contexts share experiences, best practices, and lessons learned. This form of collaboration can lead to more contextually relevant solutions and mutual learning, fostering capacity building and innovation.
2. **International Training and Fellowship Programs:** Participate in international training programs, workshops, and fellowships that focus on critical areas such as health leadership, epidemiology, and public health management. These programs help build local expertise, enabling countries to design and implement effective health policies and programs.
3. **Research Collaboration and Data Sharing:** Foster research collaboration with international academic institutions, research centers, and think tanks. Joint research projects and data-sharing agreements can accelerate the generation of evidence needed to inform policy decisions and address emerging health challenges.

Addressing Global Health Challenges Through Collaboration

Many health challenges, such as infectious disease outbreaks, antimicrobial resistance, and climate-related health threats, transcend national borders. Effective collaboration in global health security, pandemic preparedness, and coordinated research efforts can enhance collective responses to shared threats. Nigeria must actively engage in regional and global health governance platforms to ensure representation and inclusion in global health decision-making [3, 4].

Recommendation: Collaborate with international partners to address global health challenges that transcend national borders, such as pandemics, antimicrobial resistance (AMR), and climate change. Collective action is essential for tackling these issues, as they require coordinated efforts and shared resources. The action steps are as outlined below [3, 4]:

Action Steps:

1. **Pandemic Preparedness and Response:** Strengthen pandemic preparedness and response capacities through international collaboration. Engage in global efforts to develop and implement pandemic response plans, share

epidemiological data, and participate in joint exercises and simulations. This approach ensures a coordinated and effective response to pandemics, minimising their impact on public health.

2. **Combating Antimicrobial Resistance:** Partner with international organisations and countries to combat antimicrobial resistance (AMR), a growing global threat. Collaborative efforts should focus on promoting the rational use of antibiotics, supporting research into new treatments, and strengthening surveillance systems to monitor and respond to AMR.
3. **Mitigating the Health Impacts of Climate Change:** Work with global partners to address the health impacts of climate change, which disproportionately affect vulnerable populations in developing countries. International collaborations can support the development of climate-resilient health systems, promote sustainable practices, and provide funding for adaptation and mitigation efforts.

Enhancing Policy Coherence and Alignment

Disjointed policies between international donors and national health strategies often lead to inefficiencies and duplication of efforts. Ensuring policy coherence requires better alignment between foreign assistance programs and national priorities, harmonization of donor interventions, and the integration of global health initiatives within Nigeria's broader development framework [3, 4].

Recommendation: Ensure that international collaborations align with national health priorities and policies to maximize their impact and sustainability. Policy coherence and alignment are critical for integrating global initiatives into national health strategies effectively. The action steps are as outlined below [3, 4]:

Action Steps:

1. **Align International Support with National Health Plans:** Ensure that international support is aligned with national health plans and priorities. This can be achieved by involving national stakeholders in the planning and implementation of international projects, ensuring that they complement and strengthen existing health initiatives.
2. **Strengthen Coordination Mechanisms:** Establish coordination mechanisms to manage international partnerships and collaborations effectively. This includes creating a dedicated unit within the Ministry of Health to oversee international relations, ensuring that all partnerships are aligned with national goals and avoiding duplication of efforts.
3. **Monitor and Evaluate the Impact of Collaborations:** Implement monitoring and evaluation systems to assess the impact of international collaborations on

national health outcomes. Regular evaluations can help identify areas of improvement, ensure accountability, and demonstrate the value of these partnerships to both national and international stakeholders.

Promoting Global Solidarity and Mutual Learning

A strong global health system depends on mutual learning and equitable partnerships rather than one-sided aid relationships. Nigeria and other developing nations must transition from being passive aid recipients to active contributors to the global health knowledge pool. Strengthening south-south cooperation, engaging in policy dialogues, and advocating for fairer global health governance structures are critical for fostering a more balanced and equitable global health landscape [3, 4].

Recommendation: Foster a spirit of global solidarity and mutual learning through international partnerships, recognising that health challenges are interconnected and that shared solutions benefit all countries. Collaboration should be based on mutual respect, equity, and the recognition of shared goals. The action steps are as outlined below [3, 4]:

Action Steps:

1. **Engage in Global Health Diplomacy:** Actively participate in global health diplomacy efforts, advocating for the interests of developing nations in international forums. This includes contributing to global discussions on health equity, access to medicines, and the right to health, ensuring that the voices of low- and middle-income countries are heard.
2. **Promote Mutual Learning Opportunities:** Encourage the exchange of knowledge and experiences between countries, recognizing that all nations have valuable lessons to share. This can include hosting international conferences, participating in global health networks, and supporting cross-country learning visits.
3. **Support Global Health Solidarity Initiatives:** Contribute to global health solidarity initiatives, such as the COVID-19 Vaccines Global Access (COVAX) facility, which aims to ensure equitable access to vaccines worldwide. By participating in such initiatives, countries can demonstrate their commitment to global health equity and contribute to the collective effort to improve health outcomes for all.

CONCLUSION

International partnerships and collaborations play a pivotal role in the sustainable transformation of health systems. By engaging with global partners, Nigeria and other developing nations can access the resources, knowledge, and support needed to overcome their health challenges. These collaborations not only strengthen national health systems but also contribute to global health security and equity. As the world becomes increasingly interconnected, the importance of international partnerships in health will continue to grow, making them a key component of any strategy for sustainable health transformation.

STRENGTHENING HEALTH SYSTEMS FOR FUTURE CHALLENGES

In the face of evolving global health threats, strengthening health systems is imperative to ensure resilience, adaptability, and sustainability. As Nigeria and other developing nations navigate the complexities of modern public health, building robust health systems capable of withstanding future challenges is crucial. This section explores the key strategies for enhancing health systems to address both current and emerging health issues, ensuring that they are equipped to protect and improve public health outcomes in the years to come [5, 6].

Building Resilient Health Infrastructure

Future-proofing Nigeria's health system requires long-term investments in infrastructure that can withstand emerging health threats, including pandemics and climate-induced health emergencies. A focus on climate-resilient healthcare facilities, smart hospital designs, and sustainable supply chains can enhance system durability and preparedness [5, 6].

Recommendation: Invest in health infrastructure that can withstand emergencies and provide continuous, high-quality care across all regions. Resilient infrastructure is the foundation of a strong health system, capable of delivering services even in the face of natural disasters, pandemics, and other crises. The action steps are as outlined below [5, 6]:

Action Steps:

1. **Upgrade Healthcare Facilities:** Modernise healthcare facilities with a focus on durability, accessibility, and the ability to scale services during emergencies. This includes building and refurbishing hospitals, clinics, and laboratories to meet international standards, ensuring they are equipped to handle increased patient loads and complex cases during crises.
2. **Strengthen Supply Chains:** Develop robust supply chains for medical supplies, medicines, and equipment to ensure uninterrupted service delivery, even during emergencies. This involves creating strategic stockpiles, establi-

shing reliable distribution networks, and implementing advanced logistics systems to manage resources effectively.

3. **Promote Energy and Water Security:** Ensure healthcare facilities have reliable access to clean water and electricity, which are critical for maintaining operations. Investing in renewable energy sources, such as solar power, and ensuring adequate water storage and filtration systems can enhance the resilience of health facilities, particularly in remote and underserved areas.

Enhancing Workforce Capacity and Flexibility

Health workforce planning must account for shifting disease patterns, technological advancements, and evolving patient needs. Building a flexible workforce means fostering interdisciplinary collaboration, upskilling health workers in emerging areas such as digital health, and adopting adaptable staffing models that allow for rapid response to health crises [5, 6].

Recommendation: Expand and empower the health workforce to meet the demands of a rapidly changing health landscape. A well-trained, adequately staffed, and flexible health workforce is essential for delivering quality care and responding effectively to new challenges. The action steps are as outlined below [5, 6]:

Action Steps:

1. **Invest in Health Education and Training:** Strengthen health education institutions to produce a steady pipeline of skilled healthcare professionals. This includes increasing the capacity of medical schools, nursing colleges, and allied health training programs, as well as providing continuous professional development opportunities for existing workers.
2. **Promote Task-Shifting and Multi-Skilling:** Implement task-shifting strategies, where non-physician healthcare workers are trained to perform specific tasks traditionally done by doctors. This approach can help address workforce shortages and improve service delivery efficiency. Additionally, promote multi-skilling to enable health workers to adapt to various roles and responsibilities, particularly in emergencies.
3. **Enhance Workforce Retention:** Develop strategies to retain health workers, particularly in rural and underserved areas. This includes offering competitive salaries, providing safe and supportive working environments, and creating opportunities for career advancement. Retention strategies should also focus on addressing the physical and mental well-being of health workers, ensuring they are equipped to handle the stresses of their roles.

Leveraging Technology for Health System Strengthening

Digital transformation is reshaping healthcare delivery, from electronic health records and artificial intelligence diagnostics to remote patient monitoring. Investing in digital infrastructure, improving internet connectivity in rural areas, and fostering e-health innovation will be essential in optimizing healthcare delivery [5, 6].

Recommendation: Harness the power of technology to enhance health system efficiency, improve service delivery, and facilitate data-driven decision-making. Technological innovation is a critical enabler of health system strengthening, offering tools and solutions to address emerging challenges. The action steps are as outlined below [5, 6]:

Action Steps:

1. **Implement Health Information Systems:** Develop and deploy integrated Health Information Systems (HIS) that allow for real-time data collection, analysis, and sharing across all levels of the health system. HIS can improve patient care, streamline operations, and support evidence-based decision-making, enabling health systems to respond more effectively to emerging challenges.
2. **Expand Telemedicine and Digital Health Solutions:** Scale up telemedicine services to expand access to healthcare, particularly in remote and underserved areas. Digital health solutions, such as mobile health (mHealth) apps and Electronic Health Records (EHRs), can enhance patient engagement, improve care coordination, and reduce the burden on physical healthcare facilities.
3. **Promote Innovation in Medical Technologies:** Encourage the development and adoption of innovative medical technologies, such as point-of-care diagnostics, wearable health monitors, and artificial intelligence-driven tools. These technologies can improve disease detection, enable personalised treatment, and enhance the overall efficiency of health systems.

Strengthening Health System Governance and Leadership

Effective governance ensures that health policies translate into meaningful action. Strong leadership at national and sub-national levels is necessary to drive reform, enhance accountability, and sustain political commitment to healthcare improvements. Leadership training for health administrators and greater citizen participation in health governance can further reinforce system accountability [5, 6].

Recommendation: Improve governance and leadership within health systems to ensure accountability, transparency, and strategic direction. Strong governance is critical for coordinating efforts, optimising resources, and driving continuous improvement in health service delivery. The action steps are as outlined below [5, 6]:

Action Steps:

1. **Enhance Policy and Regulatory Frameworks:** Update and strengthen health policies and regulatory frameworks to reflect current and future health challenges. This includes setting clear guidelines for service delivery, quality standards, and accountability mechanisms, ensuring that health systems operate efficiently and ethically.
2. **Foster Leadership Development:** Invest in leadership development programs for health sector managers and policymakers. Effective leadership is essential for navigating complex health challenges, making strategic decisions, and motivating health workers. Leadership programs should focus on building skills in strategic planning, crisis management, and stakeholder engagement.
3. **Promote Multi-Sectoral Coordination:** Establish mechanisms for multi-sectoral coordination, bringing together various government departments, non-governmental organisations, and private sector partners. This approach ensures a holistic and integrated response to health challenges, leveraging the strengths and resources of all stakeholders.

Ensuring Financial Sustainability and Equity

Long-term health financing strategies must prioritise efficiency, financial protection mechanisms, and equitable resource distribution. Strengthening national health insurance schemes, reducing reliance on external funding, and implementing innovative financing models such as social health insurance and result-based funding will help secure sustainable financing [5, 6].

Recommendation: Secure long-term financial sustainability and promote equity in health financing to ensure that health systems can deliver quality care to all populations, regardless of their socio-economic status. Financial resilience is key to sustaining health system improvements and achieving Universal Health Coverage (UHC). The action steps are as outlined below [5, 6]:

Action Steps:

1. **Diversify Health Financing Sources:** Explore innovative financing mechanisms, such as public-private partnerships, health insurance schemes, and

international funding opportunities, to diversify the sources of health financing. This approach reduces reliance on a single funding source and enhances financial stability.

2. **Implement Pro-Poor Financing Policies:** Design and implement pro-poor health financing policies that protect vulnerable populations from financial hardship. This includes expanding access to health insurance, reducing out-o--pocket payments, and subsidising healthcare costs for low-income families.
3. **Strengthen Financial Management Systems:** Improve financial management systems within the health sector to ensure efficient use of resources and prevent wastage. This involves implementing robust budgeting, accounting, and auditing processes, as well as building the capacity of health managers in financial management.

Adapting to Emerging Global Health Threats

The future of public health in Nigeria will be shaped by emerging threats such as antimicrobial resistance, new infectious diseases, and the impact of climate change. Health systems must be agile enough to respond to these evolving challenges by integrating surveillance mechanisms, fostering cross-sectoral collaboration, and investing in emergency preparedness [5, 6].

Recommendation: Continuously adapt health systems to address emerging global health threats, such as pandemics, antimicrobial resistance (AMR), and climate change. A proactive and adaptive approach is necessary to protect public health in an increasingly interconnected and rapidly changing world. The action steps are as outlined below [5, 6]:

Action Steps:

1. **Enhance Pandemic Preparedness:** Develop and regularly update pandemic preparedness plans, ensuring that health systems are equipped to respond swiftly and effectively to future outbreaks. This includes investing in early warning systems, stockpiling essential supplies, and conducting regular training and simulations for health workers.
2. **Address Antimicrobial Resistance (AMR):** Implement strategies to combat antimicrobial resistance, including promoting the rational use of antibiotics, strengthening infection prevention and control measures, and supporting research into new treatments. AMR poses a significant threat to global health, and coordinated action is essential to mitigate its impact.
3. **Mitigate the Health Impacts of Climate Change:** Develop climate-resilient health systems capable of withstanding the impacts of climate change, such as extreme weather events, vector-borne diseases, and food insecurity. This

involves integrating climate adaptation strategies into health planning, building climate-resilient infrastructure, and promoting sustainable practices within the health sector.

CONCLUSION

Strengthening health systems for future challenges is a critical component of sustainable health transformation. By building resilient infrastructure, enhancing workforce capacity, leveraging technology, improving governance, ensuring financial sustainability, and adapting to emerging threats, Nigeria and other developing nations can create health systems that are capable of protecting and improving public health outcomes in the face of an uncertain future. These efforts will not only enhance national health security but also contribute to global health equity and resilience, ensuring that all populations can access the care they need, now and in the future.

SUSTAINABLE DEVELOPMENT GOALS AND HEALTH

The Sustainable Development Goals (SDGs), adopted by the United Nations in 2015, represent a universal call to action to end poverty, protect the planet, and ensure that all people enjoy peace and prosperity by 2030. Health is a central component of the SDGs, with Goal 3 specifically dedicated to ensuring healthy lives and promoting well-being for all at all ages. However, health is interconnected with many other goals, highlighting the importance of a holistic approach to achieving sustainable development. The integration of these goals into national planning frameworks offers a roadmap to monitor progress and for accountability purposes. This section explores the critical role of health in the SDGs and how health systems can be strengthened to contribute to their attainment [7]. Though the focus is on SDGs 3, it is critical to mention that Nigeria's health transformation agenda aligns closely with SDGs 3 and 17, and the integration of these goals into national planning frameworks offers a roadmap for progress monitoring and accountability.

- **SDG 3** – *Ensure healthy lives and promote well-being for all at all ages.*
- **SDG 17** – *Strengthen the means of implementation and revitalise global partnerships for sustainable development.*

SDG 3: Ensure Healthy Lives and Promote Well-Being for All

Overview of SDG 3

SDG 3 aims to ensure healthy lives and promote well-being across the lifespan by addressing key health challenges such as maternal and child mortality, communicable and non-communicable diseases, substance abuse, and road traffic accidents. The goal also emphasises the importance of universal health coverage (UHC), access to quality essential health services, and financial risk protection [7].

Key Targets under SDG 3:

1. **Reducing Maternal and Child Mortality:** Achieve a global reduction in maternal mortality to less than 70 per 100,000 live births and end preventable deaths of newborns and children under 5 years of age.
2. **Combatting Communicable Diseases:** End the epidemics of AIDS, tuberculosis, malaria, and neglected tropical diseases, and combat hepatitis, water-borne diseases, and other communicable diseases.
3. **Addressing Non-Communicable Diseases (NCDs):** Reduce by one-third premature mortality from non-communicable diseases through prevention, treatment, and the promotion of mental health and well-being.
4. **Universal Health Coverage (UHC):** Achieve universal health coverage, including access to quality essential health services, medicines, and vaccines for all, while ensuring financial protection for those in need.

Challenges in Achieving SDG 3: Despite significant progress in global health, many challenges remain, particularly in developing nations like Nigeria. These include weak health systems, inadequate funding, poor access to health services, and the growing burden of non-communicable diseases. Achieving SDG 3 will require concerted efforts to strengthen health systems, address social determinants of health, and mobilise resources effectively [7].

Health as a Cross-Cutting Theme in the SDGs

Interlinkages between Health and Other SDGs

Health is intrinsically linked to many other SDGs, underscoring the importance of an integrated approach to sustainable development. Key interlinkages include [7, 8]:

1. **SDG 1: No Poverty:** Good health is essential for economic productivity and poverty reduction. Illness and injury can push families into poverty, making access to affordable healthcare and social protection systems crucial for breaking the cycle of poverty.
2. **SDG 2: Zero Hunger:** Nutrition and health are deeply connected, with malnutrition contributing to poor health outcomes, especially in children.

ving food security and improved nutrition is essential for reducing mortality and morbidity rates.

3. **SDG 4: Quality Education:** Health and education are mutually reinforcing, as healthy children are more likely to attend school and perform better academically. Conversely, education promotes health literacy, enabling individuals to make informed health decisions.
4. **SDG 5: Gender Equality:** Gender equality is critical for improving health outcomes, particularly for women and girls. Ensuring access to sexual and reproductive health services and addressing gender-based violence are key to achieving both gender equality and better health outcomes.
5. **SDG 6: Clean Water and Sanitation:** Access to clean water and sanitation is fundamental to preventing water-borne diseases and promoting overall health. Efforts to improve water quality and sanitation infrastructure directly contribute to better health outcomes.
6. **SDG 13: Climate Action:** Climate change has significant health implications, including increased incidence of vector-borne diseases, heat-related illnesses, and food insecurity. Strengthening health systems to respond to climate-related health risks is essential for safeguarding public health.

Strategies for Aligning Health Systems with the SDGs

Health outcomes are shaped not only by the delivery of healthcare services but also by a complex web of interrelated social, economic, and environmental factors. Thus, aligning with the SDGs requires a paradigm shift, from a narrow, disease-specific approach to a broader, integrated, and equity-focused strategy. This entails rethinking how health policies are formulated, financed, implemented, and monitored, with a strong emphasis on inclusivity, accountability, and inter-sectoral collaboration. The key strategies for operationalizing the SDG agenda within national health systems include [7, 8]:

Integrating SDG Targets into National Health Strategies

To effectively contribute to the SDGs, national health strategies must be aligned with the specific targets of SDG 3 and related goals. This involves setting clear objectives, identifying priority areas, and ensuring that health policies are designed to address the broader determinants of health.

Promoting Multi-Sectoral Collaboration

Achieving the SDGs requires collaboration across sectors, including health, education, agriculture, environment, and finance. Multi-sectoral approaches that address the social, economic, and environmental determinants of health are critical for achieving sustainable health outcomes.

Mobilizing Resources for SDG Implementation

Sufficient and sustainable financing is crucial for achieving health-related SDG targets. Governments, international organizations, and the private sector must work together to mobilize resources, ensure efficient allocation, and reduce financial barriers to accessing healthcare.

Strengthening Health Data and Monitoring Systems

Accurate data is essential for tracking progress toward the SDGs and informing policy decisions. Strengthening health information systems and ensuring the availability of disaggregated data will enable better monitoring of health outcomes and equity.

CONCLUSION

The SDGs provide a comprehensive framework for addressing the complex and interrelated challenges of health and development. By aligning health systems with the SDGs, Nigeria and other developing nations can make significant strides in improving public health, reducing inequalities, and achieving sustainable development. The integration of health into the broader development agenda is not only essential for achieving SDG 3 but also for realizing the vision of a healthier, more equitable, and prosperous world by 2030.

THE FUTURE OF PUBLIC HEALTH IN NIGERIA AND DEVELOPING NATIONS

As the world continues to evolve in the face of new challenges and opportunities, the future of public health in Nigeria and other developing nations will be shaped by a complex interplay of social, economic, environmental, and technological factors. The journey toward sustainable health transformation requires a forward-looking approach, one that anticipates emerging health threats, leverages innovative solutions, and builds resilient health systems capable of adapting to changing circumstances. This section explores the key trends, challenges, and opportunities that will define the future of public health in Nigeria and developing nations, offering a roadmap for achieving lasting health improvements [9, 10].

Emerging Health Threats

The landscape of global health is rapidly evolving, with new and re-emerging threats challenging existing systems and preparedness efforts. From pandemics like COVID-19 to climate-induced health risks, antimicrobial resistance, and the rise of non-communicable diseases, nations must remain vigilant and adaptive. In developing contexts such as Nigeria, the convergence of weak infrastructure, population pressures, and socio-political instability exacerbates vulnerability. This subsection explores the nature of emerging health threats and underscores the need for agile, anticipatory strategies to detect, prevent, and respond to these challenges [9, 10].

Non-Communicable Diseases (NCDs)

While communicable diseases have historically been the primary focus of public health efforts in developing nations, the rising burden of Non-Communicable Diseases (NCDs) presents a significant challenge. Conditions such as cardiovascular diseases, diabetes, cancers, and chronic respiratory diseases are increasingly affecting populations in Nigeria and other developing countries, driven by factors such as urbanization, changing lifestyles, and aging populations. Addressing the dual burden of communicable and non-communicable diseases will require integrated approaches that emphasise prevention, early detection, and management of NCDs alongside continued efforts to control infectious diseases.

Climate Change and Environmental Health

Climate change poses a growing threat to public health, particularly in vulnerable regions like sub-Saharan Africa. Rising temperatures, changing precipitation patterns, and extreme weather events are contributing to the spread of vector-borne diseases, food and water insecurity, and the displacement of populations. The future of public health will depend on the ability of health systems to respond to climate-related health risks, promote environmental sustainability, and build resilience against the impacts of climate change.

Pandemics and Global Health Security

The COVID-19 pandemic has underscored the importance of global health security and the need for robust preparedness and response mechanisms. Future pandemics are inevitable, and developing nations must invest in strengthening their surveillance, early warning, and response systems. This includes building laboratory capacity, training health workers, and fostering international collaborations to detect and contain outbreaks before they escalate into global health emergencies.

Leveraging Technological Innovations

Technological innovations hold immense promise in transforming public health delivery, improving access, and enhancing efficiency. From digital health platforms and telemedicine to data analytics and artificial intelligence, technology is reshaping how health systems operate. In low-resource settings, these tools can bridge gaps in service delivery and empower communities with timely information and services. This subsection examines how adopting and scaling up appropriate technologies can strengthen health systems, foster innovation, and drive progress toward equitable health outcomes [9, 10].

Digital Health Solutions

The rapid advancement of digital technology offers unprecedented opportunities to revolutionise healthcare delivery in developing nations. Mobile health (mHealth) applications, telemedicine, and Electronic Health Records (EHRs) are transforming the way healthcare is accessed and delivered, particularly in remote and underserved areas. The future of public health will be increasingly digital, with technology playing a central role in improving access to care, enhancing health literacy, and enabling data-driven decision-making.

Artificial Intelligence and Data Analytics

Artificial Intelligence (AI) and data analytics have the potential to transform public health by enabling more accurate disease prediction, personalised medicine, and efficient resource allocation. In Nigeria and other developing nations, AI can be used to optimise health interventions, identify disease hotspots, and monitor health trends in real time. The integration of AI into public health strategies will be crucial for addressing complex health challenges and achieving better health outcomes.

Genomics and Precision Medicine

Advances in genomics and precision medicine are opening new frontiers in the prevention, diagnosis, and treatment of diseases. While these technologies are still in their infancy in many developing nations, the future holds the promise of personalised healthcare tailored to the genetic profiles of individuals. Investment in genomics research and the development of precision medicine infrastructure will be key to harnessing these innovations for the benefit of populations in Nigeria and beyond.

Building Resilient Health Systems

Resilience is the cornerstone of a responsive and sustainable health system. It refers to the capacity to withstand, adapt to, and recover from shocks, whether health emergencies, economic downturns, or political crises. In Nigeria and similar contexts, strengthening resilience requires investments in infrastructure, workforce capacity, supply chain integrity, and governance mechanisms. This subsection delves into the essential components of resilient health systems and outlines strategies for enhancing preparedness, continuity, and adaptability in the face of disruptions [9, 10].

Health Workforce Development

A strong and well-trained health workforce is the backbone of any resilient health system. The future of public health in Nigeria and developing nations will depend on the ability to recruit, train, and retain skilled health professionals across all levels of care. This includes investing in medical education, continuous professional development, and creating an enabling environment that supports health workers in delivering quality care.

Universal Health Coverage (UHC)

Achieving universal health coverage (UHC) remains a critical goal for ensuring that all individuals have access to the healthcare services they need without facing financial hardship. The future of public health will require continued efforts to expand coverage, improve the quality of care, and address barriers to access, particularly for marginalized and vulnerable populations. UHC will also necessitate innovative financing mechanisms and the efficient use of resources to ensure sustainability.

Health System Governance and Accountability

Good governance and accountability are essential for building trust in health systems and ensuring that resources are used effectively to improve health outcomes. The future of public health will require strong leadership, transparent decision-making processes, and robust accountability mechanisms to address corruption, inefficiency, and inequities in healthcare delivery. Strengthening governance at all levels, from local health facilities to national health ministries, will be key to achieving sustainable health improvements.

Harnessing the Power of Communities

Communities are not just beneficiaries of health interventions; they are powerful agents of change. Engaging communities in the design, implementation, and evaluation of health programs fosters trust, ownership, and sustainability. In contexts marked by diversity and decentralized governance, community engagement is especially crucial for addressing health inequities and ensuring culturally appropriate solutions. This subsection highlights the importance of community-led approaches and illustrates how participatory models can amplify impact and resilience [9, 10].

Community Engagement and Participation

Communities are at the heart of public health, and their active participation is crucial for the success of health initiatives. The future of public health in Nigeria and developing nations will depend on empowering communities to take ownership of their health and well-being. This involves fostering partnerships between health authorities and communities, promoting health literacy, and supporting community-driven health initiatives. Engaging communities in the design, implementation, and evaluation of health programs will ensure that interventions are culturally relevant, sustainable, and responsive to local needs.

Addressing Social Determinants of Health

Health is influenced by a wide range of social, economic, and environmental factors, collectively known as the social determinants of health. The future of public health will require a comprehensive approach that addresses these determinants, including poverty, education, housing, and access to clean water and sanitation. By tackling the root causes of health inequities, developing nations can create conditions that support healthier lives and reduce the burden of disease.

CONCLUSION

The future of public health in Nigeria and other developing nations is full of both challenges and opportunities. As these nations navigate the complexities of emerging health threats, technological advancements, and evolving societal needs, the key to success lies in building resilient, adaptive, and equitable health systems. By leveraging innovations, strengthening governance, and fostering community engagement, developing nations can achieve sustainable health improvements that benefit all citizens. The road ahead will require visionary leadership, strategic investments, and a commitment to collaboration at all levels. With the right strategies in place, the future of public health holds the promise of a healthier, more equitable world for generations to come.

CALL TO ACTION: MOBILISING FOR HEALTH TRANSFORMATION

It is pertinent to say that the future of health in Nigeria depends on collective courage, of policymakers to act, of academia to innovate, and of civil society to demand accountability. However, achieving a lasting transformation would require the following:

- **Policymakers** should invest consistently in systems that serve the poor and vulnerable.

- **Academia and researchers** should generate local evidence to guide reforms.
- **Civil society and the media** must advocate for transparency, equity, and inclusiveness in health delivery.

Thus, as we stand at the crossroads of an unprecedented opportunity to transform public health in Nigeria and other developing nations, the time for decisive action is now. The challenges are immense, ranging from systemic corruption and weak governance to emerging health threats and the complex social determinants of health. Yet, with these challenges come opportunities for innovation, collaboration, and the realisation of a healthier future for all. This section serves as a call to action, urging all stakeholders, governments, international partners, civil society, the private sector, and communities to come together in a concerted effort to achieve lasting health transformation [11, 12].

The Urgency of Health Transformation

The call for health transformation is more pressing than ever. Persistent inequities, fragile systems, and the increasing complexity of health challenges demand bold, systemic change. For Nigeria and other developing nations, the opportunity lies in reimagining public health through a lens of equity, innovation, and sustainability. This subsection introduces the critical need for transformation, emphasising why incremental adjustments are no longer sufficient and why a fundamental shift in priorities and structures is essential to meet future demands [11].

Addressing Persistent Health Inequities

Health inequities remain a significant barrier to achieving universal health coverage and improving health outcomes in developing nations. Disparities in access to healthcare, quality of services, and health outcomes are often rooted in poverty, geographic location, gender, and other social determinants. There is an urgent need to address these inequities by prioritizing the needs of the most vulnerable populations and ensuring that health interventions are inclusive, equitable, and accessible to all.

Responding to Emerging Health Threats

The rapid emergence of new health threats, such as pandemics, antimicrobial resistance, and the rising burden of non-communicable diseases, demands swift and coordinated action. The global health landscape is changing, and developing nations must be prepared to respond to these challenges with resilience and agility. This requires strengthening health systems, enhancing surveillance and early detection capabilities, and fostering global collaborations to ensure that no nation is left behind in the fight against emerging health threats.

Harnessing Technological Innovations

Technological advancements hold immense potential to revolutionize healthcare delivery and improve health outcomes in developing nations. From digital health solutions and artificial intelligence to genomics and precision medicine, these innovations offer new ways to overcome traditional barriers to healthcare access and quality. However, realizing the full potential of these technologies requires strategic investments, capacity building, and the integration of technology into national health strategies.

Mobilizing Key Stakeholders

Transformative change in health cannot be achieved by the health sector alone. Governments, civil society, development partners, private sector actors, academia, and communities each play pivotal roles in shaping and sustaining health reforms. Effective stakeholder mobilization ensures a shared vision, coordinated action, and inclusive governance. This subsection explores mechanisms for identifying, engaging, and empowering stakeholders to drive a united front for health transformation, highlighting the value of partnerships and collective ownership [11, 12].

Government Leadership and Commitment

Governments play a critical role in shaping the future of public health. Strong political will, visionary leadership, and sustained commitment to health are essential for driving the reforms needed to transform health systems. Governments must prioritize health in national agendas, allocate adequate resources, and ensure that policies are evidence-based, inclusive, and responsive to the needs of their populations. By leading the charge for health transformation, governments can create an enabling environment that fosters collaboration and innovation.

International Partnerships and Collaborations

Global health challenges require global solutions. International partnerships and collaborations are vital for mobilizing the resources, expertise, and knowledge needed to tackle complex health issues. Developing nations must continue to engage with international organizations, donor agencies, and other global health actors to build strong, resilient health systems. These partnerships should be rooted in mutual respect, shared responsibility, and a commitment to achieving common goals.

The Role of Civil Society and Communities

Civil society organizations and communities are powerful agents of change in public health. They bring unique perspectives, advocate for the rights of marginalized populations, and hold governments accountable for their commitments. Empowering civil society and communities to actively participate in health governance, policy-making, and program implementation is crucial for ensuring that health interventions are responsive to the needs of the people they are designed to serve. By mobilising grassroots movements and fostering community engagement, we can create a groundswell of support for health transformation.

Private Sector Engagement

The private sector has a key role to play in driving health innovation, improving service delivery, and expanding access to healthcare. Public-private partnerships can unlock new resources, technologies, and expertise that are essential for scaling up health interventions. The private sector should be encouraged to invest in health, not only as a corporate social responsibility initiative but as a strategic business opportunity that contributes to the overall well-being and economic growth of society.

Building Momentum for Sustainable Change

Sustained progress requires more than policy declarations; it demands momentum built on political will, institutional capacity, and continuous public engagement. Change is a process, not an event, and maintaining momentum means institutionalising reforms, monitoring progress, and celebrating milestones. This subsection focuses on how to embed health transformation within national development frameworks, reinforce accountability, and ensure that progress is not only achieved but sustained across political cycles and leadership transitions [11 - 13].

Advocacy and Public Awareness

Raising public awareness about the importance of health and the need for transformation is critical for building momentum and garnering support for health initiatives. Advocacy efforts should focus on educating the public, policymakers, and stakeholders about the challenges facing public health and the benefits of proposed solutions. By creating a shared vision for health transformation, we can inspire collective action and ensure that health remains a top priority on national and global agendas.

Sustaining Political and Financial Commitments

Achieving long-term health transformation requires sustained political and financial commitments from governments, donors, and other stakeholders. Health must be viewed as an investment in the future, one that yields significant returns in terms of economic growth, social stability, and improved quality of life. Governments and donors should prioritize health financing, ensure the efficient use of resources, and commit to long-term funding strategies that support the scaling up of successful health interventions.

Innovation and Adaptation

The path to health transformation is not linear, and challenges will inevitably arise along the way. To stay on course, stakeholders must embrace innovation and be willing to adapt to changing circumstances. This involves fostering a culture of continuous learning, encouraging experimentation, and scaling up successful innovations. By remaining flexible and open to new ideas, we can overcome obstacles and seize opportunities to drive progress in public health.

CONCLUSION

Transforming public health in Nigeria and other developing nations hinges on our collective ability to rise to the challenges of today and tomorrow. Health transformation is not the responsibility of a single entity; it requires the concerted efforts of governments, international partners, civil society, the private sector, and communities working together toward a common goal. The call to action is clear: we must mobilise now, with urgency and determination, to create a healthier, more equitable world for all. By uniting our strengths, leveraging our resources, and committing to sustainable change, we can achieve the vision of a transformed public health landscape, one where every individual has the opportunity to lead a healthy, fulfilling life. The time to act is now, and the future of public health depends on the decisions we make today.

REFERENCES

[1] World Health Organisation. (2018). WHO guideline on health policy and system support to optimise community health worker programmes. Geneva: WHO. Retrieved from: https://www.who.int

[2] Chan M. Ten years in public health, 2007–2017: Report by Dr Margaret Chan, Director-General, World Health Organisation. Geneva: WHO 2017.

[3] Kickbusch I, Reddy KS. Global health governance – the next political revolution. Public Health 2015; 129(7): 838-42.
[http://dx.doi.org/10.1016/j.puhe.2015.04.014] [PMID: 26040216]

[4] United Nations Development Programme. (2019). Partnerships for the goals: UNDP's work on SDG 17. New York: UNDP. Available from: https://www.undp.org

[5] Kruk ME, Ling EJ, Bitton A, *et al.* Building resilient health systems: a proposal for a resilience index. BMJ 2017; 357: j2323.
[http://dx.doi.org/10.1136/bmj.j2323] [PMID: 28536191]

[6] World Health Organisation. (2007). Everybody's business - Strengthening health systems to improve health outcomes. Washington, DC: World Bank. Retrieved from: https://www.who.int

[7] United Nations. (2015). Transforming our world: The 2030 Agenda for Sustainable Development. New York: United Nations. Retrieved from: https://sdgs.un.org

[8] Sachs JD. From millennium development goals to sustainable development goals. Lancet 2012; 379(9832): 2206-11.
[http://dx.doi.org/10.1016/S0140-6736(12)60685-0] [PMID: 22682467]

[9] Frenk J, Moon S. Governance challenges in global health. N Engl J Med 2013; 368(10): 936-42.
[http://dx.doi.org/10.1056/NEJMra1109339] [PMID: 23465103]

[10] United Nations Children's Fund (UNICEF). (2019). State of the world's children 2019: Children, food and nutrition—Growing well in a changing world. New York: UNICEF. Retrieved from: https://www.unicef.org

[11] Marmot M, Friel S, Bell R, Houweling TAJ, Taylor S. Closing the gap in a generation: health equity through action on the social determinants of health. Lancet 2008; 372(9650): 1661-9.
[http://dx.doi.org/10.1016/S0140-6736(08)61690-6] [PMID: 18994664]

[12] Global Health Council. (2021). New Global Health Council Report Calls for Redefining Global Health Security. Washington, DC: Global Health Council. Retrieved from: https://globalhealth.org

[13] Saleh J-EA. Resilient Communities: Navigating Public Health Challenges in Developing Nations. Bentham Science Publishers 2025.
[http://dx.doi.org/10.2174/97898153056091250101]

SUBJECT INDEX

A

B

C

Jalal-Eddeen Abubakar Saleh

D

E

F

G

O

P

Q

R

S

T

U

V

W

Z

www.ingramcontent.com/pod-product-compliance
Lightning Source LLC
LaVergne TN
LVHW070946210926
848482LV00002B/112